Primary Health Care 2000

Primary Health Care 2000

John Fry OBE MD FRCS FRCGP
General Practitioner,
Beckenham, Kent

John C. Hasler OBE MD FRCGP
Regional Postgraduate Adviser and
Clinical Lecturer in General Practice,
University of Oxford

FOREWORD BY
Leo A. Kaprio MD MPH DrPH
Regional Director Emeritus and Special
Adviser to Director General, World Health
Organization

CHURCHILL LIVINGSTONE
EDINBURGH LONDON MELBOURNE AND NEW YORK 1986

CHURCHILL LIVINGSTONE
Medical Division of Longman Group Limited

Distributed in the United States of America by
Churchill Livingstone Inc., 1560 Broadway, New
York, N.Y. 10036, and by associated companies,
branches and representatives throughout the world.

First published 1986

ISBN 0 443 03313 3

British Library Cataloguing in Publication Data
Fry, John, 1922–
   Primary health care 2000.
   1. Medical care
   I. Title   II. Hasler, John C.
   362.1   RA393

Library of Congress Cataloging-in-Publication Data
Main entry under title:
Primary health care 2000.

   1. Community health services. 2. Community health
services — Case studies. I. Fry, John. II. Hasler,
John. [DNLM: 1. Primary Health Care — trends.
W 84.6 P9528]
RA425.P757   1985   362.1'0425   85-19480
ISBN 0-443-03315-3

Printed in Great Britain by
Butler & Tanner Ltd, Frome and London

Foreword

Over the last 40 years or so, since the end of the Second World War, we have watched the countries of the world become more and more interdependent. In the international organizations we have seen our membership growing, territory after territory becoming politically independent and joining the United Nations, or any of its specialized agencies such as the World Health Organization. There are practically no old-style colonies left, but of course there remains the problem that many people in a number of countries lack human rights and political freedom.

The same is true of the right to health. For many the means and opportunities to maintain and improve their health, or to be treated or assisted when sick and suffering, are inadequate. Considerable numbers of people go without decent health care, education and food, and all these factors contribute to poor health.

The World Health Organization regularly puts out information on these facts, and the international community has long been aware of the generally poor state of health in the world. It was therefore no surprise that the governments of the world finally decided, at the World Health Assembly in 1977, that something much more effective had to be done, and the now well known resolution on 'Health for All by the Year 2000' was adopted. It was recognized that the misery of ill-health could not continue, because it impeded economic, social and cultural development and could even considerably influence political tension between north and south.

Then, as a practical step, the 1978 WHO/UNICEF Conference at Alma-Ata recommended in its Declaration that primary health care should be the method by which the health of the people should be improved. Moreover this philosophy was seen to apply not only to the developing 'third world' countries, which of course deserve top priority, but also to the industrialized countries; many of the latter already have severe health problems and others could have such problems before the year 2000 unless steps are taken to prevent them.

According to the Declaration of Alma-Ata, primary health care is:

> . . . essential health care . . . made universally accessible to individuals and families in the community through their full participation and at a cost that the community and country can afford . . . It forms an integral part both of the country's health system, of which it is the central function and main focus, and of the overall social and economic development of the community.

In the industrialized countries of the world, *primary medical care* has been available through general practitioners, polyclinics and other similar institutions for a long time. It has been part of their historical development that they have taken for granted. Hospital casualty services, too, have often been the first contact with the health system, and not only in emergencies but also for less critical complaints. The last few decades, however, have witnessed a move towards highly specialized, hospital-based services and, even in countries with a very strong tradition, primary medical care has lost prestige and clients.

Even before the Alma-Ata Conference, a renaissance in primary medical care had begun among general practitioners with the advent of health centres. The reasons for this were quite clear: hospitals had become too technical, too dehumanized and too expensive. When the World Health Organization began to emphasize the primary health care approach, therefore, it found Europe, and also Japan, the United States and other industrialized countries, ready to discuss the right medical and economic balance between hospital inpatient services and medical care in the community. In many countries this raised the question of the new roles of general practitioners, nurses, midwives and other people involved in local medical care.

The Alma-Ata Conference brought a new approach to this discussion. Primary health care is *not* the equivalent of primary medical care. There is a strong additional dimension of health promotion, disease prevention, maintaining the health of chronic patients and the handicapped, rehabilitation and mental health. Guaranteeing proper sanitary conditions and pollution control in the community is also part of primary health care activities. The co-operation of social workers, teachers, local industrial leaders, trade union groups, voluntary workers, transport authorities, and of course the local political authorities — that is, all who can influence people's health at the local level — is a crucial requirement for primary health care. Finally and most important are the people themselves as individuals, families and groups of interested people. These may include groups concerned with the environment, road safety, accident prevention or the problems of alcohol and drug abuse, or consumer association, such as those for diabetics or the parents of mentally retarded children. Co-operation among all of these interested parties is essential for proper primary health care. This list is given only as an example, and it does not include all potential situations in different countries, but it is long enough to demonstrate how complex the network of primary health care activities in a community can be. It also shows the importance of the *general practitioner* being prepared to be one of the leaders of this large team, caring for people's health in the local community.

There are very different challenges for this type of broad primary health care approach depending on the type of community, for example rural communities, small towns, middle-size industrial centres or huge metropolitan areas. In 1983 the European industrialized countries — and some countries outside Europe — were represented at the Conference on Primary Health Care in Industrialized Countries, held in Bordeaux, to take stock of what was happening, or what had happened, in the 5 years since the Alma-Ata Conference. It was quite clear that in the very complex, heavily structured industrialized countries change would come slowly, but it was also demonstrated that more and more discussion continues to take place, and that more and more experiments are being made. It is very clear that most governments prefer to encourage development at the local community level to balance the enormous cost of keeping the hospital system going. Hospitals are still needed of course, but they will have to improve their technologies and capacities. It is also clear that they have to serve the type of patient who actually needs them, and that a very large amount of both medical and health care has to take place in the community.

Various models and approaches are being developed in individual countries. In some, the medical associations and general practitioners have kept themselves somewhat aloof from these developments, but happily we very often find the best and most practical proposals coming from those who, for decades, have had experience of what happens at the local community level.

On the worldwide level, the World Health Organization strongly supports the building up of primary health care networks in developing countries, so as to be able to handle such problems as immunization, nutrition, family planning, the care of children and mothers, the proper use of drugs, and safe water supplies. These priority programmes for improving health and reducing risks should form a primary care network that will bring a relatively rapid improvement in health conditions. UNICEF and WHO hope to achieve this in countries where the general state of health is still very bad and is heavily influenced by infectious diseases and bad nutritional and sanitary conditions.

Everywhere, general practitioners, and the various types of auxiliary worker at the primary health care level, have a very important role to play in living with the people, educating them, and having cultural contact with the population for whom they work and who have the right to participate in the further development of their own health conditions.

1986   Leo A. Kaprio

Declaration of Alma-Ata 1978:
Primary health care VII

Primary health care:

1. Reflects and evolves from the economic conditions and socio-cultural and political characteristics of the country and its communities and is based on the application of the relevant results of social, biomedical and health services research and public health experience;

2. addresses the main health problems in the community, providing promotive, preventive, curative and rehabilitative services accordingly;

3. includes at least: education concerning prevailing health problems and the methods of preventing and controlling them; promotion of food supply and proper nutrition; an adequate supply of safe water and basic sanitation; maternal and child health care, including family planning; immunization against major infectious diseases; prevention and control of locally endemic diseases; appropriate treatment of common diseases and injuries; and provision of essential drugs.

4. involves, in addition to the health sector, all related sectors and aspects of national and community development, in particular agriculture, animal husbandry, food industry, education, housing, public works, communications and other sectors; and demands the coordinated efforts of all those sectors;

5. requires and promotes maximum community and individual self-reliance and participation in the planning, organization, operation and control of primary health care, making fullest use of local national and other available resources; and to this end develops through appropriate education the ability of communities to participate;

6. should be sustained by integrated, functional and mutually-supportive referral systems, leading to the progressive importance of comprehensive health care for all, and giving priority to those most in need;

7. relies, at local and referral levels, on health workers, including physicians, nurses, midwives, auxiliaries and community workers as applicable, as well as traditional practitioners as needed, suitably trained socially and technically to work as a health team and to respond to the expressed health needs of the community.

Contributors X

R. John Bennison MA, MB, MChir, D(Obst)RCOG, FRCGP
General practitioner, Hatfield Broad Oak, Essex

William Dodd MB, ChB, MRCGP
Senior Consultant, Riyadh Al Kharj Hospital Programme Riyadh Armed
Forces Hospital, Riyadh, Kingdom of Saudi Arabia

V. W. Michael Drury OBE, MB, ChB, MRCS, FRCGP
Professor of General Practice, University of Birmingham

Wesley E. Fabb MB, BS, FRACGP, FCGP(Hon), FFGP(SA)(Hon),
MCFPC(Hon)
National Director, Family Medicine Programme, Royal Australian
College of General Practitioners, Jolimont, Victoria, Australia

Boris Michael Fehler MB, BCh(Wits), DCH(RCPS)(Eng),
MFGP(SA), FRCGP
General Practice Tutor, University of Witwatersrand, South Africa

George Samuel Fehrsen BA, MB, BCh(CT), MFGP(SA)
Professor and Head of Department of Family Medicine, University of
South Africa, Medunsa, RSA

Victor L. Fernandez MB, BS(Malaya), FRCGP(Singapore)
President, College of General Practitioners, Singapore

Godfrey Fowler MA, BM, FRCGP, DRCOG, DCH
General Practitioner, Oxford; Clinical Reader in General Practice,
Oxford University; and Fellow, Balliol College, Oxford

Clive Froggatt MB, MRCGP
Member of WONCA 86 Organising Committee; Principal in General
Practice, Cheltenham; and Hospital Practitioner, Gloucestershire Child
Guidance Service

John Fry OBE MD, FRCS, FRCGP
General Practitioner, Beckenham, Kent

Eric Gambrill MB, BS, FRCGP, DRCOG
General Practitioner, Crawley, Sussex; Associate Adviser in General
Practice, University of London; and Associate Professor, Department of
Community Medicine, Baylor College of Medicine, Houston, Texas, USA

John P. Geyman MD
Professor and Chairman, Department of Family Medicine, University of
Washington, Seattle, Washington, USA

John Hasler OBE, MD, FRCGP
Regional Postgraduate Adviser and Clinical Lecturer in General Practice,
University of Oxford

Brian Hennen MA MD CCFP FCFP
Professor and Head of Department of Family Medicine, Dalhousie
University, Halifax, Nova Scotia, Canada

John Horder CBE, FRCP, FRCGP, FRCPsych
Visiting Professor, Royal Free Hospital Medical School; and Visiting
Fellow, The King's Fund College, London

Leela De A. Karunaratne MB, BS, DCH (Ceylon), FRCGP
General Practitioner and Head of Department of Family Medicine,
North Colombo Medical College, Sri Lanka

Pertti Kekki MD, ScD, DCM(Ed)
Professor of General Practice, University of Helsinki; and Permanent
Adviser on Organization and Development of Primary Health Care, The
National Board of Health, Finland

David H. H. Metcalfe MB, BChir, MFCM, FRCGP
Professor and Head of Department of General Practice, Manchester
University

David Morley MA, MD, FRCP, DCH
Professor of Tropical Child Health, Institute of Child Health, London

R. T. Mossop MB, ChB (UCT), FCGP (R), AFCM (SA) (Hon)
Chairman, Department of Community Medicine, University of Zimbabwe;
and President, College of Primary Care Physicians of Zimbabwe

C. Andrew Pearson OBE, MB, ChB, DTM, FMCGP(Nigeria)
Former Director of Training, Faculty of General Medical Practice,
National Postgraduate Medical College, Nigeria

Max R. Polliack MPH, FRCGP
Chairman, Department of Family Medicine, Tel Aviv University
Medical School, Israel

Peter Pritchard MA, MB, FRCGP, DCH
General Practitioner, Oxfordshire

Sir John Reid MD, DSc, FRCP, FFCM
Chief Medical Officer, Scottish Home and Health Department,
Edinburgh

J. G. Richards MB, ChB, FRCP(Ed), FRACP, FRNZCGP
Associate Professor of General Practice, School of Medicine, Auckland,
New Zealand

T. Michael Ryan MA (Oxon), PhD (Wales)
Research Assistant in Social Administration, University of Manchester;
and Lecturer in Social Adminstration, University College of Swansea

Ruth Sidel PhD
Professor of Sociology, Hunter College, City University of New York,
USA

Victor W. Sidel MD
Distinguished University Professor of Social Medicine, Montefiore
Medical Center and Albert Einstein College of Medicine, New York,
USA

Harald Siem MD, MPH
Medical Officer, Department of Public Health and Community
Medicine, Oslo Municipality, Norway

G. A. C. Stratfold MB, ChB, MCGP(Zimbabwe)
General Practitioner; and Honorary Secretary, College of General
Practice, Zimbabwe

Jan C. van Es MD, FRCGP(Hon)
Professor of General Practice, Free University, Amsterdam; and Chief
Editor, Medisch Contact, The Netherlands

Contents

PART ONE

Common issues

Alma-Ata and after — the background

WORLD HEALTH ORGANIZATION

The World Health Organization (WHO) is a specialized agency within the United Nations family and is the supreme co-ordinating authority for all aspects of international health. There is no matter relating to health with which it is not concerned — from prevention to cure, care and rehabilitation; from the control of communicable disease to problems of mental health; from publication of the *International Classification of Diseases* to the setting of standards for products such as antibiotics, biological substances and diagnostic reagents; and from the production of authoritative guidance in books of the *Technical Report Series* to a range of publications designed for members of the public.

Health cannot, of course, be looked at in isolation from other parts of the social fabric of nations. The level of general education of a populace is relevant to securing and maintaining good health. The economic condition of a state and of its people plays a crucial role. An adequate supply of potable water is essential, as is an effective system of sewage disposal. Nutrition is of deep relevance to health. The list is endless and calls for close linkage between health and other relevant services at national and international levels. In the latter context it is the responsibility of WHO to liaise with a wide range of official bodies, such as the World Bank, the Food and Agriculture Organization (FAO), the United Nations Development Programme (UNDP), the United Nations Children's Fund (UNICEF), the United Nations Environmental Programme (UNEP), and also with many other international, governmental and non-governmental organizations whose responsibilities touch directly or indirectly on the broad field of health.

WHO is sometimes mistakenly thought of as being primarily an aid-giving body whereas, as has been pointed out, its prime task is a co-ordinating one, and it acts essentially as a co-operative of all its member states, with strong emphasis on the exchange of technical information between them. The total budget of WHO, raised by assessments on member states, is modest, currently amounting only to some $250 million per annum, supplemented by an approximately equal sum from governmental or other voluntary donations. These limited funds are spent in accordance with successive two-yearly programme budgets, which are comprised of broad programmes with defined objectives, approaches towards attaining them, and plans of action for doing so.

The work of WHO has been remarkably successful in many fields, ranging from the dramatic eradication of smallpox from the world, a task which called for close and effective co-operation between member states and their Organization, to the more prosaic but nonetheless important publication of comprehensive statistics covering many aspects of health and health services throughout the world. In a recent survey (Franck et al 1982) of the opinions of senior diplomats on aspects of the United Nations system, it is significant that WHO, together with UNICEF, led the field in terms of their perceived success compared with other intergovernmental organizations associated with the UN.

The policy of WHO is determined by the annual *World Health Assembly*, which is attended by delegations, usually led by ministers, from all 164 member states. Decisions are commonly arrived at by consensus but, when matters come to a vote, it is on the basis of one vote per member state, irrespective of its population or amount of contribution to WHO's budget. It would be unrealistic to claim that WHO is a non-political body, as that would be impossible for any organization which includes nations from one end of the political spectrum to the other, in addition to which it is true, both internationally and nationally, that health, taken in its broadest sense, must always ultimately involve major political considerations. Having said that, however, it is equally true to say that WHO is one of the least political of the United Nations specialized agencies, rightly concentrating its main efforts on its vast range of technical activities.

Each World Health Assembly, in the course of debating its substantial agenda, passes a series of resolutions defining its policies and often allocating responsibilities for carrying out their various components. Such resolutions may be in general terms or may be highly specific, and they frequently link back to earlier resolutions, thus enabling continuity in the evolution of the Organization's philosophy to be traced from successive records of the Assembly and of the Executive Board.

The *Executive Board* is comprised of 31 persons 'technically qualified in the field of health', each being nominated by his or her member state, the countries in question having been elected by the Assembly so as to secure an equitable geographical distribution. Members serve on the Board in their individual expert capacities as nominees and not as delegates of their countries. The Board acts as the executive organ of the Assembly as well as, where appropriate, taking its own initiatives. It thus works closely, on the one hand, with the Assembly and, on the other, with the Secretariat of WHO. The Secretariat is headed by the Director General, who has an international staff working at all levels, from those who represent WHO and co-ordinate its programmes in individual developing countries, through the Regional offices, to global Headquarters in Geneva.

The six *Regions of WHO* comprise those for Africa, the Americas, the Eastern Mediterranean, Europe, South-East Asia, and the Western Pacific. Each has a Regional Committee which meets annually and comprises delegates from all member states in the Region, and its Secretariat is led by a Regional Director. The Regions pay especial attention to health matters as they affect their particular geographical areas and also contribute to the evolution and carrying out of global policies as determined by the World Health Assembly.

As with all large organizations there is a state of dynamic equilibrium between its constituent components in the form of the Assembly, the Regional Committees, the Executive Board and the Secretariat. Some member states, drawing on their own national political philosophies, favour a centralist approach to the work of WHO, whilst others prefer a high degree of Regional or more peripheral delegation. Overall, however, the Organization is currently in a healthy state, with the various policy organs and the Secretariat working in a complementary manner towards the agreed collective objectives of WHO.

'Health for All'

Two closely related events of crucial significance to WHO and its member states have taken place since 1977 and have led to a major reorientation of the work of the Organization. In that year the

World Health Assembly reaffirmed WHO's constitutional objectives and went on to decide that, 'the main social target of governments and WHO in the coming decades should be the attainment by all the citizens of the world by the year 2000 of a level of health which will permit them to lead a socially and economically productive life'. The resolution called on countries to collaborate and to mobilize resources towards that end, and asked the Executive Board and the Director General to reorientate the work of WHO accordingly.

This was the starting point for what has come to be known by the somewhat ambiguous title of 'Health for all by the year 2000'. It is, in that context, interesting to note that, in responding to the Assembly's request, the January 1978 meeting of the Executive Board asked its Programme Committee to propose strategies for attaining the more realistically defined objective of 'an acceptable level of health for all' by the target date.

The second major event was the Alma-Ata conference on primary health care, the lead up to which involved a series of actions on the part of the Assembly and of the Executive Board. In 1974, the Assembly reviewed the Director General's report for 1973, together with his fifth report on the world health situation. It noted the disparities in levels of development of health services between countries, and requested the Director General to report on what could be done to secure more effective co-ordination between WHO's activities and national health programmes.

The Executive Board considered the Director General's subsequent report in January 1975, noted that much of the rural population in developing countries or had little or no access to health services, and that, '. . . without prejudice to the training of physicians and of other health service personnel, priority attention should be given to primary health care at the community level . . .'. The Board then went on to pass a resolution which focussed attention on primary health care, and on prerequisite steps towards achieving it, and asked the Director General to present a further report on the subject to the forthcoming World Health Assembly. At the same time it was suggested that the Assembly might, at an appropriate stage, wish to '. . . undertake a review of the experiences of health services of various countries in providing primary health care . . .'.

The 1975 Assembly approved the revised report, passed a resolution requesting member states and the Director General to take appropriate steps to promote primary health care, and instructed the Executive Board to arrange an international conference on the subject as soon as possible. WHO subsequently received invitations from certain governments to hold the conference in their countries. In the event, the 1976 Assembly agreed that the conference should be held in the USSR and, having heard a statement from the representative of UNICEF, also agreed that the event should be co-sponsored by WHO and that body.

The scene was thus set for the historic conference on primary health care, held at Alma-Ata, the capital of the Kazakh Soviet Socialist Republic. The conference was preceded by a series of national, regional and international meetings on primary health care held throughout the world in 1977 and 1978. The outcomes of these meetings were available to the conference, the main document for which consisted of a joint report (WHO 1978) by the Director General of WHO and the Executive Director of UNICEF, together with six regional background papers prepared by the WHO Regional Directors. A substantial number of other papers and exhibits were available to the conference, and the government of the USSR arranged for participants to see something of their approach to primary health care through a series of visits in Kazakhstan and neighbouring Republics.

The conference was attended by governmental delegations from 134 member states, together with representatives of 67 United Nations organizations, specialized agencies and non-governmental organizations in official relations with WHO and UNICEF. The notable absentee was China, which was still recovering from the upheaval of its cultural revolution, and whose relations with the USSR were strained at the time. It is also likely that, just as the Soviet Union was anxious to demonstrate to those attending the conference its particular national approach to primary health care, China did not feel, in view of its own great advances in the provision of health services, that it stood to learn much from the Soviet Union. It should be emphasized, however, that China has always been and remains one of the strongest supporters of the WHO initiative in primary health care, and that many other countries have taken the opportunity of studying its particular approach to the problem, just as those at Alma-Ata studied the Soviet Union's method.

Rediscovery of primary health care

The Alma-Ata conference provided a major boost to the process, which had begun a few years earlier, of drawing attention to, or rediscovering, primary health care. There is no doubt that many developing countries and some developed ones had continued to neglect their real health problems in favour of sporadic forays into the realm of high technology medicine. Equally, health programmes were still all too often based on 'vertical' ad hoc approaches to individual health problems, institutions or particular groups of the population. Such approaches are understandably popular with donor agencies, as it is often thereby possible to show that 'something has been done' about a specific problem, whereas the painstaking building up of a primary health care system and of the infrastructure of a comprehensive health service is a much slower and less dramatic occupation, although a more fundamental and relevant one. The situation may also be compounded by groups of health personnel whose posts and authority depend largely on the retention of specific vertical programmes which are incompatible with a system based on primary health care.

The *Alma-Ata conference* had an important role to play in establishing a clear understanding of what is meant by primary health care, as distinct from the much narrower concept of primary medical care, which is still all too often mistakenly regarded as a synonym.

The immediate outcome of the conference was the *Declaration of Alma-Ata*. International pronouncements of most kinds tend to be in terms which are generalized to a point which places them in danger of being meaningless, usually for political reasons or because of the need to avoid specificity in order to accommodate different national needs and approaches. The Declaration of Alma-Ata is in large measure an exception to that state of affairs and its 10 articles deserve repeated study.

They reaffirm health as a fundamental human right and stress existing inequalities both internationally and within countries. They emphasize the relationship between health on the one hand and social and economic development on the other. Stress is also laid on the importance of individual and collective public participation in the planning and provision of health care. The clear responsibilities of governments in relation to health are enunciated, with emphasis on primary health care as the key component, and governments are enjoined to formulate national policies, strategies and plans of action to further that approach. International interdependence in the field of health is stressed and appropriate co-operation advocated; and the Declaration ends with a call for more

resources to be devoted to health rather than to the further proliferation of armaments.

Articles VI and VII are of particular practical importance to those
concerned with the provision of primary health care. The first of
these Articles provides a concise and comprehensive definition of
such care, whilst the second, reproduced on page ix, spells out its
essential components in detail. The seven subsections of the latter
merit closer study, and the following comments are relevant:

Subsection 1. Each country must determine its own detailed
approach to primary health care, as such systems cannot simply be
transplanted in toto from the different circumstances of other
nations. The need for action based on research is indisputable, yet
there is still little relevant material available in most countries,
particularly in the crucial area of health services research.

Subsection 2. The need to define the main national health problems is obvious, but it is not always easy to ensure that they are
tackled in preference to other easier or more attractive alternatives.
Similarly, achieving an appropriate balance in the components of
primary health care, from health promotion through to rehabilitation, is usually difficult.

Subsection 3. The items listed here are basic essentials, and imply
wide political and practical considerations, which also involve the
commitments of ministries and agencies other than those traditionally responsible for 'health' in the narrower sense of that word.
Coordinating such matters at all levels is a severe challenge for developing countries and also frequently poses problems for developed
ones, where the practicalities of intersectoral co-ordination all too
often fall well short of national theory.

Subsection 4. This underlines and widens the issues of intersectoral co-ordination which have just been mentioned. Whilst must
depends on governmental structure, matters such as the pecking
order of ministries and of personalities at national and local levels
are also frequently relevant.

Subsection 5. Whilst most countries would no doubt subscribe to
the importance of public participation in relation to primary health
care, the practicalities of the situation are highly variable, ranging
from direct and universal participation at the periphery to a highly
formalized elected or nominated form of participation at a more
centralized level. There is also a wide diversity of approaches to
helping the public to understand matters relevant to the planning,
organization, operation and control of services, with variable
dividing lines being drawn between what might be respectively

described as education on the one hand and indoctrination on the other.

Subsection 6. The allocation of agreed functions to the various tiers of a comprehensive health care system can present problems in developing and in developed countries, and there is constant need to review aspects of the matter in the light of such factors as new scientific developments and the current levels of training of different types of health service personnel. A familiar example is the division of responsibility between primary care and secondary (hospital) teams in relation to successive phases of treatment of a particular disease.

Subsection 7. The concept of the primary care team is a basic one, but subject to wide variability in the light of local circumstances. It is also important to enable the members of the team to evolve their complementary roles and not to inhibit such evolution by needlessly restrictive rules and job descriptions.

Implications of WHO policy

The implications for developing countries are clear, although the attainment of the objective for the year 2000 presents an enormous challenge for most of them. Poverty still constitutes the main inhibiting factor, with its all too common consequences of malnutrition, inadequate and impure water supplies and the absence of safe disposal of sewage and refuse. Most *developing countries* lack an adequate health service infrastructure and managerial system; most do not have anything resembling effective information systems with which to measure their current health problems and monitor progress towards agreed objectives. Coherent manpower policies are still uncommon and essential vaccines and drugs frequently are unobtainable or in short supply. Some, sadly, continue to dissipate their small available resources on facilities which have no relevance to their real health needs.

Developed countries also have lessons to learn and major roles to play over the next two decades; and they are certainly not exempt from criticism in relation to some of the matters which have just been mentioned. Many have, for historical reasons, either never had effective systems of primary health or medical care, or have allowed the latter to decay, with the result that their health systems are hospital and specialist based. Such systems are most unlikely to be able to promote primary health care in the wide sense of the term which was defined at Alma-Ata; they deny patients the benefit of a single health worker who can look at the individual and the family in a comprehensive manner; and they tend to be needlessly profligate in their use of human and technical resources.

Patterns of health care in developed countries are usually the result of a process of evolution, and sometimes approaches to its provision have been perpetuated long after they have ceased to be appropriate. Such countries must ask themselves whether, if they were starting from scratch, they would really have adopted their present patterns of care. One field which is particularly worthy of study is manpower. What, at any particular stage in the development of a country's health service, should be the respective roles of doctors, nurses, other health personnel and of lay people? The answer to that question should not be a fixed one, but should permit the evolution of roles; legislation governing particular health professions should always have the prime objective of protecting the public, rather than maintaining vested professional interests and encouraging a lack of flexibility in the most appropriate and economical use of manpower.

Influencing factors at national level

Wide national political and other circumstances will have a crucial effect on countries' approaches to primary health care and to attaining the declared objective for the year 2000. Where, for example does the true balance of power lie between national, subnational and local levels and what is the nature and degree of democratic input at each of these? What is the proportion and absolute amount of the gross national product which is devoted to health, in the wide sense defined at Alma-Ata? What is the pecking order between ministries and between ministers and what is the health input to overall national planning? How strong are the power bases of the various health professions and to what extent do such factors support or militate against the primary health care approach?

Methods of financing health services are clearly relevant to the encouragement or discouragement of primary health care. No matter whether they are financed entirely by the state, covered in whole or in part by insurance, or privately provided, there is need to look at the financing system and to decide how best it can be adjusted to promote the comprehensive aims of primary health care. Governments must inevitably be involved in this process. There is also a particular need to study and resolve problems of manpower.

What numbers of each type of health personnel are required at any given time, how should they be trained and how should their respective roles be encouraged to evolve?

This, in turn leads on to the questions of the individual's responsibility for his own health and of self-care. The maintenance of health clearly calls for major efforts on the part of the individual, but that will be successful only if it is backed by collective and governmental action. It is useless teaching a villager in a developing country about a balanced diet if poverty or the absence of an effective national food policy offers no hope of being able to eat anything approaching such a diet. The prevention of water-borne disease will be achieved only as the result of collective as well as individual action. And in both developed and developing countries, the rising tide of death and suffering caused by tobacco will be brought under control only if governments have clear strategies for dealing with the subject to complement individual decisions to abjure this lethal addiction.

Self-care is likewise an essential component of all health systems. There is need to help individuals and families to understand their roles and, once again, it is necessary for health workers to determine the best use of their individual skills vis-à-vis those of members of the communities whom they serve. A balance must be struck between professional authoritarianism on the one hand and abandoning people to remedies and practices which are clearly dangerous on the other. In many developing countries one aspect of this is gradually being tackled by harnessing and gently reorienting the skills of traditional healers and birth attendants so that their work complements those of more scientifically trained personnel.

Roles of government

The World Health Organization is an intergovernmental agency and, through membership of it, countries acknowledge that they have a collective responsibility in health matters just as they have responsibilities in relation to the health of their own people. Some nations embody health as a human right in their constitutions, although sometimes that is no guarantee that practice equates with, or even approximates to, theory. In a few cases, aspects of a written constitution may even militate against a country taking action which is clearly in the interests of health.

All nations have legislation which impinges directly or indirectly on many aspects of health and health services. Such legislation ranges in its form from inflexible and precise rules on all relevant matters to more flexible approaches. Examples of the latter are to be seen in much of the United Kingdom's health legislation, which commonly deals with a subject in general terms, leaving more detailed aspects to be settled, and adjusted as necessary from time to time, by subordinate regulations.

All countries must face up to the difficult task of the allocation of what will always be finite resources to potentially infinite demand for health services, and to competing claims in terms of geography, particular groups of the population and different aspects of health care; they must similarly agree about the most appropriate balance between the centre, intermediate tiers and the periphery in relation to the determination of policy and the use of resources. These are difficult tasks, involving the need to change the distribution of resources in health budgets and fundamental considerations of the delegation of power.

Governmental attitudes and policies in relation to other aspects of the national social fabric are also relevant to health, including such matters as general education, housing, many aspects of the physical, mental and social environment, agriculture and last, but not least, the overall national economic situation.

An adequate, but not excessively complicated, data collection system is necessary in order to determine base-lines in many health matters and to monitor progress towards agreed targets. This, in turn, is part of the essential organizational and administrative infrastructure on which effective health services must be founded. The overall planning of health services clearly involves governmental responsibilities, and current WHO initiatives are concentrated on facilitating this planning process. Incremental planning, whereby a state undertakes simply to increase the numbers of particular categories of health workers or the number of hospital beds every year, is insufficient. It is the health objectives which it is proposed to attain which matter, and these should be clearly spelt out.

Much has been done by WHO and its member states since the Alma-Ata conference in 1978. By the following year the World Health Assembly was able to approve the Executive Board's initial document entitled, 'Formulating strategies for health for all by the year 2000' (WHO 1979), and the General Assembly of the United Nations, in 1979, gave its support to what was proposed. Following discussions at national and regional levels a global strategy was agreed in 1981, and a plan of action for achieving it was approved by the 1982 World Health Assembly. Since the publication of the report on the Alma-Ata conference, a series of further interlinked documents has been produced (WHO 1981a–d, 1982a) covering the development of indicators for monitoring progress, guiding principles for a managerial process for national health development, health programme evaluation and a plan of action for implementing the global strategy. Finally in this series, WHO published its seventh general programme of work covering the period 1984–1989 (WHO 1982b), indicating how the activities of the Organization should be reoriented to help member states in the implementation of primary health care as the key step towards attaining the target for the year 2000.

That target will be achieved only insofar as individual countries accept their self-imposed commitments stemming from the resolution of the 1977 World Health Assembly and the 1978 Alma-Ata conference. Action must articulate local needs into agreed national policies, strategies, and plans of action. These have to be completed in accordance with an agreed timetable for subsequent correlation with regional and global plans of action. Within a broad overall framework there is scope for countries to develop their individual approaches, depending on their needs and resources, and to assess how they can best co-operate with fellow member states faced with similar problems or from which useful lessons could be learnt. Such exchange of information and technical co-operation is one of the classical activities fostered by WHO.

Similarly, at Regional level, each of the six WHO Regions is faced with its own particular pattern of health problems and has had to take this into account in formulating its regional strategy and plan of action. The European Region, for example, is composed predominantly of developed countries, and its plan begins with a statement drawing attention to the provision of wide prerequisites for health, ranging from freedom from the fear of war to such basic matters as education, food and housing. It then makes particular features of the promotion of lifestyles conducive to health, the reduction of environmental risks and the provision of adequate and appropriate health care accessible to all.

With so vast a global task it is not realistic to expect that all 164 member states of WHO will go forward at the same pace. The results of the first monitoring exercise, which were discussed at the 1984 World Health Assembly, showed that some nations were indeed making clear progress towards defined objectives, whilst others had made but little. In some of the latter, a major inhibiting factor has been lack of political will, but other potent inhibitions have also applied in the forms of extreme poverty, war, the virtual absence of a health service infrastructure, inadequate or inappropriately trained health service manpower, and the use of scarce resources to further activities which are irrelevant to the real health needs of the countries in question.

It is premature to attempt to predict the ultimate outcome of this vast reorientation of the work of WHO and its member states, but there can be no doubt about the need for it. In its absence, WHO would certainly have continued to make progress in many individual fields of endeavour, and there is no doubting the value of such activities as the international control of communicable disease, the standardization of biological substances and the publication of expert technical advice. At both international and national levels, however, this would all too often have implied the perpetuation of ad hoc 'vertical' approaches to individual health problems instead of a comprehensive 'horizontal' one, with emphasis on primary health care as defined at Alma-Ata.

The latter is strategically the correct approach, and WHO has carefully examined its own internal functioning to prepare itself for its task. The same is happening although, as has been said, at a very variable rate, in individual member states, and it is hoped and intended that the ongoing cyclical process of planning and monitoring at national, regional and global levels will prove a stimulus to continuing and accelerating action over the remaining 15 years of the present century. Cynics decried the agreement by WHO and its member states to rid the world of smallpox, but that was successfully accomplished. The project for achieving an acceptable level of health for all inhabitants of the world through national approaches based on primary health care is, admittedly, a vastly greater challenge, but cynicism directed towards the objective in question must be shown, in the fullness of time, to have been equally misplaced.

The overall responsibility for action rests with WHO and its member states but, if it is to succeed, it must go much deeper, to involve communities and individuals. That presents a huge challenge to developing and developed countries alike. It also presents a particular opportunity and duty for health workers of all kinds to examine their roles and modify them as necessary in the interests of the communities and individuals they serve. They should provide leadership of a facilitating rather than a prescriptive kind, and they should analyse and reanalyse the lessons to be learnt from the Declaration of Alma-Ata and all that is now beginning to stem from it.

The views expressed in this paper are personal and do not purport to be those of the World Health Organization.

REFERENCES

Franck T M, Renninger J P, Tikhomirov V B 1982 Diplomats' views on the United Nations system: an attitude survey. United Nations Institute for Training and Research, New York
WHO 1978 Alma-Ata 1978: Primary health care. WHO, Geneva
WHO 1979 Formulating strategies for health for all by the year 2000. WHO, Geneva
WHO 1981a Global strategy for health for all by the year 2000, WHO, Geneva
WHO 1981b Development of indicators for monitoring progress towards health for all by the year 2000. WHO, Geneva
WHO 1981c Managerial process for national health development. WHO, Geneva
WHO 1981d Health programme evaluation: guiding principles. WHO, Geneva
WHO 1982a Plan of action for implementing the global strategy for health for all. WHO, Geneva
WHO 1982b Seventh general programme of work covering the period 1984–1989. WHO, Geneva

Primary health care seen from a general practice

In this chapter I shall discuss these four questions:

1. How does general medical practice or family practice — the element in medical care for which the World Organization of National Colleges and Academies provides a world-wide link — relate in meaning to 'primary health care' — the main object of current policy for the World Health Organization and the main subject of this book?

2. Why has this subject moved from neglect to renewed interest?

3. Is 'primary health care' acceptable? Realistic?

4. What particular challenges does it offer to WONCA, to general practitioners and family physicians?

These four questions will be addressed in sequence.

1. How does 'general medical practice' or 'family practice' relate in meaning to 'primary health care'?

All these terms, and others, are in use in different parts of the world. They have in common the contrast with specialist medical care and secondary medical care, even if the boundary is less clear in many countries than, for example, in the United Kingdom. The contrast is well-expressed in these World Health Organization definitions:

Primary care:

> . . . frontline medical care; as a rule not limited to patients in specific age groups; the field of practice where the patient usually makes his first contact with the physician and has direct access to him or her.

Secondary care:

> . . . care requiring attention of a special nature, usually more sophisticated and complicated than could be handled by the general practitioner.

(WHO 1974)

But beside their common meaning, there are also significant differences implied in the words 'general practice', 'family practice',
'primary medical care' and 'primary health care'. The most
obvious differences are in the groups of people actively involved.
'General practice' traditionally implies a doctor and a doctor's role
with sick individuals. 'Family practice', in current American usage,
likewise focusses on the doctor, but stresses the relation of individuals to their family. 'Primary *medical* care' has come to imply, at
least in the United Kingdom, workers other than doctors — mainly
nurses, public health nurses, dentists, ophthalmic opticians, and
others — any professional in fact to whom people have direct
access. 'Primary *health* care', in current World Health Organization usage, also involves all these professions, but stresses in
addition the participation of people, non-professionals, people
without special training, not merely as voluntary health workers,
but as citizens. No-one can live without some experience of health
and illness and some concern for them. This emphasis is clear in
Article VII. 5 of the Alma Ata Declaration:

> . . .primary health care requires and promotes maximum community
> and individual self-reliance and participation in the planning, organ-
> isation, operation and control (of primary health care) . . ..
>
> (WHO 1978)

It is not difficult to see another difference implied by these
different terms — they move in emphasis from concern with the
care and cure of ill people, towards preventing illness, self-care and
a greater concern for living healthily.

There are themes here which apply to all countries. But there are
great variations both between and within countries. No one country
presents a perfect, real-life example of 'primary health care' as the
Alma Ata Declaration describes its many features. It is after all an
ideal to aim for, an ideal which governments and professions in
different countries view with varying degrees of enthusiasm,
according as it is close to or far from their own ideals. It is defined
in Article VI of the Declaration. The definition is discussed in the
third section of this chapter.

2. Why has this subject moved from neglect to renewed interest worldwide?

The Declaration itself (VII. 1) points out that primary health care
reflects and evolves from the economic conditions and sociocultural
and political characteristics of a country and its communities. It is

difficult, therefore, for anyone writing on the subject to divorce himself from what is familiar in his own country — and particularly for a writer whose training and experience has been mainly in active general practice in one relatively developed country.

But a course of events experienced in the United Kingdom in the last 50 years has been paralleled in many other countries, if not in all. This short review of recent history will therefore focus on the country with which I am most familiar.

The general practitioner, mainstay of the system of medical care, found himself isolated. As a species he faced even the possibility of extinction, except as a survival in remote rural districts. How could one doctor pretend to cover all tasks or master knowledge now expanding at an ever faster rate? From the joint historical roots of apothecary (shopkeeper compounding and selling medicines) and surgeon, the name and role of 'general practitioner' came into use in the early 19th century (Loudon 1983). But specialization in medicine was already growing before that century was out. By 1950 it seemed obvious to many leaders of opinion that the future of medicine must lie wholly in specialization backed by technology. A patient would have direct access to specialist; inevitably the role of the general doctor would disappear. The great therapeutic advances at that time seemed to provide convincing evidence.

This logical process went furthest in Sweden and the United States; in the latter country the proportion of full-time specialists rose from 16% in 1931 to 77% in 1969 (Stevens 1971). In the United Kingdom other factors stemmed the trend; the National Health Service offered registration with a personal doctor to every citizen and reinforced the tradition by which specialist care was normally reached only by referral from a general practitioner. In most other European countries the position was intermediate between that of the United States and the United Kingdom. In France, for instance, in 1975 (Guidevaux M et al) 30% of patients were seeing specialists by direct access.

Why then are there signs that this trend is changing in all countries? Why are the United States and Sweden now training more general practitioners? Why is the European Economic Community now agreeing a directive on the training of general practitioners? Above all, why does the World Health Organization see primary health care, rather than the further development of specialties, as the key to the attainment of a level of health which will permit people to lead a socially and economically productive life? (Declaration, Article V).

There is more than one reason. The escalating costs of medical care are probably the most powerful at present. Costs are greatest in countries where access to specialists and secondary hospital care is direct.

Table 2.1   Access to specialist physicians and the cost of health care

	Percentage of GNP Spent on Health Care
Countries with direct uncontrolled access by the patient to the specialist	
West Germany	9.4
United States	8.7
Sweden	8.5
France	7.9
Countries with direct access to specialists, but where patients will have to pay the difference between the specialist and general-practitioner rates of fee	
Austria	7.3
Canada	7.1
Italy	7.1
Switzerland	6.9
Countries where access to the specialist is normally by referral from the primary-care physician	
Netherlands	7.9
United Kingdom	6.1

Sources: Chiefly Simanis J G 1975 *National Health Systems in Eight Countries*, DHEW, Washington D.C., for referral patterns, supplemented by enquiries in the countries concerned (Maxwell 1981).

Maxwell has suggested that control over access to specialists is a key variable in determining the cost of a health service. Control is maximal in a two-tier system where the specialist is normally reached by referral.

But it is also clear that increasing specialization and the fragmentation which goes with it throw into sharper relief the need for a personal doctor who provides a broad scope, ready access, coordination and continuity of care when the patient is at home and at work. Public opinion has played an important part in reversing the trend towards specialization in Sweden (Sjönell 1984) and the United States (Citizen's Commission 1966). In the USA this influence came into play before the present concern with costs.

Developments in the medical profession started earlier still. The American Academy of General Practice (later Family Practice) was founded in 1947; the British College (then including Australia and New Zealand) in 1952. These and other similar institutions have had a growing influence, particularly in more developed countries.

But the trend which finds new importance in personal doctoring is not identical with the trend towards primary health care. Here developments in the United Kingdom provide only some of the clues; one must look to other parts of the world for others. 'Primary health care' is not only an ideal for the future; many of its features are to be found already in different countries, but none shows all.

In the United Kingdom only a minority of doctors now work alone. Most work in groups of three or more. They also work in teams with nurses and public health nurses, under the title 'primary care' or 'domiciliary' teams. Social workers, mainly a separate service, are sometimes included in the team, which increasingly works from a single location. More recently there has been a concerted effort to increase the preventive activity of this team, in response to changes in disease prevalence (Royal College of General Practitioners 1982 1983 and 1984) and to increase the participation of people generally in health and health services, in response to growing public knowledge of medicine and growing understanding of the relevance of lifestyles to illness.

Concern for prevention, self-care, healthy living and participation by the population has been a prominent feature of health services in countries of East Europe. So has concern for health services at the place of work. It is unlikely to have been mere chance which attached the name Alma Ata to the primary care initiatives of the World Health Organisation.

3. Is 'primary health care' acceptable? Realistic?

Article VI defines 'primary health care' in three sentences. But these sentences are highly concentrated, because they reflect a concept which contains many elements. These are separated and explained in more detail in the separate clauses of Article VII. The whole concept is proposed as an ideal towards which all countries could now work, however different their starting points. Are the various elements in the ideal compatible with the objectives of the World Organization of National Colleges and Academic Associations of Family Medicine/General Practice? Are they acceptable to general practitioners and family physicians?

> Essential health care — an integral part of the country's health system — it's central function and main focus. . . . The first level of contact of individuals, the family and community with the national health system and the first element of a continuing health care process. . . . It brings health care as close as possible to where people

> live and work. . . . It addresses the main health problems in the community, providing promotive, preventive, curative and rehabilitative services. . . . It is based on practical, scientifically sound and socially acceptable methods and technology.

For any general practitioner or family physician who experienced the isolation and neglect described earlier in this chapter, these descriptions are not merely acceptable, but most welcome encouragement. Indeed they might be alternative expressions of the objectives of WONCA or of such statements about the job of the general practitioner as the 'Leeuwenhorst' definition, at present accepted in the United Kingdom and several other European countries (Leeuwenhorst 1974). But there is more in these Articles:

> . . . primary health care is universally acceptable to individuals and families in the community at every stage of their development. . . . It requires and promotes maximum community and individual self-reliance and participation in the planning, organization, operation and control of care. . . . At a cost that the community and country can afford to maintain. . . . An integral part not only of the country's health system but also of the overall social and economic development of the community. . . . Involves, in addition to the health sector, all related sectors and aspects of national and community development (e.g. food industry education, etc.); and demands the co-ordinated efforts of all those sectors. . . . Gives priority to those most in need. . . . Sustained by integrative and mutually supportive referral systems, it relies on physicians, nurses, midwives, auxiliaries and community workers, but also on traditional practitioners, suitable trained to work as a team.

All these statements above are drawn from Articles VI and VII and they omit nothing essential which is is included in them. Although none appear incompatible with the objectives of the World Organization of National Colleges and Academics of Family Medicine/General Practice (WONCA) those in the last paragraph extend beyond the ground which WONCA covers. Even among these none would be unacceptable in the United Kingdom today. Whether or not general practitioners and family physicians in other countries would reject some particular aspect may well become apparent in subsequent chapters of this book. Worthwhile ideals are often formidable and hard to attain. 'Primary health care' is formidable because of the range of tasks which it covers. There are several elements in it which must be hard for any country to attain, harder for some than others, even assuming an effort to do so. John Reid has provided examples in the previous chapter. Difficulties particularly affecting general practitioners are considered in the next section of this chapter.

Meanwhile, so far from seeing general practitioners as sole agents for carrying out these tasks, the Declaration envisages team work by many health professions, backed by referral to specialist services and by co-ordination of health with other relevant departments at the level of local and central government. Moreover the frontline has moved forward. 'Self-reliance, self-determination, participation' all refer to non-professionals, people as individuals in families, who all experience health and illness and must at times therefore take the brunt of the battle.' Clearly general practitioners find a central place in this scheme, but only in so far as they reject past isolation and accept less familiar roles as organizers, co-ordinators and teachers. For them the challenge of primary health care is to achieve these changes without abandoning the essentials of personal doctoring — broad scope, ready access and continuity of care.

4. What particular challenges does 'primary health care' offer to WONCA and to the general practitioners and family physicians whom it represents?

The objectives of WONCA are:
a. To promote and monitor high standards of general/family practice through education and research.
b. To foster communication and understanding among general practitioners/family physicians.
c. To represent the academic and research activities of general practitioners/family physicians to other world organizations.
d. To stimulate the development of the educational and research organizations of general practitioners/family physicians.

There are now 30 national members in the organization. All individual members of national member organizations can regard themselves as belonging to the world organization (Game 1983).

Although most governments have endorsed the Alma Ata Declaration, it does not have the force of obligation. In any case general practitioners/family physicians in many countries are individually free to decide for themselves whether they agree with its principles and whether they wish to work towards them.

It is my belief that individuals and institutions concerned to promote high standards of general practice and family medicine should endorse these principles, in the confidence that they will forward the objectives in pursuit of which high standards are needed — the promotion of health and the prevention, care and cure of illness.

WONCA has already done valuable work in the international exchange of information and ideas. This diminishes national prejudice and encourages reflection about systems and methods which are less familiar. Moreover, WONCA links members of a professional group, which is bound to be influential in helping or hindering 'primary health care', but it is not the only one or the most important. The danger for WONCA could lie in the prejudices of a limited professional group, acting on a narrow concept of health care and reluctant to share responsibility with others. WONCA's definition of primary care (primary health care) (WONCA 1981) illustrates this problem at its root:

> Health care emphasizes responsibility for the patient, beginning at the time of the first encounter and continuing thereafter. This includes overall management and co-ordination of health care such as appropriate use of consultants, specialists and other health care resources. In addition maintenance of continuity on a long-term basis, including co-ordination of secondary and tertiary care is required.

This is a doctor-centred definition — 'responsibility for . . . .' 'first encounter . . .' 'management . . .'. It could possibly be read to include care by nurses, but it is certainly not patient-centred. It puts the emphasis on what health professionals can do rather than on what people can do for themselves. It seems to stem from a particular era in the development of one part of the medical profession, described in the second section of this article. It is more limited than the Alma Ata definition and could prove incompatible.

But there is no problem of compatibility with the World Health Organization in WONCA's special concern with research and education. There is too little research in primary health care in all countries, compared with other fields of medicine. Ignorance and illusions abound. Meanwhile the influence of primary health care is negligible in the medical schools of many countries; it is insufficient even in those where, in the form of general practice, it features routinely in the curriculum. WONCA has greater cause for satisfaction in the development of specific postgraduate training for doctors who have chosen a career in primary care. Moreover, there has been a remarkable growth in the annual number of papers, journals and books about the subject (there were practically none in 1950). The recent emphasis in continuing education on the general practitioner's own clinical problems and performance promises a revitalizing influence of great importance.

The challenge of the Alma Ata Declaration to WONCA lies

mainly therefore outside and beyond the education of general prac-
titioners/family physicians and research into their field of work.

As an organization originating in more developed countries and
with a membership still derived predominantly from them, can it
accept that Alma Ata applies to all countries and not merely to those
which have less resources? Can it accept that a 'level of health which
will permit a socially and economically productive life' is a worthwhile aim which has not been attained even in more developed
countries? Will WONCA influence its constituent Colleges and
Academies and its individual members to question the assumptions
of a medical school training and the traditional roles of doctors,
nurses and patients? Will its members wish to influence WONCA?

Can general practioners/family physicians fully accept the responsibility of carrying out 'the central function and being the main
focus' of a country's health system? What does that imply for their
relation with specialists and secondary care — is the specialist to
be leader or helper, father or brother, someone better at doing the
same job or equal colleague in doing one which is different?

Are general practitioners/family physicians really willing to
provide care where people live and work? At times when they need
it? With personal continuity, when this matters? Good care in
deprived areas, rural areas or the unattractive centre of industrial
cities?

Will they take the steps needed to organize preventive work —
immunizations, active detection of unsuspected disorders,
persistent attention to harmful life-styles? Will they themselves set
an example, for instance in balancing medical work, family life and
leisure, or in the use of alcohol? Will they help others to learn, so
that self-care can more often replace their own active interventions?

Can they accept that some tasks are better done by nurses, social
workers or counsellors than by doctors? That teamwork offers
chances of growth, but needs to be cultivated? Can they accept that
more patients may wish to be active partners, not only in their own
care but in organizing it for others? That their ideas, comments and
co-operation are much more often a help than a hindrance? How
far can they fulfil a role which demands such a variety of interpersonal skills and such flexibility in their application?

These are the sort of questions which the Declaration raises for
a doctor working in Western Europe. Different ones will challenge
those who work in countries where trained professionals, equipment, drugs and money are scarce or absent. Such countries are
likely to form a larger proportion of the membership of WONCA

in future and their problems will concern it increasingly. Its founding members have valuable experience to offer, but they may also be able to learn, about, for instance, what matters most in medical care and what can properly be achieved by simpler methods. No country can now escape the conflict between the increasing demands and costs of health care and what its people can afford.

Conclusion

'Primary health care', as defined by the Alma Ata Declaration, is a wider concept than general practice/family medicine, requiring that doctors in this field look again at their traditional role and consider certain changes. But it does not challenge the need for doctors, nurses and others whose remit is broad, who are readily accessible and provide continuity in personal care. Indeed, it stresses their value.

REFERENCES

Citizens' Commission on Graduate Medical Education 1966 The graduate education of physicians. American Medical Association, Chicago

Game D A 1983 Why WONCA? Journal of the Royal College of General Practitioners 33: 131–133

Guidevaux M et al 1975 Les Malades en Medecine libérale. INSERM, Paris

Hogarth J 1975 Glossary of health care terminology. WHO Regional Office for Europe, Copenhagen

Leeuwenhorst Working Party 1974 The general practitioner in Europe. In: Royal College of General Practitioners (1978) Some aims for training in general practice. Occasional paper 6. Royal College of General Practitioners, London

Loudon I S L 1983 The origin of the general practitioner. Journal of the Royal College of General Practitioners 33: 13–18

Maxwell R J 1981 Health and wealth. Lexington Books, Lexington, Massachusetts

Sjönell G 1984 Relationship between use of increased primary health care and other outpatient care in a Swedish urban area. Sundbyberg, Stockholm

Stevens R 1971 American medicine and the public Interest. Yale University Press New Haven and London

Royal College of General Practitioners 1982 Healthier Children. Thinking Prevention. Report from General Practice. Occasional Paper 22. Royal College of General Practitioners, London

Royal College of General Practitioners 1983 Promoting prevention. Report from General Practice. Occasional Paper 22. Royal College of General Practitioners, London

Royal College of General Practitioners 1984 Combined reports on prevention. Reports from General Practice 18–21. Royal College of General Practitioners, London

World Organization of National Colleges, Academies and Academic Associations
   of General Practitioners/Family Physicians 1981 An international glossary for
   primary care. Jouranl of Family Practice 13: 671–681
World Health Organization 1974 in Hogarth 1975 op cit
World Health Organization 1978 Alma Ata 1978. Primary health care. Report of
   the International Conference. World Health Organization, Geneva

Economics, politics and society

Primary health care: Reflects and evolves from the economic conditions and sociocultural and political characteristics of the country and its communities as is based on the application of the relevant results of social, biomedical and health services research and public health experience.

(Alma-Ata 1978)

Primary health care

Primary health care, general practice, family medicine, or whatever title is given, is inextricably involved in the economics and politics of society of all countries no matter what is the system of provision of health and medical care.

It is useful to recall the basic reasons for such involvements.

Primary health care is an essential level of care in any and every national health system.

Primary health care has its own special features and characteristics and its own specific core of knowledge and skills developed from experience, practice and research.

The national health system of a country is part of a wider welfare service provided for the people.

The welfare services are part of a greater society and include provision of work opportunities, housing and shelter, food and water, sanitation, education, transport, assistance for the needy and fair shares of national wealth and resources.

Society requires 'politics', in the widest sense, to create and achieve a good life for its people.

Politics involve responsibilities, leadership, priorities, equable allocations of resources, rationing and concern with value for money'.

Systems of health care

Each national system of health care is unique but the same. It is unique because each has developed through a slow process of evolution over a long time or been created *de novo* by revolution. Some countries have no recognizable system.

Each national system is rooted in national history that is involved in political and cultural philosophies and beliefs. Some are based on extreme socialistic views, others on free-enterprise with individuals and families responsible for their own care and its costs, most appear to e somewhere between these extremes.

National health systems may be influenced by geography and climate, by religious principles and by education and skills of the people. However, the greatest influencing factor is national wealth, based on sound economics, and plentiful resources.

Division of countries into 'developed' and 'developing' is artificial. It is factors, such as have been noted, that are responsible for differences.

All health systems have the same needs and requirements. There have to be four basic levels of care. Self-care, primary professional care, general specialist care and superspecialist care. Each level has to have its own understandable and acceptable roles supported by resources, organisation, education, training, support and supervision. Each system has to decide how each level should operate and how each should relate to the others. The movements between each level such as decisions of individuals to seek primary professional care, the referrals between primary care, general specialist care and super specialist care are important influences on efficiency, effectiveness and economics of the system.

The types of health systems can be classified in various ways but probably the most practical is to relate them in terms of economics. That is, how hospitals, practices, doctors, nurses and others are paid and for what and from where and how does the money come.

Thus, there are completely *socialized health systems* in USSR, Eastern Europe, Cuba and China. There are incompletely socialized systems in United Kingdom and the Scandinavian countries.

There are systems based on a variety of *prepaid health insurance schemes* as in USA, Canada, West Germany, Australia and Japan.

There are systems that combine socialized, insurance and private fees systems into *'public-private mix'* as in France and Netherlands. However, it must be stated honestly that some form of public-private exists in all systems. Everywhere it is possible, even in USSR and China, to opt out of the public system and obtain some private medical care. (See McLachlan & Maynard 1982 for a comprehensive review.)

Then there are countries that have no system of health care apart from basic public health services.These are the poor countries of the world, where national resources are no more than at subsistence level and who can spend very little on health services.

Thus within the web of modern society there is an intertwining web that enmeshes primary health care with economics, politics and society in various degrees.

(For a good description of primary care systems, see Stephen 1979).

GENERAL ISSUE

Economics

Health care is expensive and has to be paid for. The proportions of a developed country's wealth that is spend on health services is between 5 and 10% of its gross national product (GNP) (Fig. 3.1)

There is a direct relationship between national wealth and the amounts spent on health. The wealthier the country the more it spends.

In developed countries between 5 and 10% of the health budgets is spent on primary health services and this is unrelated to the type of system.

Primary medical care is cheap because it requires less expensive technologies, manpower and capital expenditure than hospitals.

Expenditure on health care is directly related to the number of doctors per population. The more doctors there are, the more expensive is health care (Abel-Smith 1984).

The cost of primary medical care relates also to the ways in which the doctors are paid. Systems where payment of family doctors is by salary or capitation fees cost less than those where payment is by fees for items of services (Abel-Smith 1984).

Medical politics is much involved with negotiations of rates of pay of doctors. The average income of family doctors tend to follow

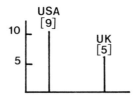

Fig. 3.1 Health expenditure as percentage of GNP in 1979 in various countries. (Office of Health Economics Compendium, 1981, Table 1.2.)

national wealth, although paradoxically in poor countries the few doctors in practice can command high fees from those few who can afford them.

There is no such thing as a 'free health service'. They all cost much money. This is obviously apparent where the public pays fees for services or premiums for health insurance politices, but not so where the doctor is paid by salary or capitation fees.

The annual per capita expenditure, for every man, woman and child, in 1979 ranged from £400 in Sweden and USA to less than £100 in Italy (Fig. 3.2).

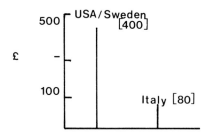

Fig. 3.2 Per capita expenditure on health in 1979 in various countries. (Office of Health Economics Compendium, 1981, Table 1.2.)

Thus for a family of parents and 2 young children the expenditure in 1979 in Sweden and USA was £1600 and of this about £150 was spent on primary health care.

The money for health care comes largely from national government taxes and from health insurance schemes. Only a small proportion comes from private fees from patients. The cost of health now is too great for any family to have to meet alone. There has to be direct or indirect government subsidies. Therefore, it is inevitable that health care is part of party politics.

With high and rising costs of health care, those involved in paying for it — governments and health insurance agencies — are increasingly concerned with value for their money. They seek effective, efficient and economic services.

Questions are being asked but few answers are available on what is useful and beneficial in health care and what is less than useful or beneficial.

The value and benefits of modern medical technologies and procedures are being doubted (Aaron & Schwartz 1984). They compared costs, prevalence and outcome of selected procedures in

USA and UK, such as dialysis and renal transplantation, chemo-therapy and radiotherapy for cancer, hip replacement, coronary artery surgery, CT scanners and diagnostic X-rays. They believe that many of these procedures are not cost-effective and their wide-spread use must be controlled.

Search for economies in health care must lead to more and better health services research, audits and self-check exercises to attempt to measure quality as well as quantity of care. Logically, incentives for better care and disincentives for poor care might follow.

Politics

'Politics' involves national and local governments, but it also involves professional bodies, representing medical and paramedical professions, too.

Government involvement

As noted, this is now inevitable because of its subsidization of health care financially and because of the needs for planning and use of resources to ensure fair and equable distribution and allo-cation. Such forward planning may involve controls, directives, cuts and rationing leading to conflicts with the medical profession and the public. Democratic governments are anxious to retain the support of voters by ensuring their satisfaction with their health services. This may rate as a higher priority than keeping doctors happy.

Professional bodies

Medical associations, colleges and academies that represent doctors sooner or later will clash with governments in their negotiations. Among issues that are of concern are:

1. Maintenance of clinical freedom and independence.
2. Assurance of high standards and quality. These require adequate resources and facilities for practice, education and training. Such resources and facilities require government finance.
3. Regulation, control and direction of the medical profession is necessary, in keeping with appropriate freedom and independence, but such functions are best carried out by the profession itself rather than by outside bodies and agencies.

4. Conditions of service and remuneration must be negotiated with governments or health insurance agencies.

A major dilemma is how can, and should, political bodies representing the profession become involved in such decisions and in accepting responsibilities for planning better health services in line with national resources.

Society

The public naturally are most interested and concerned in the primary health care that they receive. Their 'wants' are for good health in a better and longer life.

They want both quality and quantity. They seek primary health care that is readily available and accessible; that is affordable at costs that all can meet; personal and continuous, so that patients and doctor come to know each other over years of contact; and of a quality that ensures cure, relief, comfort and prevention.

Public expectations are increasing with desire for more involvement and participation in the health process. The roles, processes and outcomes of traditional medical practice are being questioned and assessed. There is growing public interest in, and use of, non-traditional systems such as homeopathy, naturopathy, acupuncture, chiropractice and others. The development of the holistic movement that encompasses care of the 'whole' person signifies public disenchantment with some features of modern medicine.

The medical profession in general, and primary health care in particular, must heed these signals and review its public relations and services.

SOME FACTS OF ECONOMIC MEDICAL LIFE

There are some facts that have to be accepted as real and inevitable in providing health care.

1. Escalating costs are reaching *finite limits*. Expenditure on health services everywhere has assumed rates of infinite growth.

2. *'Wants'* of services by patients and of facilities by doctors are always going to be greater than *'needs'* as calculated by planners and administrators, and these will always exceed the *resources* that are available.

3. The challenge has to be how to make the *best use of available resources*.

4. *'Value for money'* the keywords of providers implies the applications of audits to checks on quantity of resources needed and on the quality of care provided, as demonstrated by outcomes using controlled trials and other methods.

5. Neither *health nor health services* can ever be shared equally. There are *inequalities* in standards of health among social classes, occupational groups and families. There are inequalities in distribution of resources between countries and regions within a country.

6. Attempts have to be made to try and achieve *fairer shares*. This will lead to *rationing* of services in some areas and disciplines.

7. There has to be a *balance* between *controls* and *directives* by health authorities and professional freedom-independence.

8. In the end there have to be some *incentives and disincentives* for public and profession to live within limits of available resources.

THE BRITISH NATIONAL HEALTH SERVICE (NHS) — A CASE HISTORY

As a more specific illustrative example of the influence of society, politics and economics, some details and facts are appropriate.

1. The NHS is *part of a large welfare system*.

2. It is *available to all* and is utilized at some time by the whole population.

3. In *any year approximately 80% of the population will use it* on one or more occasion, this is made up of:

    a. 65% who will consult their general practitioners

    b. 12% of the population who will be admitted to hospital (hospitalized) on one or more occasions

    c. 18% of the population who will be newly referred to hospital and specialists (consultants) by general practitioners

    d. 20% who will attend hospital accident-emergency departments

(There is overlap between these groups and therefore the totals are over 100%) (Fry et al 1984)

4. The *NHS is government controlled*. It cost over £17 000 million in 1984, that is 6% of GNP. This is the same proportion as for defence and for education. In addition, the cost of social services is another 12% of GNP. It is significant that about one-fifth of wealth/income is spent on health and social services. Therefore, its expenditure and services must be responsible to Parliament, that is, the elected representatives of the people.

5. The *government's agent is the Department of Health and Social Security*. Health is one of its responsibilities. There are three parts — hospital services, general practitioner and allied services, and community services.

6. *Family Practitioner Committees* are the administrative bodies for general practice. Each covers a population of about 250 000 involving over 100 general practitioners.

7. *General practitioners* are independent contractors within NHS, contracted to provide services to those who are 'registered' with them. They are free to organize their work and services as they wish, but are responsible for standards of their services. General practitioners are paid by a mixture — capitation fees, fees for services, basic allowances and reimbursement for premises and staff employed.

Society

The NHS is widely acceptable — 98% of the population are registered with general practitioners; 7% of the population, in addition, subscribe to private insurance schemes for private hospital care, chiefly for minor or moderate 'cold surgical procedures'.

There is general satisfaction with the NHS but there are about 8000 complaints about doctors each year referred to:
1. General Medical Council (1000) (professional conduct)
2. Family practitioner committees (700) (services provided by general practitioners)
3. Hospital doctors (6300) (care provided in hospitals)

Complaints about general practitioners include bad manners, failure to visit at home, unsatisfactory appointment systems and inadequate care (Fry, Brooks and McColl 1984).

Politics

As noted, government involvement in health services is unavoidable because of the huge amount of public money involved.

On the *government side* the bodies involved are the national Department of Health and Social Security (in England), the regional health authorities and the district health authorities (chiefly for hospital services) and family practitioner committees (FPC) (for general practice).

The *profession* is represented by a number of groups in its negotiations, discussions and collaboration with government:

1. The *British Medical Association* (BMA) represents the whole profession (65% of all practising doctors are members).

2. The political branch of BMA that negotiates for general practice is the *General Medical Services Committee.*

3. The *Royal College of General Practitioners* is the academic body of general practice — one-third of general practitioners are members and fellows.

4. *Local medical committees* are elected by general practitioners in FPC areas and they deal with local issues.

5. The *General Medical Council* is an independent statutory body concerned with educational standards and conduct of all doctors.

Although there are many groups involved they work well together to achieve results.

Economics

The *population* of the United Kingdom is 56 million. In 1985 the cost of the NHS was over £17 000 million, or £300 per capita.

The *costs of the NHS* have been escalating (Fig. 3.3).

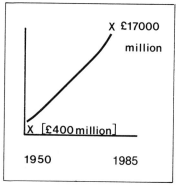

Fig. 3.3 In real terms, allowing for inflation, the cost of the NHS increased fourfold from 1950 to 1985.

Where the money comes from

Almost all funding of the NHS comes from central government through general taxes. 9% comes from national health insurance contributions and 3% from direct payments for prescriptions, dental treatment, spectacles and similar charges (Fig. 3.4).

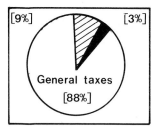

Fig. 3.4 NHS funding. (Fry et al 1984).

Where the money goes

Hospitals account for 64% of NHS costs, general practice for 6%, drugs prescribed by general practitioners 10% and other services for the rest 20%.

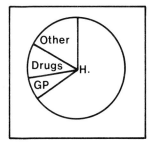

Fig. 3.5 NHS expenditure.

Costs per doctor

It has been estimated that in the year 1982–83 an *average hospital consultant* controlled £530 000 of NHS money and a *general practitioner* £80 000 (Hansard, Parliamentary questions col. 2609 and 2623, 1983–84).

However, the amounts controlled by a general practitioner are much greater and may amount up to £250 000 per GP. They are made up as follows (for 1982–83):

General practice

remuneration of GP	£20.000
drugs prescribed	£45.000
expenses	£15.000
	£80.000

Investigations (carried out for GPs at hospitals)	£7.000
Hospital services	
patients admitted to hospital	£110.000
patients seen at hospital	
outpatient departments	£25.000

These are huge costs and they show the great economic importance of the general practitioner. Since NHS costs increase correspondingly with increases in numbers of doctors, questions of medical manpower are of interest to politicians, administrators and economists.

Medical manpower

The numbers and rates of doctors in the NHS have more than doubled since 1950.

The rates per 1000 population are in Table 3.1 and the increases were greater for hospital doctors than general practitioners.

Table 3.1   Doctors in NHS (England and Wales) 1950–1981 in rates per 1000 of population (Fry et al 1984)

	1950	1981	Proportionate increase
Hospital doctors	2.7	8.4	× 3.1
General practitioners	3.4	5.0	× 1. 5
Numbers	(28 000)	(64 000)	

The numbers of NHS general practitioners have been increasing faster than the population growth and consequently the average number of persons registered per general practitioner has been decreasing (Fig. 3.6).

There are no good guidelines on manpower requirements. The number of medical students starting on their studies has varied according to national policies over the past 40 years. It seems that every 10 years there has been a pendulum swing from more students → fewer students → more students → fewer students. These ups and down have been based on recommendations of committes set up by the government and profession.

Now in the 1980s we are in a phase of believing that there are too many medical students. About 400 started their training in 1983–84 and one-half of were women.

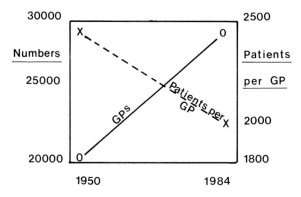

Fig. 3.6 Numbers of GPs and average numbers of patients per GP in NHS (1950–1984). (Fry et al 1984.)

It is probable that there are (at most) up to 2000 vacancies through death, retirement and new appointments in general practice each year and up to 1500 in hospital service for doctors. This suggests a surplus of 500 newly graduated doctors per year. Already there is medical unemployment and this may grow.

PRESENT PROBLEMS

There are some problems that are *common to, and shared by,* all countries and some that are particularly influenced by *national systems*, which are dealt with in Part 2. Here the common shared problems are discussed.

As the Alma-Ata Declaration noted, primary health care must relate to a country's economics, politics and society's views.

Economics

Everywhere resources available for health services are limited in money, facilities and manpower. As noted, 'wants' will always exceed 'needs' and 'resources'.

The major problem and challenge is how to make the best use of the resources that are available. Modus vivendi has to be achieved in terms of efficiency, effectiveness and economics. The question, '*Who does what best where, when, how and why?*', has to be posed and answered.

1. *Who?* Should it be a highly trained doctor, or may some tasks of primary health care be carried out as well, or perhaps even

better, by less highly and less expensively trained nurses or other paramedical workers?

2. *How many?* In addition it has to be asked how many doctors, nurses and others do we require for primary health care? The question cannot be answered satisfactorily because there is no reliable data.

3. *What?* What tasks being carried out in primary health care are useful and beneficial or useless and even harmful? Here also there are no data or trails that can be applied in practice.

4. *How?* Similarly, detailed procedures in current practice have to be questioned as to whether they are the best to achieve planned goals.

5. *Where?* A re-examination is necessary of the places where health care is being carried out. It may be that some care may be better distributed between self-care in the community, primary professional care in health units and general specialists care in hospitals and elsewhere. It must not be assumed that present customs and habits are sacrosanct and unchangeable.

6. *When?* To what stages in the health processes should primary health care be aimed? Some anticipatory and preventive care has to be directed to symptomatic stages, other at early diagnosis and yet others at long-term support and follow-up.

7. *Why?* Whatever changes are being considered, explanations and good reasons must be provided for public and professions. A major problem is lack of good communication.

Politics

As noted above, government involvement in health care is necessary and has to be accepted.

Present and future dilemmas exist over concordats between governmental controls and professional freedom and independence.

Bodies representing the medical profession have to carry out a continuing negotiating dialogue without government, quasi-government and other agencies involved in the economics and financing of health care.

In the negotiations it has to be remembered that ultimately 'what is best for the patient' outweighs 'what is best for the doctor'. The problems must be faced of how to involve active patients, as well as their elected political representatives, in future planning.

Society

People now are better educated and informed on health matters than ever before and they will continue to be through media and regular educational methods. No longer can the medical profession remain a secret society, as in the past.

The profession and individual doctors have to work out ways of improving public and personal relations.

Politics is about keeping voters (society) happy and satisfied. Governments and other finding bodies are more interested in voters than in doctors.

FUTURE NEEDS

1. Primary health care has to be accepted as important and essential requiring proper and adequate finance, support and planning.

2. The amounts of such financing, support and planning have to worked out nationally and locally and must relate to needs that include education, training, facilities and services.

3. Abysmal lack of data and information based on reliable health services research makes future effective planning difficult, if not impossible.

4. It is essential that in all health care systems research is carried out to assess and measure quantity and quality and the relations between the two. What quantities are needed to achieve good quality of care?

5. It is only through reliable and acceptable researches that good planned health care can be provided. Such planned care has to consider present and future roles of patients, doctors, administrators and politicians.

6. Possible economics and improvements in primary health care may be possible by better use of manpower, of prescribing, of diagnostic and investigative procedures, of hospitals and of self-care.

7. Better primary health care in the future will only come about through closer understanding and collaboration between the people, the government and the profession and, to achieve this, demands positive leadership from all sides.

REFERENCES

Aaron H , Schwartz W B 1984 The painful prescription: rationing hospital care. The Brookings Institution, Washington DC
Abel-Smith B 1984 Cost containment in health care: and study of 12 European countries. Bedford Square Press, London
Fry J, Brooks D, McColl I 1984 NHS data book. MTP, Lancaster
McLachlan G, Maynard A (eds) 1982 The public/private mix for health: the relevance and effects of change. Nuffield Procincial Hospitals Trust, London
Stephen W J 1979 An analysis of primary medical care-an international study. Cambridge University Press, Cambridge

Perspectives

HEALTH AND DISEASE

Both health and disease are difficult to define and even more difficult to quantify or measure. *Health*, says the WHO, is more than an absence of disease: it is complete mental and physical well-being. That sounds grand, but is not helpful for two reasons. Firstly, no one will attain health as defined in that way, and secondly, 'well-being' as such is almost equally difficult to define. René Dubos in his book *Man Adapting* (1965) proferred a much more useful definition: 'Health is the ability to adapt your environment, or, if necessary, to adapt to it'. In other words, health is the ability to go to where the food is, to come in out of the cold, to extend the house, to go to University, and so on. The extent to which a person or groups of people are capable of adapting their environment or adapting to it is observable and often measurable. Health should be seen in terms of abilities and, by the same token, potentials for improving one's own lot, one's family's lot, and one's group or community's lot. Thus it can be seen to correlate with the concept of 'personal space': the area of one's life over which one has control. Experiences such as illness, or poverty, or hunger, diminish that space by constraining the width of choices about one's life that one can make. So does an unhappy marriage, or finding oneself in the wrong job.

Disease' is often used as the generic term for pathology, or pathological processes, in contradistinction to 'illness', which is the subjective experience of the sufferer. Hence the use of the expression 'disease centred teaching v. person centred teaching', or 'disease centred care v. person centred care'. This is too widespread a usage to abandon, but it is worth noting that some writers use 'disease' as a much more global statement of the patient's condition: their ease is diminished.

From this it can be seen that health and disease are not, in fact, opposites or conceptual alternatives, because the concept of health is much broader, and disease is only one of the things that may diminish it. It is important to draw this distinction because otherwise it is easy to confuse objectives. Curing or ameliorating disease can only contribute some components of health and even if totally successful cannot secure complete health. If the medical task is to do with the cure, amelioration or prevention of disease, and it is, then it is important to realize that even unqualified success doesn't secure 'complete health' for the individual or population to whom that care is directed. Failure to observe this distinction has serious consequences because it creates erroneous expectations. If you are unable to adapt to your environment, that is, if your personal space is cramped, your health is diminished and you are likely to look to the medical profession for help. If it is disease which is impinging on your ability to adapt, or on your personal space, then this is an appropriate route toward help. If, however, what is diminishing your health is actually poverty, or an unhappy marriage, or some other social problem, then there is a grave risk that such action will 'medicalize' the problem. There may well be collusion: if a personal problem can be ascribed to disease, it is somebody else's (the doctor's) job to do something about it, whereas if the problem is due to poor relationships, then the onus is on the individual to do something about it. Doctors, because of their training, are more comfortable with situations that they can see as disease requiring them to take definitive action than problems which cannot be interpreted in those terms and which are not susceptible to the usual range of interventions available to them. They tend, therefore, to collude with the patient and provide the problem with a medical label and the patient with a prescription. It is important to recognize that the patient's personal space has been further diminished by having to share it to some extent with the health professional!

CULTURALLY DETERMINED CONCEPTS

The way in which health and disease are understood and interpreted in different cultures and different groups within any one culture varies widely.

In western culture it has been shown that some see health as an asset and as a right. It is an essential part of their life equipment and can be capitalized on in seeking social advancement. When such people become ill they tend to seek care early and quite aggressively, because any loss of health is seen as a bar to further social success. (Interestingly, among people with all the social advantages, health is becoming an end in itself and the 'man who has everything' not only abjures the enjoyments of tobacco, alcohol and good food, but punishes himself on the jogging track!)

At the other end of the social scale health is seen as just one more of those things that is nice if you have it, but can't be expected to be doled out equally to everybody. Plenty of studies have shown that disadvantaged people *expect* to feel tired, to have backache, to suffer from headaches, cough, and indigestion: these are part of their lot in life. Everybody is like it, what can you expect? Diminution in their health, therefore, does not act in the same way as a spur to action, but merely is added to the catalogue of disadvantage and suffering.

In any case their 'life agenda' is much more crowded with matters of immediate concern. Medical care may be some way off, may be expensive, will cost loss of wages or interfere with time that needs to be spent searching for work or food or shelter. Ironically, therefore, those most likely to be unhealthy, to suffer disease, are the least likely to seek help or, at any rate, to seek it early.

Interestingly, doctors' intolerance of, and anger about, patients who enter care late is not mirrored in their own care-seeking behaviour, which is often bizarre. Some of this is perhaps due to pressure of their own life agenda: they can't make time to be ill themselves. They share the well known pattern of illness, with senior executives, of only being ill on holiday or at weekends. But this is compounded by a morbid fear of being thought by their colleagues, from whom they seek help, to be weak or neurotic. Curiously, their higher level of knowledge than ordinary lay people does not contribute to more rational behaviour. They often recognize that their symptoms must be those of serious physical illness but fail to present for care. Despite their extra knowledge, they share much of their behaviour with the rest of humanity, to whom, of course, they belong. Lay people, too, fear to be thought neurotic, fear to be thought to be wasting the doctor's time, even in North America where they are paying the doctor well for his time!. Underlying both sets of behaviour, of course, is the unwillingness to sacrifice autonomy — some introspection might provide insights!

It may be objected that this sort of behaviour by doctors, who in most countries are at the top of the social tree, belies the earlier statement that socially advantaged people see health as an asset and, at any diminution of it, enter care early. If this is so, it may just be a function of the specialist knowledge held by the doctor both about disease processes and his or her colleague's attitudes; on the other hand it might be argued that doctors are not upwardly socially mobile, because they are already in the top stratum of society both in terms of wealth and esteem, and therefore ill health is not seen as a bar to further progress.

If there are significant differences in attitudes to health and the seeking of care between advantaged and disadvantaged people within one culture, one might expect much wider differences between cultures. Bice and Kalimo (1971) examined attitudes in South America, Scandinavia, Eastern Europe, The Balkans, North America, and Great Britain and found that, with regard to six concepts, there was little difference. They measured people's attitudes to the perceived availability of care, their scepticism about effectiveness of care, their scepticism about doctors, their feelings about being dependent when ill, their tendency to use services for physical problems, and their tendency to use services for psychosocial problems. The similarities far outweighed differences despite radically different health care delivery systems.

Much work has been done, notably by Becker and his associates (1977), on 'health belief systems', basing their work on psychological and behavioural theory which postulates that behaviour is controlled not only by the expectation of benefit, but also by the probability of achieving that benefit and by an assessment of the seriousness of the risk associated with the disease in question.

Obviously, if the perceived risk is low, or the perceived probability of benefit is low, then care-seeking and compliance will also be low. Hence the necessity for doctors to elucidate the health beliefs of their patients, not only in their role as health educators but in their day-to-day practice. More recently theories have been advanced about 'locus of control'. If one sees oneself in control of one's own life, able to make decisions about it, and believing that one can do positive things about one's health and disease, behaviour will be different from the situation in which one believes that one is controlled by outside forces and even that disease may be sent as a punishment. The locus of control idea is particularly important in less sophisticated (in Western terms) societies where disease as a phenomenon has been incorporated into socioreligious belief systems. The New Testament provides plenty of examples.

We can begin to differentiate, therefore, between those persons whose social and cultural circumstances predict early entry into care, compliance with treatment, and acceptance of preventive measures and advice on the one hand, and those who, constrained by the same forces and circumstances, are likely to enter care late, comply poorly with treatment, and be resistant to preventive measures and advice. Our own reaction as doctors to the latter needs careful examination. We have our own psychological quirks. We have had to learn to live with failure, with frustration, with uncertainty, and compensate for this by a tendency towards activism, optimism, and impatience with doubt. It is very easy for us, therefore, to impinge on, and further diminish, the personal space of people who haven't got much anyway. Jealous of our own autonomy we may be insufficiently careful of others. We may not align our priorities for the patient with their own life priorities. Faced with a down and out vagrant, sleeping rough, and feeding off scraps, are we justified in advising him to stop smoking fag ends, one of the few pleasures available to him, for the sake for prolonging an unenjoyable life? In some other areas of enthusiastic prevention there may be even less evidence of effectiveness on a population basis as a justification for intervention. Ivan Illich [1982] has accused us of medicalizing health.

Who are then at risk? Obviously, late entry into care and poor compliance with both treatment and prevention carry avoidable risks, and, therefore, those persons whose station in life or circumstances predict such behaviours, run those risks. These are people to whom society has vouchsafed little personal space or whose life agendas are crowded. Perhaps this is the meaning of Rahe's [1977] work on life events. Interestingly, before his death, J Cassels [personal communication] suggested that sound personal relationships in the home and at work exerted a protective effect even from high life event scores. This could be equated with a modicum of extra personal space.

Most people, if not all, are, at some time or another, in jeopardy of disease or trauma. Identifiable excessive dangers may allow certain groups of people to be characterized as 'at risk', and therefore identified as the targets for, or recipients of, specific interventions. It must not be forgotten, however, that not all members of such groups will succumb, even if no intervention is undertaken, and that, conversely, members of the public outside those groups may be affected. Not only must the identification of risk factors be valid, but the differentiation between those at risk and the rest must be reliable. To be labelled as 'at risk' and made the target of some preventive intervention is to be made in some way out of the ordinary and this may be in itself diminish personal space. Even then, the expected benefit for the group has to be compared with the sporadic incidence in the rest of the population when trying to decide on whether the strategy is justifiable in cost benefit terms.

Risk factors that can be used to indentify such groups may be genetic, geographical, environmental, behavioural, occupational, economic or cultural. Within each category it is easy to propose targets for intervention: sickle cell disease, malaria, lead poisoning, lung cancer, bladder cancer, malnutrition, hypovitaminosis, respectively. Equally, however, other risk factors can be identified in each category that are not only less susceptible to medical intervention, but are more likely to invade people's personal space, for example, sexually transmitted diseases, or refusal of blood transfusion by Jehovah's witnesses.

The equation that has to be solved, therefore, before an identified 'at risk group' is subjected to a medical intervention, not only involves 'hard' data about probabilities, effectiveness, and monetary costs, but the 'softer' but no less important considerations of personal costs in being labelled, and of loss of personal space. The surprising thing is not that the 'soft' considerations are usually ignored, but that the 'hard' data are often defective when population initiatives are launched. Here too we are vulnerable to 'collusion': in the face of manifest problems the people, directly, through pressure groups, or through their politicians press for action, and their doctors and health administrators prefer to be 'doing something about it' and to be seen to be doing so. Obviously, some population medicine initiatives have been highly successful: the eradication of smallpox is a brilliant example. By and large, however, the record is disappointing, either because the intervention proposed was less effective than hoped, or less acceptable. In other words, 'the population voted with their feet'. As an example, cervical cytology screening in the UK, even though the at risk group was clearly identifiable, has barely altered the death rate.

The most effective interventions to improve health have not, of course, been medical but social and environmental: better education, better housing, less poverty, better nutrition, safety at work, clean water, safe sewage disposal, etc. All of these can be seen not only in terms of physical hygiene, but as gains in personal space.

Population-base interventions in response to identified risk factors pose serious problems, not only of cost effectiveness and therefore of resource allocation, but in the realms of ethics and

mandate: did these people *ask* us to enter their lives? But identification of such risks in the individual *is* an important part of the
primary care physician's job. Where that doctor has a defined population it may be possible to identify such individuals as members
of a group, and negotiate with them in terms of offering a preventive initiative *as part of* of comprehensive care. Nevertheless, the
considerations discussed above still apply. Given that these people
are at risk, what are the strategies available to the doctor to achieve
more effective care? Elucidation of health beliefs and locus of
control ideas allow him or her to present the plan for care in a more
person centred, sensitive, and relevant fashion. The plan itself may
be modified to provide more respect for the patient's autonomy,
and its priorities more in line with the patients. The wind is
tempered to the shorn lamb!

This calls for a high level of skill, as does the need to recognize
small deviations from normal health, and to elucidate, with the
patient, the real nature of the problem. While these skills may be,
and often are, found in other health care workers, their shorter
training, smaller knowledge base, and position in the hierarchy
make it difficult for them to exercise them. For this reason there
is much to be said, when it is feasible in terms of finance and
trained manpower, for deploying properly trained doctors as 'first
contact' health workers. In developing countries, as literacy and
sophistication grows, expectations rise, and the ordinary people can
be seen to seek doctors for first contact care, often bypassing high
quality health facilities manned by health assistants, nurses etc. In
order that such doctors can be effective, they should delegate much
follow-up and preventive care to other health workers who are not
only quite capable of discharging such tasks, but are usually better
than doctors at doing so!

Even when the problem is sensitively elucidated, defined in terms
that are culturally and personally appropriate, and the agreed
management plan acceptable and effective, the benefit must be
seen, in total health terms, to be limited. The patient's personal
space, his or her ability to adapt the environment, is diminished not
only by disease, as we have seen, but by the social ills of poverty,
unemployment, poor housing, occupational and environmental
hazards, and poor education. As long as Medicine sees its role
mainly as reactive, waiting to pick up the pieces, waiting till the
patient presents for care, then it will and can do nothing to ameli-
orate these risk factors.

PRESENT PROBLEMS

Underlying the emergence of what could be called 'the culture of health' in any given society will, of course, be its general experience of health and disease; for example, a society that has had to endure a very high infant mortality rate tends to maintain a high birth rate, as replacements. It is the common experience of health in the developing world that the infant mortality rate comes down before people can be convinced that they can lower their fertility rate, and the result is a population explosion.

Illnesses common in a society generate their own culture and folklore, their own interpretations and expectations. Western doctors are often puzzled by, and even irritated by, the concern of people from the Indian subcontinent about pyrexia in their children: something that most Western mothers take in their stride. It is easy to forget that in much of the world 'fever' is the herald of malaria, always serious, and potentially lethal. Sometimes 'sophisticated' societies lose vitality, lose certain capabilities. It is difficult for those of us living in 'advanced' societies to understand the feelings of these for whom death is a commonplace family event, yet you have only got to look at the graveyards around our churches to see, by what has been called graveyard epidemiology, that death in infancy, young adulthood and childbirth were commonplace before the turn of the century. These were still the common experience of our grandparents, yet now we have lost the social and emotional strategies which allowed them to cope. Today a child's death is much more difficult for the family to bear because it is such an unheard of event. Responses to sudden changes in patterns of morbidity and mortality may be inappropriate. We have already given as an example the failure of people to curb their fertility rate as infant mortality drops.

Sometimes the contribution of medical technology is misinterpreted and made the focus of hope and investment when the benefit has really come from sanitary engineering. In most developing countries money invested in public health works, immunization and infant nutrition projects, will make a much greater contribution to the health of that society than will the erection, equipment and staffing of expensive specialist hospitals. This, however, is an olympian view and it might be difficult, in the face of established illness, to defend it, when the wherewithal to treat and sometimes cure that illness is available to some people elsewhere. Nations, like people, must have their autonomy, they must be allowed to make choices.

Perhaps the role of medicine should be to make sure at least that these are as well informed choices as possible. There are certainly, in some parts of the world, grotesque anomalies. There are countries in which children with heart murmurs can have cardiac catheterization but where there is no basic immunization programme!

Such situations are, of course, indefensible: why do they come about? Partly, because there is a tendency for any ruling class, whatever its politics to seek advantages for itself; one of these advantages is the sort of health care that they perceive to suit their needs. This tendency may be compounded by two malignant forces. The first of these is the irresponsible and cynical exploitation of such countries by the providers of medical technology and even packaged medical care, hospitals, equipment, doctors and nurses in one deal. As commercial organizations these are looking to maximize the profits for their shareholders and there is far more to be gained from the installation of a Western-type teaching hospital than from the provision of a network of peripheral clinics, staffed by health assistants, and equipped with little more than baby scales and plastic syringes. The other circumstances which tends to push developing countries in this direction is the development of private medical practice, reasonable enough if there is no other way of getting the doctors paid. But this tends to concentrate the doctors around those places where there are enough people with enough money to pay for their services rather than distributing them evenly across the whole population.

These forces tend to produce a 'top down' specialist-orientated curative service in the capital and the major cities of a country while leaving the small towns, villages and country districts denuded of effective health care. But the politicians and the leaders of such countries are not the only ones to subscribe to these beliefs, and there are plenty of examples of poor country people actually bypassing village clinics and seeking care in the outpatient departments of urban hospitals, which are neither staffed nor equipped to cope with undifferentiated need. This compounds a further problem, which is that the long and demanding medical training, while it may recruit people from a fairly wide social spectrum, turns out doctors who are, by definition, of the upper class with the social aspirations of that class. Not for them the outback, the backward villages, or the shabbier corners of the big towns. That is not what they have worked for, nor is it what they, or their parents, invested so much money in. Few go back to the community from which they came. They have become fish too big for the pool they left to go to medical school. Of course you don't have to go to a developing country to see maldistribution of doctors! The United States is a classic example: during the 1970s there were many towns with a population of 20 000 or less who could not get a doctor to go there or to stay. One study showed that no doctor would stay in a town smaller than the one in which his wife grew up.

FUTURE NEEDS

The establishment of effective primary care in any country demands clear public understanding of the role of the generalist in dealing with undifferentiated need cheaply, effectively, and locally; adequate investment by government whether as direct employer or merely provider of the infrastructure, premises, supporting staff, equipment, and administration; and a modus vivendi with specialists. The latter is particularly difficult to achieve for three reasons.

Firstly, the specialists have subjected themselves to longer training and more examinations and feel themselves better qualified: they believe they can provide better care and therefore should do so. Secondly, they have the technology, the impressive equipment, potent treatments and strong magic that often resonate with the patient's health beliefs. Thirdly, they may be in direct economic competition with the primary care generalists.

It is fair to say that the huge upheaval of enthusiasm and excitement that characterized the family medicine movement in the United States in the late 1960s and early 1970s seems to have been contained by the backlash from primary care internal medicine, primary care paediatrics and primary care obstetrics/gynaecology. We, therefore, reach the paradox that the generation of health, to which primary care could make a greater contribution, because it can deal with disease, *and* risk, in ways which protect 'space' and enhance adaptibility, is frustrated by the power and competitiveness of those branches of medicine whose task is much more narrow. Money is spent on the wrong things, decision-making is in the hands of the wrong people, resources are invested in the wrong places. Systems tend to be set up which are relatively insensitive to the population's health beliefs and therefore less able to provide care which will be appropriately used. That care will tend not to value autonomy and self-reliance, but to create dependence and limit autonomy. Look at the difference between an inpatient and somebody going to a GP's surgery.

What has to be changed by 2000 A.D. to achieve 'health for all'? Firstly, services must meet needs and must be designed to meet *real* needs. Needs, therefore, must be clearly understood and quantified before planning can start. Such plans must make some concessions to human frailty. An idealistic but rigid plan, which might be seen to be holding a country back, must be diluted with some of the 'luxuries'. Meanwhile, since people's understanding of health and disease and expectations of care are the strongest predictors of the way in which they will use health services, these provide a target for education. Information must be provided so that people can make informed choices and have more self-confidence in their own independence, autonomy and self-care. Primary care, as a speciality, must generate its own expertise and its own academic credibility, both within the world of medical education and within the world of politics. Medicine, as a component of society, must be prepared to relinquish the purely reactive role if it is to contribute to more than the absence or control of disease: it must be prepared to take social action on behalf of the people for whom it cares to improve their physical, social and psychological environment. In this way it can contribute to a modicum of health for all by the year 2000.

REFERENCES

Bice T, Kalimo E 1971 Comparisons of health related attitudes — a cross national factor analytic study. Social Sciences Medicine 5: 283–318
Becker M et al 1977 The health belief model and predictor of dietary compliance — a field experiment. Journal of Health and Social Behaviour 18: 348–366
Illich I 1982 Keynote speech. Royal College of General Practitioners/Canadian College of Family Physicians, Spring Meeting, Dublin
Rahe R H 1977 Epidemiological studies of life change and illness. In: Lipowski Z J, Lipsit D R, Whybrow P C (eds) Psychosomatic medicine: current trends and clinical applications. Oxford University Press, New York

Needs

The variations in the pattern of health and disease that occur throughout the world are such that almost any effort to classify or categorize 'needs' is bound to be crude. The history, the culture, environment, social, political and economic factors affecting need differ so greatly that individuals have difficulty in identifying the relative weights to apply to each when evaluating the system within a country in which they spend a whole lifetime let alone a country viewed as a visitor. In the end every community, national or local produces its own patterns of health and disease.

Money, affluence and disease

This chapter must, therefore, consist of broad generalizations and a convenient, and usual, starting point is to begin with the relationships between money and disease. In every country both birth rate and death rate are inversely proportional to the gross national product per capita and at the the same time the expenditure on health services is directly proportional to the gross national product (Omran 1975). This confirms on the international scale what has

Table 5.1 (Abstracted from 1977 World Population Data Sheet of the Population Reference Bureau Inc.)

Region	Population mid-1977 (millions)	Birth rate	Death rate	Rate of natural increase	Infant mortality	GNP/ capita US $
Africa	423	45	19	2.6	154	400
Asia	2325	32	12	2.0	116	530
N. America	240	15	9	0.6	16	7020
Latin America	336	36	9	2.7	78	1030
Europe	478	15	10	0.4	22	4090
USSR	259	18	9	0.9	28	2620
Oceania	22	22	9	1.3	55	4490

Table 5.2   Three major causes of death by age (infancy excluded) in less developed countries, 1970s (WHO)

Age	1st cause	2nd cause	3rd cause
1–4	Influenza & pneumonia	Gastroenterides	Accident
5–14	Accidents	Influenza & pneumonia	Malignancy
15–44	Accidents	Tuberculosis	Malignancy
45–64	Heart disease	Malignancy	Vascular lesion
65 +	Heart disease	Vascular lesion	Malignancy

Table 5.3   Three major causes of death by age (infancy excluded) in developed countries, 1970s (WHO)

Age	1st cause	2nd cause	3rd cause
1–4	Accidents	Influenza & pneumonia	Congenital malformation
5–14	Accidents	Malignancy	Congenital malformation
15–44	Accidents	Malignancy	Heart disease
45–64	Malignancy	Heart disease	Vascular lesions
65 +	Heart disease	Vascular lesion	Malignancy

been known to occur within the border of a country, that those with the greatest need have the least health care resources available (Table 5.1).

In any list of the major health problems faced by the world five headings would appear; accidents, cancer, cardiovascular disease, infections and parasitic disease and malnutrition. But there is a relatively sharp division between affluent societies, in which cancer and cardiovascular disease would be prominent, and poor countries, in which accidents, infections and malnutrition would be the major features (Table 5.2 and 5.3).

Half the people in the poorest 36 countries in the world, making up nearly one-third of the population of the world, suffer from malnourishment. They are the countries with the highest birth and death rates so the effect is most upon mothers and small children.

Health quality factors

The shift from the disease spectrum of the poor country to that of the rich country depends little upon the quality of health care. It is almost entirely dependent upon social conditions although clearly these have a major inter-relationship with other factors. Clean water supply, efficient waste disposal, food supply, the size and distribution of the population and the quality of housing and communication are more important than the number of health care personnel, hospital beds or the availability of drugs. The relationship between infections and parasitic disease and malnutrition is synergistic and both may sap the efforts of the individual to take other steps to protect himself. Whilst accidents and trauma figure high in the list of causes of ill-health in both rich and poor countries the aetiology of each is very different. In rich countries, impact with cars, moving machinery and electricity are major elements, whereas in poor countries it is the use of simple hand-tools, burns and the effect of natural disasters — flood, fire and earthquake — on inadequately sheltered people that are most important.

Certain other broad generalizations can be made whilst categorizing health needs. Firstly, as a poor country becomes more affluent there is a shift towards urbanization which itself changes the health care needs of the community. Secondly, within the high birth and death rate of the poor country there is a very high early childhood mortality rate. Factors leading to this include the pressures that large families make upon scarce resources, the shorter birth interval rate leading to early weaning and thus malnutrition and the inability of a pregnant or nursing mother to offer the required degree of protection to her other children. Lastly, there is the undoubted fact that the gap between the rich and poor countries in terms of health status is widening.

Uncertainties on improvements

An historical examination of health status in affluent societies shows that there has been a shift from 'poor' society status of morbidity that has taken about two centuries to occur. It could be argued that a similar change will occur to current 'poor' status countries, but in a much shorter time.

This may not occur because countries are more interdependant, the cultural effects are different today than they were in the 18th century, modern technology introduces new factors and the supply of food and resources available in these societies may be much less because of their rapidly increasing populations. There are also local geographical variants, e.g. in cancer, a high rate of bladder cancer is associated with schistosomiasis in Egypt, oropharyngeal cancer is associated with chewing the betel nut and other substances in Thailand, oesophageal cancer in Iran and gastric cancer in Japan may have a local dietary cause. The same sort of local cultural variations may be found in all of the major disease groups we are discussing.

Three models

Omran (1975), in discussing the epidemiological transition that is taking place alongside the demographic and socioeconomic transitions, has described three main models. The classic historical model of most of the developed countries, taking place over a period of two centuries and associated with better food and better sanitation and a sharp decline in bacteriological infection, is characterized by a gradual decline from high mortality and high fertility to low mortality and low fertility. Secondly, the accelerated model of rapidly modernizing countries such as Japan, in which these processes occur over less than 100 years and in which the key factor seems to be fertility control. Lastly, the delayed model in the developing countries with a substantial decline in mortality in the last 50 years, but a very slow decline in fertility giving rise to a large population increase.

PRIORITIES OF NEEDS

In 1972 WHO invited its member states to reply to a series of questions about the inter-relationship of health care programmes and socioeconomic development (WHO 1974). The areas of high priority identified by the respondents were:
  1. The prevention and control of disease, especially communicable disease.
  2. Personal health care for rural populations, and deprived sections of the community.
  3. Maternal and child health services
  4. Education and training of health care personnel.
  5. Environmental health services.

1. The prevention and control of disease, especially communicable disease and environmental health services

The health needs of a population, in terms of preventive services, are too inextricably mixed to allow a clear separation between environmental control and personal preventive services. Environmental control is rarely the responsibility of doctors providing

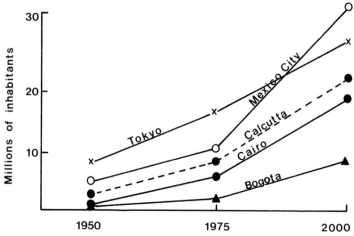

Fig. 5.1 Projected populations of some urban agglomerations 1950–2000. (From United Nations 1975 Working paper, Population division.)

primary and personal care, but in many areas the distinction between prevention and treatment are blurred. The variety of environmental controls possible is great and, in general, is better applied as a country becomes more wealthy and more urbanized, although the dense conglomeration of people in urban areas produces its own set of environmental hazards. It is a truism that the sanitary engineer has made a greater contribution towards the reduction of morbidity and mortality than the doctor and the top priority in terms of need has to be accorded to clean water, sanitation and waste disposal, but as a country becomes wealthier the contribution that doctors have to make to environmental health becomes greater and becomes a factor that doctors use to promote positive health. Fluoride added to water, iodine added to salt, lead removed from petrol and sulphur dioxide from chimney emissions, legislation against smoking and for seat belts and crash helmets and, more recently still, radiation emission controls, are examples. It is also a prime medical responsibility when there is competition for scarce resources to identify priority areas of prevention *viz-a-viz* treatment.

Environmental hazards, though severe in overcrowded slums of the third world, are currently worst in rural areas. Increasing trends towards urbanization will shift the major health and social problems to underprivileged urban centres (Fig. 5.1).

It is in the personal prevention of communicable disease, primarily by immunization, that the primary health care worker begins to play a major role. At present fewer than 10% of the 80 million children born each year in the poor countries are immunized against infectious disease (WHO 1979). Over 5 million children under 5 die each year from infections and another 5 million are blinded, crippled or otherwise permanently handicapped. The chief killers are measles, whooping cough and neonatal tetanus and the leading crippler is poliomyelitis. Effective prevention has to capture the minds of people as well as their bodies. Gandhi played a major part in the control of malaria in India by persuading people that it was right to kill the mosquito. Unfortunately, prevention of disease has always played a secondary role to treatment. The reasons are partly attitudinal, neither patients nor doctors think preventively and tend to consider health only when ill-health comes; partly educational, in that medical schools afford prevention a low priority in teaching, and partly financial, in that rewards are highest for treating sickness. In free enterprise countries the majority of immunizations against acute communicable disease are given by private physicians, often as part of the routine surveillance of young infants. The medical attention given to births affords the entry point into personal preventive services for the infant but it still requires considerable organization to achieve high population immunization levels. In some countries vaccines are supplied free to doctors and fees paid for procedures. In others special health workers are seconded to work alongside, and even in wealthy countries there are parallel programmes based on clinics which cater for the less wealthy. The clinic system becomes dominant as a country becomes less affluent and is the only way in which personal preventive services can be applied in a poor country. However, even in Western Europe the great majority of immunizations are carried out in public clinics because of their wider acceptance by all income levels.

Prevention and control of disease need:

a. Increasing attention to the environment in all countries

b. A steadily expanding programme of communicable disease control

c. An attitudinal shift amongst all health workers toward preventive medicine.

2. Personal health care, especially for rural populations and deprived sections of the community

There is a need in every system of health care to have a person to whom the patient, whether sick or well, can turn to first for help.

Such a person provides both a response to an existing health problem presented and also initiates personal care to prevent illness occurring. It requires a high level of trust between the individual and the health carer. In the past, this has been easy in relatively static communities, now increasing mobility of populations makes it more difficult. The structure and function of the family influences the health patterns of the individual and the community and is the best way of supporting self-care. Most problems affecting health are dealt with within the family and only a few, less than one-quarter in the UK, are taken to the medical system. Within the family, the mother is the primary health care worker, even though she has little access to professional information or technical resources, but has much practical experience.

Patterns are changing. Wars and famines, political upheavals, population migration and changing patterns of women's work have led to decline of family support for its members, particularly in poor countries. Thus, in periurban areas of developing countries, 40% of people aged 20 have only one parent alive and a further 8% will have lost both parents. In developed countries 9 out of 10 20-year-olds have both parents alive (WHO 1978).

Between 1976 and 2000 the world's population is expected to increase from around 4 billion to more than 6 billion (United Nations 1980). There will thus be 2 billion more people seeking access to personal primary health care.

If we could assume that the resources available to primary health care would increase proportionally with this population growth then it might be possible to envisage many of the needs being met, but it is apparent that nowhere is this likely to happen. The key needs that patients have of primary care are accessibility, availability and continuity of care. Secondary requirements are an effective referral system, where necessary, to more specialized services and assurances of the standards of the care provided.

Accessability of primary care depends on numbers of health care workers, their distribution and transport services. In poor countries it depends also on the acceptability of the form of health care. For example, in one instance a city educated nurse who spent several months in a village could not persuade a single woman to have a tubal ligation, whereas an illiterate 'dai' from the same village was able to persuade 75 women during the same period (United Nations 1980).

It has been customary to believe that the number of physicians must rise in order to improve the quality of health care. This re-

Table 5.4 Life expectancy at birth (from Sixth report on the world health situation, WHO)

	Developed countries	Developing countries	Difference in years
1950	65	42	23
1975	72	55	17
2000	75–80	65–70	10

sulted in policies after the end of World War II that steadily increased the output of doctors in all countries. The numbers of primary care doctors required to meet needs depends on many different factors; the way in which doctors are paid and the amount of money there is to pay them, the patterns of use of other health workers, and on the demands. Doctors are expensive and are a major drain on resources. Doctors are capable of delegating much of their work to workers trained in other ways, who are much less expensive to employ.

Increasing the numbers of physicians does little to correct problems of maldistribution. Doctors tend to be sucked into hospital-based secondary care and, in poorer countries, they concentrate in more affluent urban areas.

New approaches are required to change the health manpower profile and make better use of auxiliary staff in new roles and functions. The number of health care workers involved in primary care is likely to increase but fewer of them will be doctors.

Life expectancy at birth is the best single measure of the level of health of a population. Table 5.4 shows the projected values for the year 2000 and indicates how population needs will have come closer together.

The major needs of the world's population for personal health care, especially for deprived populations, are:
a. Easy access to an acceptably trained primary health care worker
b. Greater attention to health education and self-help
c. An effective referral system for secondary care.

3. Maternal and child health

24% of the world's population are women of reproductive age and another 36% are children below the age of 15. Whilst maternal, infant and child mortalities are crude measures of health, they are more reliable at present than available measures of morbidity. 10% of the 122 million infants born each year die before the age of 1 year and another 4% before the age of 5, but the risk of dying before adolescence in a rich country is about 1 in 40, in poor regions it is as high as 1 in 2 (UN/WHO 1980). Maternal mortality shows similar variation, from 5–10 per 100 000 live births in rural areas of poor countries where nearly half the deaths amongst women aged 15–30 are due to maternal mortality.

The commonest causes of death in mothers in poor countries are postpartum haemorrhage, often associated with anaemia due to malnutrition and infection, and sepsis. The commonest causes of perinatal mortality include malnutrition, the diarrhoeal diseases, respiratory infection and tetanus which can cause up to 10% of all deaths.

All these causes are inter-related compounded from effects of uncontrolled fertility, poor nutrition and infections, which themselves derive from socioeconomic factors including a lack of primary health care. At one time, the solution to the medical aspects of these problems was seen to be modelled on the institutional care given within developed countries, but it is now apparent that this is impossible.

Primary care, attuned to local needs and local resources and aimed at increasing self-help and community participation often using locally trained village health workers, is a major need. This has to be supported by a good secondary referral system for problems which cannot be met in the primary care arena. Such a pattern of care obviates the performance of inappropriate activities, especially in prenatal care, which use up large amounts of scarce resources. If such techniques are aimed particularly at individuals and groups who are at greatest risk, it implies that in poor as well as rich countries basic levels of care will be applied to all, and more skilled care for people at greatest risk.

In developed countries the same reordering of priorities is required. In both rich and poor countries the maintenance of breast feeding is the single most effective defence against malnutrition and infection and, whereas in poor countries iron, folate or vitamin deficiency may be the most important factors, in rich countries malnutrition of affluence leads to obesity, cardiovascular disease, arthritis and diabetes.

The major needs of mothers and children are for:
a. Increasing education to support self care
b. Primary care integrating maternity care, child health care and family planning
c. Effective and accessible referral systems to secondary care.

The impact that fertility control has upon the health status of mothers and children is of key importance. New methods available and making these widely accessible is a major need. It is now estimated that nearly 40% of the world's population, excluding Russia and China, use some form of contraception regularly. Regional variations range from 60% in developed countries to 3% in West Africa (WHO 1979). In the year 2000 it will be just over 200 years since Malthus published his essay about the perils of increasing population and, although food production is much greater than he predicted, it is now recognized that there are limits and that large populations face hazards other than hunger.

4. Education and training of health care personnel

Reference has already been made to problems caused by an increase in the number of physicians. Between 1955 and 1975 nearly 500 new medical schools were established in the world, an increase of 78% in number. Once again, regional variations were great. Brazil had a growth rate of 230% and the UK of 15%. The rapid growth in the poorer countries combined with more liberal entry requirements has led, in some instances, to excessively large classes sometimes containing hundreds of students of whom the majority will have no opportunity to practise. The actual training of doctors and other health care workers is inappropriate for the needs of the population.

The combination of these two factors has led to gross maldistribution with too many doctors in urban areas, whereas in rural areas of the same country there is a great shortage. The concept of doctors supported by a fairly large cadre of nurses is common in wealthier countries. In many of the poorer countries there are strong cultural and economic forces operating against the employment of nurses. Thus, apart from the inequalities in the supply of doctors, there are equal or even greater inequalities in the supply of all health workers. In 1976 nearly 10% of the world's population were looked after by health care workers at a rate of less than 1 to every 2000 of the population, whereas at the upper range of the scale 10% were being looked after by 1 worker to every 100 of the population. In poor countries there were only 2–3 health workers per doctor, in wealthier countries there were nearly 5. Most of the problems in the deprived areas of the world derive from the fact that a smaller proportion of a smaller total budget is spent on health care than in wealthier countries. Given that health care is very labour intensive and that up to 80% of the health budget may be spent in salaries, there is little left over. The economic problems of the richer countries are also beginning to bear down on the wages and salary component of health budgets leading people to look much more critically at cost effectiveness. Given that a doctor is unable to function effectively without a major input from other health workers, the relative proportions of different workers become a key issue. Consideration of the productivity of other workers, whose training and utilization are much less costly than those of doctors, suggests that in poor and rich parts of the world much too great emphasis has been placed upon numbers of doctors.

The needs of the world in terms of health manpower for primary care can be summarized as:

a. Health care workers trained appropriately for their tasks
b. Distribution of health workers according to local need
c. Integration of the activities of doctors and other health workers.

REFERENCES

Djukanovich V, Mach E P 1975 Alternative approaches to meeting basic health needs in developing countries. WHO, Geneva
Omran A R 1975 Community medicine in developing countries. New York. Springer Publishing Company
UN 1980 Population by sex and age for regions 1950–2000 (document ESA/P/WP.60) United Nations Population Division,
UN/WHO 1980 Recent levels and trends in mortality. UN/WHO, New York and Geneva
WHO 1974 In: Public health papers. WHO, Geneva
WHO 1978 Health and the family. Studies on the demography of family life cycles and their health implications. WHO, Geneva
WHO 1979 Sixth report on the world health situation (1973–77), part 1. WHO, Geneva
WHO 1979 World Health Statistics Quarterly 32

Prevention

THE FENCE OR THE AMBULANCE

'Twas a dangerous cliff, as they freely confessed
Though to walk near its crest was so pleasant:
But over its terrible edge there had slipped
A duke and many a peasant;
So the people said something would have to be done,
But their projects did not all tally:
Some said, 'Put a fence round the edge of the cliff';
Some, 'An ambulance down in the valley'.

But the cry for the ambulance carried the day,
For it spread to the neighbouring city;
A fence may be useful or not, it is true,
But each heart became brimful of pity
For those who had slipped o'er that dangerous cliff,
And the dwellers in highway and alley
Gave pounds or gave pence, not to put up a fence
But an ambulance down in the valley.

"For the cliff is alright if you're careful", they said;
"And if folks ever slip or are dropping,
It isn't the slipping that hurts them so much
As the shock down below — when they're stopping".
So day after day when these mishaps occurred,
Quick forth would the rescuers sally,
To pick up the victims who fell off the cliff
With their ambulance down in the valley.

Then an old man remarked, "It's a marvel to me
That people give far more attention
To repairing results than to stopping the cause
When they'd much better aim at prevention;
Let us stop at its source all this mischief", cried he
"Come, neighbours and friends, let us rally;
If the cliff we will fence, we might almost dispense
With the ambulance down in the valley."

MALINES (1953)

INTRODUCTION

Prevention, by which is meant health promotion and maintenance as well as disease prevention, is an important general theme underlying the goal of 'Health for all by the year 2000'. Prevention is the challenge of today to achieve a better tomorrow.

The historical perspective

Prevention is not new: far from it. The decline in morbidity and mortality in developed countries during the last hundred years (and in developing countries more recently) has been attributable largely to developments in public health and preventive medicine rather than in the treatment of established disease. These developments were environmental improvements — the provision of pure water, the disposal of sewage, improved nutrition, better housing and enhanced life conditions generally. All of these contributed to the decline in infections, the major killers historically in developed countries and currently in the developing ones. The dramatic fall in tuberculosis, for example, long preceded the discovery of specific preventive measures or of antituberculous drugs (McKeown 1976).

While it is true that medical interventions played some part — though some would dispute this (Illich 1974) — it has been preventive activities, such as immunization, antenatal care and contraception, which have made the major impact, rather than therapeutic miracles.

But the economic developments which have led to these environmental improvements seem in turn to have resulted in the adoption of faulty lifestyles and premature death (Trowell & Burkitt 1981). The big killers today in developed countries (and increasingly in the developing ones) — heart attacks, cancer and strokes — appear to some extent at least to be attributable to aspects of human behaviour. Tobacco smoking is a major cause of heart attacks and cancer and it has been estimated (Doll & Peto 1981) that, together, tobacco, alcohol and some aspects of diet account for about two-thirds of cancer deaths.

The revival of interest in preventive medicine in the closing decades of the 20th century acknowledges, therefore, that the major challenge now lies in achieving changes in human behaviour rather than the external environment. This revival has been encouraged by the painful recognition that, in spite of the enormous progress in recent decades in the development of new therapeutic tech-

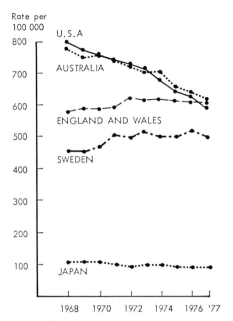

Fig. 6.1 Ischaemic heart disease mortality rates 1968–77, males 35–74 years. Age-adjusted rates/100 000

niques, the law of diminishing returns and the pressures of economic stringency limit the potential for the cure of disease.

There are indications that changing habits may in some countries be contributing to a decline in these behaviourally-determined diseases. As illustrated in Figure 6.1, mortality from ischaemic heart disease fell by about 25% between 1968 and 1978 in the USA, while remaining relatively unchanged in Britain. The rates in the two countries now are similar.

While the causes of this fall are debated, the evidence suggests that it is due not so much to reduced case fatality (attributable to treatment) but to a reduction in the incidence of heart attacks, attributable in varying degrees to reduction in smoking, dietary changes, including reduction in fat consumption, increased exercise and improved detection and management of high blood pressure.

Critics argue that there is no gain if prevention merely postpones mortality and increases the number of elderly disabled. But preventing disease reduces disability, or at least postpones it, as well as premature death. Moreover, evidence suggests that the natural biological lifespan is relatively fixed at about 80 years and

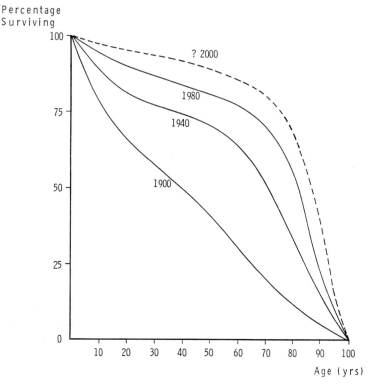

Fig. 6.2 Human survival curves for the years 1900, 1940 and 1980 and that projected for the year 2000

that the effect of prevention (and treatment) is to 'rectangularize' the human survival curve (see Fig. 6.2) by reducing premature death and allowing more people to achieve a full lifespan.

Non-medical factors

Just as, historically, prevention depended on educational, economic, social and political developments, so future achievements in prevention are likely to be determined as much by these factors as by strictly medical ones. In Britain in the 19th century improvements in water supplies and sewage disposal required legislation and recently a British health minister acknowledged that:

> . . . the solution of many of today's medical problems will be found not in the research laboratories of our hospitals, but in our Parlia-

ments. For the prospective patient, the answer may not be the incision at the operating table, but prevention by decision at the Cabinet table.

Community involvement

The importance of participation of people in their own health care is emphasized in the Alma-Ata Declaration. Health care providers have a responsibility to:

> . . . increase individual and community capabilities for involvement and self-reliance in health and to promote healthy behaviour, particularly regarding family health and nutrition, environmental health, healthy-lifestyles and disease prevention and control.
>
> (WHO 1982)

Paternalistic health care is outmoded. Changing disease patterns, rising expectations and new relationships between health care providers and consumers necessitate a shift from medical 'intervention' to 'facilitation': to a partnership between health professionals and lay people. This is especially true in relation to prevention. This implies greater emphasis on individuals', families' and communities' own health perceptions, beliefs, expectations, needs and activities. Encouragement rather than coercion must be the approach.

Prevention versus cure

Although, according to the adage, 'prevention is better than cure', they are not alternatives but complementary. The danger of polarization of attitudes and activities between prevention on the one hand and treatment on the other must be averted. But at the same time the present imbalance in favour of sophisticated technological 'cures' must be corrected.

The concept of 'anticipatory care', which combines health promotion and maintenance, disease prevention, treatment and continuing care emphasizes their essential unity.

WHAT IS PREVENTABLE?

A number of reports from international bodies (WHO 1979), governments (DHSS 1976) and professional organizations (RCP 1984, RCGP 1981a) have identified the considerable preventive potential currently available.

This is in spite of the critical scrutiny to which claims for preventability have, and rightly so, been a subject. Efforts must be concentrated on measures which are of proven benefit and economically viable, as well as practicable and acceptable to providers and recipients.

Infections

As pointed out in the introduction, the major influences on health are socioeconomic and other 'non-medical' factors. These are of special significance in relation to infections (and infestations), though immunization (and to a lesser extent prophylactic antibiotics and other forms of medication) also play an important part.

Taking immunization, there are still gaps between capability and achievement even in developed countries. Measles, for example, has been virtually eradicated from the USA where a level of immunization of more than 90% has been achieved, whereas Britain with its immunization rate of only just over 50% still experiences more than 100 000 cases and about 20 measles deaths annually. Likewise, rubella is a preventable infectious disease which currently causes many avoidable tragedies in the shape of congenitally malformed infants resulting from pregnancy rubella in non-immune women.

Cardiovascular disease

The most important cause of premature death in developed countries (and an increasingly important one in developing ones) is arterial disease — essentially heart attacks and strokes. Together, in Britain, they account for almost half of all deaths between middle age and retirement and heart attacks alone for roughly half of all male deaths in this age group.

One of five recent reports on aspects of prevention, published by the Royal College of General Practitioners (RCGP 1981b) concludes that, 'about half of all strokes and a quarter of all deaths from coronary heart disease in people under the age of 70 are probably preventable by the application of existing knowledge'. This is the major preventive challenge for primary care in the developed countries. Moreover, the spread of this 'modern epidemic' of cardiovascular disease — consequent on the adoption of 'western-lifestyles' — to developing countries requires urgent limitation of this problem.

Risk factors

Aspects of lifestyle, on a population basis at least, are clearly associated with the development of coronary heart disease. Smoking, high blood pressure, faulty diets (including an excess intake of fat, especially of the 'saturated' variety), high alcohol intake and lack of exercise have all been shown with varying degrees of certainty to cause this disease. Moreover, removal of, or reduction in, these 'risk factors' has been shown to reduce the incidence of the disease. Herein lies the scope for prevention (WHO 1982b).

Smoking. The World Health Organization has described tobacco smoking as an 'epidemic' and as the most important cause of preventable disease and premature death. It has declared that 'control of smoking could do more than any other single action in the field of preventive medicine'. Annually, about 100 000 deaths in Britain and almost half a million in the USA are attributable to tobacco.

Smoking is estimated to be responsible for 25% of coronary heart disease deaths in men under the age of 65 years as well as 75% of deaths from chronic airways disease and 90% of lung cancer deaths.

High blood pressure. This is also a major risk factor for heart attacks and, more especially, for strokes. As with smoking, the evidence, that control of the risk limits the disease, is overwhelming and the case for detection and treatment of a blood pressure above a level of 180/100 is now beyond reasonable doubt.

Diet. This is the third major risk factor contributing to arterial disease. But although the epidemiological evidence relating coronary heart disease mortality to saturated fat intake is strong, it is less clear that lowering the intake of fat reduces the incidence of this disease. Nevertheless, there is increasing agreement that, although the evidence falls short of proof, reduction in saturated fat consumption will reduce the risk of heart attacks and should be pursued (DHSS 1984).

Moreover, there is no doubt that control of obesity is a desirable objective and that, in achieving this, a reduction in energy intake involving a decrease in fat, especially saturated fat, consumption (and an increase in dietary fibre) is important.

Other cardiovascular risk factors. Evidence relating risk factors, such as lack of exercise, stress and personality type to coronary heart disease is less clear and the benefit of 'controlling' these risk factors is even less certain. However, on more general grounds, there is a case for increasing the general level of exercise in the community and for control of stress.

Furthermore, those with a family history of premature cardio-vascular disease, or who themselves have diabetes, warrant special consideration in relation to the risk factors of smoking, high blood pressure and diet.

Cancer

Cancer is second only to cardiovascular disease as a cause of death in developed countries, accounting for about a quarter of all deaths. Many of these are probably preventable in the light of the estimate by Doll and Peto (1981) that about a third of all cancer deaths are attributable to tobacco and that, taken together, tobacco, alcohol and aspects of 'Western' diet probably account for more than two-thirds of cancer deaths.

Screening for cancer by the detection of precancerous conditions or early stages of the disease has proved generally disappointing. Although the benefits of early detection (by cervical cytology) and management of premalignant changes in the cervix uteri are now undisputed, the costs and benefits of screening for breast cancer, the commonest female malignancy in developed countries (but soon to be overtaken by lung cancer) are far from clear.

Contrary to popular belief, factors in the external environment are relatively trivial causes of cancer.

Doll (1983) estimates that 'pollution' causes not more than 1% of all fatal cancers, so that pollution control, however desirable on other grounds, is unlikely to contribute significantly to cancer prevention.

Trauma

The remaining important cause of premature death offering oppor-tunities for prevention is physical injury. Its importance lies not so much in the number of accidental deaths occurring but in the high proportion of them affecting the young. Accidents in the home, on the roads and at work are frequently preventable. Alcohol plays a part in many of them. Education about risk reduction and legis-lation (for example, about drinking and driving and about the wearing of seat belts) are important factors in prevention.

Contraception and antenatal care

The importance of contraception and antenatal care as preventive activities deserves emphasis and is frequently forgotten. Both are well established aspects of primary care and have made major contributions to reductions in maternal and infant morbidity and mortality.

But despite the ready availability of reliable and safe contraception, there are in Britain, for example, more than 125 000 pregnancy terminations annually which clearly indicates a major discrepancy between need and use. The preventive potential and effectives of postcoital contraception needs also to be emphasized.

Antenatal screening has been a major determinant of decline in perinatal mortality and routine antenatal care was, together with immunization, one of the first preventive activities to be widely adopted in primary care. To routine and regular maternal examinations have recently been added tests which detect a variety of fetal abnormalities so that (given the acceptance of pregnancy termination) the birth of many deformed or handicapped infants can now be avoided.

HOW CAN PREVENTION BE ACHIEVED?

Prevention can be pursued at a number of different levels — international, national, regional, district, local, practice population or individual. But the underlying principles and considerations are the same.

Some general principles

There is continuing debate about the costs and benefits of preventive medicine — between 'evangelists', on the one hand, who enthusiastically promote preventive action, and 'agnostics' on the other, who are sceptical of preventive measures. There are, indeed, many uncertainties about the effectiveness of prevention, not least because the value of preventive measures is often difficult to prove. One reason for this is that there may well be a long time lag between the implementation of the measure and the possible demonstration of its effect. But there are also uncertainties about much therapeutics!

However, it is important that the scientific basis for a preventive procedure, including its evaluation, should be clearly established before it is pursued. The essential criteria for 'screening' have been clearly established (Nuffield Provincial Hospitals Trust 1968) and rigorous appraisal of the effectiveness and cost-benefit balance are necessary. Research has demonstrated limited areas only of proven benefit and has dampened early overenthusiasm for 'multiphasic screening'. But, in addition to accepted preventive practices like immunization, contraception and antenatal care, the case for preventive intervention in some other important areas is now proven beyond reasonable doubt; these include:

1. Avoidance and cessation of tobacco smoking.

2. Detection and management of blood pressure above certain levels.

3. Avoidance and control of obesity, limitation of fat (especially saturated fat) consumption and encouragement of fibre-rich carbohydrate intake.

4. Detection and management of premalignant changes by cervical cytology.

'Mass' vesus 'high risk' strategies

There is also much discussion of the so-called 'mass strategy' and 'high risk' approaches to prevention. The former necessitates preventive measures in the population as a whole because although preventable events occur more frequently in those at 'high risk', in absolute terms most of these events happen in the large majority who are at relatively low risk rather than the comparatively few 'high risk' individuals.

The 'high risk' strategy on the other hand requires identification of those at greater risk than others and the concentration of preventive activities on them because of the likely greater benefit in relation to cost and effort.

Although these approaches are often proposed as alternatives they are in face complementary and should be viewed together.

Some definitions

Methods of prevention are often classified into primary, secondary and tertiary. Simple definitions of these and of the associated terms screening and case finding may be helpful.

Primary prevention

This is the ideal form of prevention, namely avoidance or removal of the cause, and is one of the major aims of health education. Being a non-smoker, or stopping smoking, is an example.

Secondary prevention

This involves presymptomatic detection of 'risk factors', or of the disease itself at an early preclinical stage. *Screening* — the sifting of an apparently healthy population to identify those at risk of, or with, preclinical features of a disease — is generally synonymous with secondary prevention. *Case finding* is a form of screening in which this 'doctor-initiated' activity is limited to the *opportunistic* approach. It is less 'aggressive', more acceptable and more effective than population screening and it is the 'screening' method appropriate to primary care. Detection of hypertension or of premalignant changes in the cervix uteri are examples of secondary prevention.

Tertiary prevention

This is the management of established disease to prevent complications and limit disability or handicap. It is, of course, just another name for careful treatment, management and follow up. Proper supervision of patients with diabetes is an example of tertiary prevention.

THE ROLE OF PRIMARY CARE

Special characteristics

Primary care is a unique situation in relation to prevention because:
1. It has extensive access to the population as a whole
2. Contacts are frequent
3. All types of people use it, including those 'at risk'
4. Contacts are largely patient-initiated
5. Patients consulting expect advice
6. Primary care doctors are credible and trusted
7. Communication is one-to-one
8. Anxiety and fear of disease may motivate behaviour change
9. The team approach can provide support and help
10. Each primary care team may care for an identifiable population

These assets are especially characteristic of British National Health Service general practice, with its defined lists of patients, two-thirds of whom consult at least once a year (and on average three to four times a year) and almost all of whom are seen at least once every five years.

But although the derivation of the word doctor implies a teaching role (latin: *docere*, i.e. to teach), the shift from the traditional approach of symptom-relief and disease management to one of teacher (health promotion) and active interventionist (disease prevention) involves a philosophical change for most doctors. The 'medical shopkeeper' (Hart 1981) approach, orientated to pharmacological magic, is deeply engrained by medical education and practice. The management of 'at risk', asymptomatic people is generally accorded a low priority and 'mass' prevention strategies an even lower one.

The consultation opportunity

The exceptional potential of a primary care consultation (Stott & Davis 1979) for opportunistic health promotion and disease prevention is illustrated in Figure 6.3.

A Management of presenting problems	B Modification of help-seeking behaviour
C Management of continuing problems	D Opportunistic health promotion

Fig. 6.3 The exceptional potential in each primary care consultation

The conventional tasks are those of diagnosis and management of symptoms the patient presents (and perhaps of any known pre-existing disease). But to these may be added 'modification of help-seeking behaviour' and 'opportunistic health promotion'; in other words, health education and preventive medicine.

For example, a consultation initiated by a known hypertensive patient because of a sore throat may be used not only to advise on the simple self-care of sore throats and, incidentally, to monitor the blood pressure, but also as an opportunity to ask and advise about smoking.

Moreover, these opportunities are not limited to the doctor. The potential arising from the patient-initiated contact with the doctor can be exploited for preventive purposes by other members of primary health care teams, especially nurses (Fullard et al 1984).

Health beliefs and compliance

Health behaviour is influenced by a variety of factors and important amongst them are the individual's 'health beliefs' — in particular, a degree of concern about health matters, perceived vulnerability to illness and the individual estimate of the benefits of a course of action compared with its 'costs' (Becker 1974). Likewise compliance with advice is determined by characteristics of doctor and patient and the quality of the communication between them (Ley 1976). Compliance is enhanced when the patient's views about health and disease are elicited so that advice can be given whch is appropriate and, when possible, congruent with these.

Patient leaflets

Leaflets are a useful adjunct to verbal advice. They may reinforce and supplement the spoken word, saving time, providing reference material and acting as reminders. They should be simply written and, whenever possible, personalized and handed directly to the patient. Use of such leaflets has been shown to enhance the effectiveness of advice against smoking for example (Russell et al 1979).

THE PRESENT PRIORITIES FOR PREVENTION IN PRIMARY HEALTH CARE

The priorities for prevention by the year 2000 are concerned with lifestyle. They are the control of tobacco smoking and reduction in the risk of cardiovascular disease. Although currently primarily relevant to developed countries, they are rapidly becoming increasingly important in developing countries as the 'contagion' of Western lifestyle spreads to them.

How can the primary health care meet this challenge?

Smoking

Advice and help to avoid or stop tobacco smoking is the single most important preventive activity for primary health care to undertake.

Roughly one-third of the adult population in Britain and the USA smokes tobacco — a proportion of which, although falling, still means that many millions are still at major risk of premature death because of this habit.

Surveys show that about three-quarters of smokers report wanting to stop smoking — and many succeed, most without help. But research has shown that advice from a personal doctor, reinforced with an antismoking leaflet, enhances the smoking cessation (Jamrozik et al 1984a). Simple smoking cessation advice should be given opportunistically (Fowler 1983). Nicotine chewing gum may be a useful additional aid but its effective use requires careful supervision and compliance (Jamrozik et al 1984b).

The role of primary health care in smoking cessation may be summarized as follows:

1. Routinely ask about and record patient's smoking habits.

2. Seek opportunity to inform smokers about the hazards of smoking and offer advice on stopping.

3. Offer smoking cessation advice whenever requested.

4. Give simple advice on how to stop.

5. Supplement such advice with appropriate literature consider the prescription of nicotine chewing gum.

6. Follow up patient's attempts to stop smoking.

7. Encourage non-smokers and ex-smokers not to start, particularly in children and young adults.

Doctors and other health personnel should set a good example by not smoking themselves, should prohibit smoking on health premises and should support efforts to achieve prohibition of all forms of tobacco promotion.

Cardiovascular disease

Cardiovascular disease (and in particular coronary heart disease) prevention has been identified by the World Health Organization as a high priority.

As previously indicated there are two complementary strands to this: the 'mass strategy' or population approach and the 'high-risk strategy' aimed at the more susceptible individuals. Both can be pursued though primary health care.

The population approach requires primary health care to actively promote healthy lifestyles amongst the population it serves. This means providing, for the people being cared for, health education about smoking, diet, obesity, exercise and the detection and control of high blood pressure. Research has demonstrated both the feasibility of doing this and the risk factor reduction which may follow (Pushka et al 1979, Hjermann et al 1981), though it must be admitted that some large intervention trials have failed to show significant benefit. Given the long 'incubation period' of coronary heart disease and other difficulties, the 'failure' of some of these trials is not altogether surprising. The chief benefit of detection and control of hypertension is in the reduction of the risk of cerebro-vascular disease, but it is now clear that coronary heart disease risk is also reduced by this, as well as by smoking and dietary changes.

The 'high risk' approach means identifying in a primary health care practice population those individuals at special risk. All primary health care personnel need to be involved in this and the task must be undertaken systematically and continuously. 'One off' exercises are of very limited value. All adult patients should be screened for cardiovascular disease risk factors, but especially those with a family history of premature cardiovascular disease and also those who have diabetes. Such screening should include:

1. Enquiry about smoking habit and smoking cessation advice for smokers.

2. Weighing and dietary advice, especially for those who are obese, have elevated blood lipids or who have other cardiovascular disease risk factors.

3. Recording of blood pressure and appropriate management of detected hypertension.

4. Enquiry and advice about the level of physical activity.

This is likely to be done most systematically when it is the specific task of a particular primary health care team member, such as a nurse, but the whole team should be committed to this approach.

It can be done on an opportunistic basis, in patients consulting for some other reason, and the aim should be to achieve these measures at least once every five years (repeating them more frequently, as appropriate, when they are found to be abnormal).

Implementation of such a plan has proved feasible in primary health care practices and a more detailed discussion may be found elsewhere (Fullard et al 1984).

FUTURE NEEDS

The outstanding need at the present time is for prevention to be accorded a greater degree of priority — in health policies, in the distribution of resources, in the eyes of the medical profession, in medical education and in the estimation of the public.

Having swung violently towards sophisticated technological medical intervention, the pendulum is now swinging back as a proper balance between prevention and cure is acknowledged: between self-help and professional help.

But there are many obstacles to be overcome — in public attitudes, professional resistance and political inaction.

To conclude, in the words of Dr David Owen, a prominent British politician, former Minister of Health and doctor, 'the degree to which this area has been neglected in the rush towards therapeutic and technological medicine is little short of a public scandal'.

THE SPECIAL NEEDS OF DEVELOPING COUNTRIES

Although 'developed' and 'developing' countries have much in common in relation to prevention, the developing ones also have their own special problems. These are often similar to the ones which were at one time important in Western countries but which, in Britain in the 19th century for example, were overcome by the application of public health measures. As illustrated in Figure 6.4, infection remains the most important single cause of mortality in developing countries whereas in the developed ones circulatory diseases have taken over from infections as the prime cause of death.

Poverty is a major underlying cause of disease generally and accounts for many of the special health problems of developing countries. It prevents the acquisition of such basic ingredients of health as adequate nutrition and living conditions, safe drinking water and essential sanitation. Amelioration of poverty must therefore be one of the primary aims of any preventive medicine programme. The average per capita expenditure on health in developing countries is less than 5% of that in the developed ones and, to make matters worse, improvements in health care provision in developing countries have often taken the form of sophisticated hospital-based specialist care for a privileged tiny urban elite, ignoring the basic health needs of the majority of the population.

'Health for all' demands a broadly based approach to prevention,

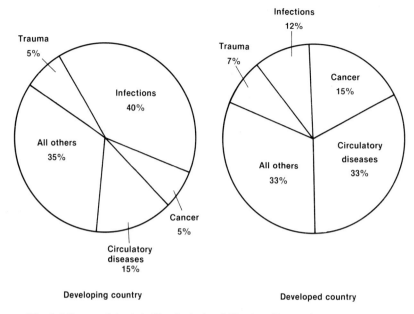

Fig. 6.4 Causes of death in 'developing' and 'developed' countries

with emphasis on the community rather than the hospital, on prevention for the majority rather than a cure for the few, on community involvement and participation rather than the creation of dependence on professional health personnel. It requires education of people about health matters and above all political commitment to the provision of 'health for all' and especially the essential provision of comprehensive preventive services.

An example of this sort of commitment and its effective implementation is provided by China where, over the last two or three decades, major health improvements have occurred. Emphasis has been placed on cummunity-based programmes involving public education, disease prevention programmes, such as immunization which have often been compulsory, and the much publicized 'barefoot doctors'. The preventive programmes have included high levels of achievement in family planning and immunization, and have made major contributions and have made major contributions to improvements in the health of the vast population of this nation. It is, therefore, all the more tragic that these measures are now being undermined by the 'modern epidemic' of smoking-related diseases caused by the spread of the smoking contagion from the West.

Preventive strategies in developing countries must therefore place special emphasis on activities which are basic to health promotion and disease prevention. These include:

1. Improved nutrition
2. Better living conditions
3. Provision of safe water and sanitation
4. Control of infections and infestations
5. Control of fecundity and population size
6. Public health education
7. Self-care
8. Community involvement and participation
9. Emphasis on prevention rather than cure
10. Professional health services orientated to primary care rather than hospitals.

REFERENCES

Becker M H 1974 The health belief model and personal behaviour. Health Education Monograph 2: 328–335
Doll R, Peto R 1981 The causes of cancer. Oxford University Press, Oxford
Doll R 1983 Prospects for prevention. British Medical Journal 286: 445–452
Department of Health and Social Security 1976 Prevention and health: everybody's business. Her Majesty's Stationary Office, London
Department of Health and Social Security 1984 Diet and cardiovascular disease. HMSO, London
Fowler G 1983 Smoking. In: Gray M, Fowler G (eds) Preventive medicine in general practice. Oxford University Press, Oxford
Fullard E M, Fowler G, Gray J A M 1985 The Oxford prevention of heart attack and stroke project. British Medical Journal (in press)
Hart J T 1981 A new kind of doctor. Journal of Royal Society of Medicine 74: 871–883
Illich I 1974 Medical nemesis. Calder and Boyars, London
Jamrozik K, Vessey M, Fowler G, Wald N, Parker G, Van Vunakis H 1984 Controlled trial of three different anti-smoking interventions in general practice. British Medical Journal 288: 1499–1505
Jamrozik K, Fowler G, Vessey M, Wald N 1984. Placebo controlled trial of nicotine chewing gum in general practice. British Medical Journal (in press)
Ley P 1976 Towards better doctor-patient communication. In: Bennett A E (ed) Communication between doctors and patients. Nuffield Provincial Hospitals Trust and Oxford University Press, London
McKeown T 1976 The role of medicine. Dream mirage or nemsis? Nuffield Provincial Hospitals Trust, London
Malines J 1953 Journal of the Social Association 7, No. 4, 24
Nuffield Provincial Hospitals Trust 1968 Screening in medical care. Oxford University Press, Oxford
Owen, Rt Hon Dr D 1984 Medicine, morality and the market. Osler Lecture, McGill University, Montreal 4 April 1984 (personal communication)

Royal College of General Practitioners 1981a Health and prevention in primary care. RCGP, London
Royal College of General Practitioners 1981b Prevention of arterial disease in general practice. RCGP, London
Royal College of Physicians 1984 Health or smoking? Pitman, London
Russell M A H, Wilson C, Taylor C, Baker C D 1979 Effect of general practitioners' advice against smoking. British Medical Journal ii: 231–235
Stott N C H, Davis R H 1979 The exceptional potential in each primary care consultation. Journal Royal College of General Practitioners 29: 201–205
Trowell HC, Burkitt D P (eds) 1981 Western diseases: their emergence and prevention. Arnold, London
WHO 1978 Alma-Ata 1978. Primary health care: report of the international conference. World Health Organization, Geneva
WHO 1979 Controlling the smoking epidemic. World Health Organization, Geneva
WHO 1082 Seventh general programme of work concerning the period 1984–1989 ('Health for all' series number 8). World Health Organization, Geneva

FURTHER READING

Gray J A M, Fowler G 1984 Essentials of preventive medicine. Blackwell's Scientific Publications, Oxford

Participation

WHY PARTICIPATE AT ALL?

Imagine a primary health care service in which patients had complete control over all decisions without reference to doctors or nurses. Applied to the consultation this proposition would be regarded by most family doctors as absurd. They would consider themselves to be reduced to lackeys, unable to contribute their initiative, knowledge and skills to the problems of their patients. Even applied to the organization of the practice, this proposition would not be given much of a welcome.

Now imagine the obverse proposition. Doctors take all the decisions without consulting their patients. Both in the consultation and outside, patients have a wholly passive role, unable to contribute their resources, knowledge and skill to their own care or to the effectiveness of the practice. This picture is nearer to existing patterns, yet is this right? Should not the ideal arrangement be a compromise in which professionals (doctors, nurses and lay staff) and patients (or their representatives) each contribute according to the requirements of a particular situation or problem? It is time to question whether such a compromise is feasible, the nature of its benefits, and the costs.

A compromise of this kind implies flexibility, rather than taking up an authoritarian stance. This corresponds to what has been termed the adult-to-adult relationship (Harris 1973) between the patient-oriented doctor and the active patient who seeks to be independent. It is at one end of the spectrum described by Byrne and Long (1976) in *Doctors talking to patients*. At one end is the doctor-technician and at the other is the patient-oriented doctor with a more counselling style of working.

In the consultation, as in any situation of leadership, there are occasions when authority is appropriate. But management studies tend to show that subordinate-centred leadership is more effective, resulting in greater motivation and job satisfaction (Tannenbaum & Schmidt 1958). If the less authoritarian style is preferable in the boss-subordinate relationship, how much more important might it be with doctors and patients, who are, (nominally at least), equals? Is it not likely that a more participative style in the consultation and in practice management would lead to greater patient satisfaction?

A participative style in the consultation is gaining support (Pendleton et al 1984), and even has statutory backing in Sweden. But participation in the business of practice management tends to be received with strong negative reactions. 'Why should patients be involved in running my practice, or interfering in my job?'. There are firm feelings about professional territory. But just as the patient can rightly question, 'Whose health is it?', so too they may begin to question, 'Whose practice?'. Should not doctors encourage them to talk not only of 'my doctor' but also of 'my practice'? If the aim is to build a doctor-patient relationship making optimum use of patients' *and* professional resources, then a participative approach is not only preferable but essential.

The provision of primary health care, however, has other dimensions besides doctor and patient. At practice level there are nurses, other health professionals, and lay administrative staff who need to share in setting objectives and carrying out tasks. At more central levels, there is yet another party — a health bureaucracy, with different aims of those of the doctor and the patient. Different payment methods may affect the operation of the bureaucracy but a tripartite participative model is inescapable. How do patients relate to the bureaucracy? Have they any way of influencing its working?

Major social and economic changes are occurring to which primary health care must respond if it is to be effective. New demands are being made, for instance from new self-help groups and consumer organizations. At the same time, changes in government policy and organization are influencing the demands on primary health care. This may be partly due to a need for economy in times of economic scarcity, but there is also a growing realization of the key role of primary health care in society.

But first, let us return to the main question in this section — 'Why participate?'. Different people would answer this in different ways, depending on their individual style and beliefs, but a list of arguments for participation can be drawn up (see Table 7.1). Each

Table 7.1 Why participate?

Advantages to members of the community and to patients
Participation: encourages people to take an active role in maintaining or restoring their health
  discourages dependency and apathy about health
  allows the patient to make a positive contribution to the provision of neighbourhood health care
  lessens the patients' feeling of powerlessness in the face of professionals and bureaucracy
  increases the diffusion of information in the community about health and health services, so that more effective use may be made of them
  encourages people to have a stake in the service being provided, and so be prepared to support the allocation of resources for health care

Advantages to doctors and staff
1. At individual level
Participation: is part of the range of behaviour essential in the consultation
  is doing things *with* people not *to* people
  extends the role of the doctor
  helps the doctor to clarify his aims, and to respond to change

2. At the practice level
Participation: helps to clarify the aims of the practice
  provides feedback for evaluating service to patients
  helps the practice respond to change
  encourages patients to contribute to their own health and health care and supports self-help groups
  allows patients to make a positive contribution to the running of the practice
  facilitates health education, and preventive medicine
  increases the overall effectiveness of the practice
  improves doctor–patient communication and relationships
  increases job satisfaction of doctors and staff
  reduces or defuses complaints

3. At more central levels
Participation: is an essential element of democratically-based health care
  lessens professional and technical domination of health care
  helps the bureaucracy to respond to change
  encourages a more rational use of health services
  helps in choice of allocation of scarce resources
  provides an input into teaching of health care professionals at all levels
  is part of a world movement which cannot be ignored.

health professional should make their own list, and discuss it with patients, where possible. Participation, in the author's view, works to the advantage of doctors, patients and organizations, but it is not achieved without cost. Such costs are discussed on page 96.

Response to the Alma-Ata declaration

The professional responses to the Alma-Ata declaration's suggestions for more participation in developed countries has been essentially to ignore it altogether. Some dismissed it as relevant only to poorer countries with poorly developed medical services. Only a few voices spoke up on the importance of this issue. In 1979, Dr Leo Kaprio, the WHO regional director for Europe (Kaprio 1979) argued strongly for the ideal of community participation in health:

> Here, the notion of Primary Health Care (PHC) requires that the care given should involve the local community. Care should, if possible, result from community activity, or at least be a part of it in the sense that the local community takes an active, or even sponsoring, role. Locally derived priorities are served and local community resources used, as far as possible. A more subtle and more important feature, mentioned above, is that PHC is not imposed from outside and is always in harmony with the lifestyle and culture of the community. It follows that health is often defined in local, rather than 'imported' medical terms.

He then added, in relation to Europe (Kaprio 1979):

> A general problem in the European Region is that of community non-participation in medical care. In our Region the physician remains supreme in all, or most, fields of health care and the community usually respects this arrangement. However, the relationship is not a participant one, and only in a few countries does the care spring from the community in the idealistic sense in which this phase is used in PHC. More usually, the many different methods of payment, issues of confidentiality, and emphasis on the physician/patient relationship preclude extensive community involvement in medical care. However, it is not clear that this threatens the health of our populations in any significant way.

This remains true today. Participation is viewed as a threat to the professional status quo, and unnecessary in a health care system managed and delivered by dedicated professionals. Furthermore, although more cogent arguments can now be advanced for a participative approach, proof that this results in a more effective service is still lacking. This is hardly surprising, given the lack of clear and agreed objectives, and of indicators of performance, in primary health care.

The Alma-Ata statements on community participation are at the centre of professional values and beliefs, and pose a threat. The temptation by physicians to dismiss participation as irrelevant, too political or too difficult is strong. But there is a rising popular tide of demand for involvement which is reinforced by the Alma-Ata message and provides challenges for the future.

WHAT IS PARTICIPATION?

Participation is a very old idea, yet it has emerged as a new political issue (Richardson 1983a). The word has many meanings, ranging from the dictionary definition of 'taking part' in some joint action, to joint decision making, with many shades of meaning in between.

Since the beginning of the century, participation has been considered the cornerstone of democracy, but it then had a very different meaning and scope. It tended to refer to the right to vote to choose a leader; once chosen, the leader could go his own way without formally consulting his constituents, until the next election was imminent. Today, participation has been extended to include the influencing of elected leaders by individuals, pressure groups and institutions, as well as a say in decision making at individual and collective levels. But such participation presupposes that the individuals or institutions have the necessary knowledge and capability to make decisions.

Participation may involve people directly (direct participation) or it may work through complex institutions where the consumer interest is represented indirectly (Richardson 1983a). Direct participation is, one hopes, increasingly taking place between doctor and patient. At the slightly more complex levels of the patient participation group (PPG) (Pritchard 1981) or Community Health Council (CHC) (Levitt 1980) participation is less direct. Furthermore, participation may be formal or informal. At the level of the consultation or the practice, participation tends to be informal, whereas nearer to central government more formal structures are likely. Whatever the formality of the structures, the people taking part may, of course, influence each other informally. A general practitioner living in the community he serves is in a better position to benefit from informal participation than his commuter colleagues.

Participation is an active process. Its obverse is apathy. Passivity is enshrined in the concept of the sick role — that the patient wants to get well, that he or she could not get well unaided and so needs expert medical help (Robinson 1978). In exchange for submissive behaviour the patient expects to be relieved of certain social responsibilities and of the opprobrium of being ill, and also to receive benefits in cash or kind. The whole stigma of the sick-role is so repugnant to many patients that they either refuse to seek help (Hannay 1979), or prefer alternative therapies. A participatory approach to PHC might change all this.

PARTICIPATION AND POWER

Richardson (1983a) described participation at its simplest as, 'the addition of a new set of people into a particular situation'. This inevitably calls for changed relationships, and makes it likely that the new entrants to the situation will have some influence on subsequent decision making. Without some change the whole operation is, after all, pointless. Arnstein (1969) dismisses such pseudoparticipation, involving no transfer of power, as tokenism or manipulative non-participation.

If doctors deny their patients a say in decisions about their health, or even information about it, the result will be unhappiness on both sides. Some sharing of basic decisions, in other words, is helpful to a good doctor–patient relationship. The question is where to strike the balance. In the past, the balance of power was very much in favour of the general practitioner, even though his therapeutic power was limited. Now he has powerful remedies at his fingertips and high-technology services available on referral. Perhaps he should rethink his 'mystique' as a means to a power base.

Cynics may argue that nobody will give up power unless forced, but this is not borne out by the experience of patient participation. General practitioners are introducing this across the country (UK), as discussed at greater length below. For participation to be put into effect everywhere, however, not just where a band of enthusiasts chooses, some professional incentives or sanctions will be necessary. This may be viewed as preferable to having contractual changes forced upon them by public pressure.

Doctors are not alone in their reluctance to give up power; it is a natural reaction of any professional group. Nonetheless, the benefits of a more participative approach, as listed in Table 7.1, go a long way towards rewarding doctors who decide to follow this path.

Moreover, those who argue that transfer of power will result in gains for patients and losses for doctors assume a fixed amount of power and resources. Where primary health care operates as a small unit in a larger system of health care, this assumption is unwarranted. An integrated partnership of patients, doctors and staff can attract considerable resources both from community networks and from the NHS as a whole. This view is compatible with the 'open system' model of primary health care (Pritchard et al 1984).

There are many factors affecting the balance of power, some of which are listed in Table 7.2 below.

Table 7.2   The power balance

Factors increasing doctors' power	Factors restoring a more equitable balance
Greater knowledge	'Open medicine', and access to knowledge
Greater access to services	Increased information about and access to services
Professional autonomy and non-accountability	Greater accountability to users
Ownership of equity of primary care service	A greater stake in the service

'Distance' from patient, and barriers to communication, e.g.
   delay in appointments
   short consulting times
   impression of being very busy
   insensitive reception service
   inaccessibility by telephone
   few home visits
	Reduction of distance by change of attitudes and procedures, and a more open dialogue

Monopoly of decision-making	Shared decision-making, as in patient participation group

WHAT FORMS DOES PARTICIPATION TAKE IN PHC?

For many years in the United Kingdom (UK) and other democratic countries, elected and appointed lay people serving on statutory bodies have had the duty to provide health care services at various levels, with the co-operation of professionals. There is some tendency for the latter to dominate the management of these services and for lay people to have little influence. (Kaprio 1979).

To try to correct this tendency, Community Health Councils (CHCs) were set up in the UK in 1974 at district level to act on behalf of the consumer (Levitt 1980). Their role has been difficult, with scanty resources and hostile responses from health professionals. Each covering a population of a quarter to half a million, their attention has mostly focused on hospital services. Their impact on primary health care has often been favourable, but not dramatic.

Patient participation groups (PPGs) in primary health care

Since 1972, some general practices have been setting up patient participation groups (PPGs), almost always on the initiative of the doctors. The numbers have grown slowly but steadily, and there are about 100 active groups. This only represents about 1 practice in 100. Several groups have started and failed, often from lack of response from patients. PPGs vary widely in their nature and aim to respond to the unique circumstances of each practice and the population served. Their activities vary widely (Paine 1982) but can be summarized as:

1. Voice and interaction
2. Health education
3. Community and practice support
4. Special interest and self-help groups
5. Fact finding
6. Providing information
7. Fund raising

Other activities include linking the practice to community agencies, and influencing organizations outside PHC.

Wood and Metcalfe (1980) analysed the characteristics of the doctors involved in the groups, and found that they were more confident and more innovative than average. They considered that the group helped to reduce friction, increase mutual understanding, improve effectiveness, extend the general practitioner's role and act as an essential tool.

General practitioners who did not have a PPG produced diametrically opposite answers!

The initiation and survival of a PPG appears to depend very much on the goodwill and enthusiasm of the doctors, some therefore argue that groups are manipulated by doctors to provide the appearance of participation without the substance (i.e. tokenism, or non-participation in Arnstein's terms). There may be some truth in this statement, in that power voluntarily shared by the doctors, can be taken back. But if the aim is partnership, rather than delegated power or patient control, then this is realistic and achievable. A slogan of the National Association of Patient Participation is 'Partnership for Health'. This focuses on the positive and preventive features of PPGs. Some PPGs have faced up to providing a channel for complaints, and have a lay person as adjudicator or patient advocate within the practice.

Some disappointment has been expressed at the slow growth in numbers of PPGs, from 1 to 100 in 12 years. Certainly there is a long way to go before it can be said to have an influence on the overall standard of general practice. Research into its effectiveness is only just starting, and until there is positive evidence for its usefulness, many sceptics will hold back. But does not all change start in this way? The time scale for change in general practice is slow, particularly in an area involving deeply-held beliefs.

The Royal College of General Practitioners (RCGP) Patient Liaison Group

The RCGP has shown strong support for patient participation and set up a patient liaison group (RCGP 1983). Its remits were:

1. To nominate and support patient representatives in order to attend appropriate working parties, Divisional Executives and College Council.

2. To initiate new areas for discussion in Council.

3. To initiate activities in faculties and districts.

4. To review regularly how the arrangements both centrally and locally are working.

Participative evaluation and accountability

The Royal College of General Practitioners has given high priority to the introduction of a practice-based method of education and assessment which has focused on four main areas:

1. Professional values
2. Accessibility
3. Clinical competence
4. Ability to communicate (RCGP 1985).

Whereas medical audit and performance review have traditionally been confined to the area of clinical competence, the RCGP approach is equally concerned with the three other areas, in which some input from patients is essential.

Professional values may be personal to the individual doctor, or be shared by the whole profession, but they cannot be viewed in isolation from the society in which they operate. For the values to be relevant to the needs of the community, and to be able to reflect changing values in society, some interaction with patients is essential.

Accessibility is a relative term, and must be measured against norms, that can only be decided upon after negotiation with patients or their relatives. This too should be the subject of participation, both locally and nationally.

The ability to communicate must include being able to listen as well as to explain. For PHC to be effective there must be good communication in the one-to-one consultation, as well as in groups, in the PHC team, and in the management of the practice. Patients or their representatives should be able to participate in all these groups at some point.

Clinical competence. The RCGP also launched a 'Quality Initiative' in 1983, encouraging general practitioners to describe the work of their practices and monitor their progress. This is a courageous and unique move into an uncertain area of evaluation and accountability (Pritchard 1984). Ulitmately, general practitioners must be accountable to their patients and to society as well as to themselves. Many patients, would like additional safeguards to the doctor's own conscience.

Patients involvement in the process of professional accountability remains to be worked out in greater detail. A start has been made with PPGs, CHCs and Patient Liaison Groups. Methods for participative evaluation by members of local communities have been developed in conjunction with the World Health Organization (Feuerstein 1978) but have not been widely applied in developed countries.

Self-help groups

The growth in self-help and mutual-help groups in the past decade has been dramatic (Richardson & Goodman 1983). A study of such groups related to health has shown that there may be around 1500 such groups in a single district, and 1000 with a national focus. (Gann 1981). This movement is worldwide and particularly active in Europe (Hatch & Kickbusch 1983). Trojan (1983) has analysed such groups along two axes, according to whether their aims were predominantly for self-change, or for social change, and whether the groups were close to the public/professional systems or remote from them. General practitioners are likely to be more aware of those groups which aim at self-change and are close to the professional care system. The more remote groups, and those aiming at social change are likely to be viewed with suspicion or hostility. Yet all such groups are an additional resource for patients — even if they may be critical of current medical practice — and should be welcomed by general practitioners. Such groups may need support from health professionals, which has to be given with sensitivity if tender groups are not to be harmed (Richardson 1984a).

Self-help groups may be a valuable source of knowledge for doctors as well as patients. Many of them have efficient information systems and obtain the best professional advice. They may provide a useful input into the training of doctors and nursing staff in PHC.

EVALUATING PARTICIPATION

Once a structure has been established and people meet, what is the nature and quality of the process? Are the real issues discussed, or is there a smokescreen of trivia? Who makes decisions, how are they made, and which way do they usually go? Outcome measures, as always, are hard to find. That all participants should be satisfied with the process, if not the decision, is one legitimate outcome. Responses to health education is another that can be measured. Attendance for screening or preventive procedures can be counted, and changes following a participative approach measured. One can also consider whether a participative health care service works better in terms of availability, accessibility and acceptability. Improved outcomes for health would he hard to distinguish from other factors, but can be inferred if health-maintaining behaviour is changed in a favourable direction.

Participation should have an impact on doctors', as well as patients' attitudes and behaviour, and attempts can be made to study this. Does participation encourage good PHC practices, the formation of self-help groups, and mobilize more resources from outside?

These and other questions are the subject of a current major research project (Richardson 1983b).

Skills

General practitioners are increasingly being trained to communicate in the consultation, and to adopt a more counselling style so that the patient has the opportunity to participate. Communicating with staff and patients in a patient participation group or a self-help group may need additional skills. They will need confidence, but this must be tempered with humility, and a readiness to listen and admit shortcomings. A defensive attitude tends to be counter-productive. Encouraging people to complain or criticize runs counter to most people's nature, and has to be learned the hard way. The pay-off in mutual understanding and support soon reinforces this behavioural change.

To set up and maintain a PPG requires management skills which are not part of medical training. Even an experienced practice manager can find it a difficult task (Pritchard 1983).

Resources

Participation costs money but can also generate resources. Some PPGs raise money for their own activities (sometimes large-scale) and for improvements in the practice: some exert pressure on outside bodies to release resources or maintain services. But participation may need help in getting started, until the point of self-sufficiency is reached. Health authorities have been reluctant to give financial support to PPGs (apart from limited health education or research projects) in spite of a clear recommendation by the Royal Commission on the Health Service (DHSS 1979).

BARRIERS TO PARTICIPATION, AND COSTS

Do general practitioners want patients to be active, self-reliant and responsible? Or do they prefer them to be obedient, compliant and respectful — silently accepting the decisions made for them by their expert advisers? The latter view was nearer the norm in British general practice 60 years ago. For instance, Dr John Pickles, father of Dr William Pickles the first President of the (now) Royal College of General Practitioners, is supposed to have said of patients who ask questions, 'I can always bluff them. If they ask me what's wrong with them, I say to them, 'That's my business. Do as I tell you and take your medicine and you'll get better' (Pemberton 1972).

This view is echoed today by a journalist who gives a bleak description of doctors dispensing charity to passive but resentful patients (Toynbee 1984). The barriers of fixed professional attitudes and anxieties about loss of control are probably the most formidable and resistant to change. Only long-term education and public pressure can bring about change.

The development of a large National Health Service with its inevitable bureaucracy is aimed at providing a service to the public, but may be hampered by its very size and complexity, and the professional polarization which it engenders. Individual and public interest may be lost in the expediency of day-to-day management.

Where complaints procedures are insensitive or ineffective, patients may have recourse to law, which immediately stifles communication and inhibits an open participatory system. This is a vicious circle, in that participation at an earlier stage can defuse complaints or bring them to a satisfactory conclusion.

Participation is a mechanism for predicting and facilitating change, so that by avoiding participation, the change process may be inhibited until irresistible forces build up. The increasing resort to alternative or unorthodox therapy is an example of a failure of health care services to inspire confidence and to perceive a need, so that people vote with their feet.

Other barriers to participation have been mentioned, such as lack of skills in communication and management, as well as lack of energy and enthusiasm for meeting change half way, rather than waiting to be carried with the tide.

These barriers are indicative of the cost of participation to individuals who try to introduce it. The key question is whether the investment of time, energy and money is justified by the results. General practitioners and patients involved in participation have mostly responded positively, and consider the patient participation group an 'essential tool'.

One criticism of participation is that it is mostly confined to articulate and relatively healthy middle class people. There is some substance in this, but it obscures the issue that the less accessible people are to participation, the more likely they are to need it. For example, groups like the mentally ill, the very poor, young people and the elderly housebound may be difficult to reach except at considerable cost. This is a challenge to participation groups of which they are well aware and try to meet.

At more central levels, the financial cost of participative institutions like Community Health Councils is often called in question. But how can participation be costed? Does it have to be economically viable, or is it accepted as part of our system of values? To deny participation is to undervalue people's autonomy, as well as their own potential contribution to their health and care (Vuori 1985).

WHAT OF THE FUTURE? TARGETS FOR 2000

General practitioners are not keen on planning ahead. They mostly are concerned with short-term goals, such as getting through the day without too many crises. The NHS planning system is concerned mostly with hospital-based services, and strategic planning of PHC is rudimentary or absent.

Looking 5 years ahead may be the practical time span achievable in general practice, so to look over 15 years ahead is less precise, but important. In the ideal practice of 2000 A.D., the knowledge gap between doctor and patient will be narrower and the emphasis will be on skills and attitudes. The doctor will have skills in understanding the patient's real concerns, not only the symptoms presented. Society will have changed radically, and doctors will need increased insight into the forces at work and the stresses produced. Closer links will be needed with community and social agencies than exist at present. Communication and social skills will be more necessary if family doctors are to remain in the mainstream of society, not peripheral technicians. Participation will be an essential part of this two-way communication.

Targets

Can some targets be set up for achieving acceptable levels of participation by a given time? Each country and health care system will need its own targets. The European Office of the World Health Organization has suggested that: *'By 1985, all countries will ensure effective and representative community participation at all levels of health care organization and development'*.

Setting up detailed targets is not easy. A start can be made by promoting effective participative methods and encouraging their adoption.

Formal participation is more amenable to planning and target setting, and to evaluation of the effectiveness of institutions like CHCs and Health Authorities in achieving participation. Performance indicators need to be developed.

Central government and administration cannot escape scrutiny of its level of participation.

Suggestions for action are:

1. Neighbourhood level

Each practice as part of a group of professionals supported by volunteers, working from shared premises, serving a population of 10–20 000. Close links with other social agencies which are relevant to health (e.g. social services, housing, education, employment and youth service). The practice centre a focus for supporting self-help groups related to health. A community participation group based on the centre with a central role in co-ordinating community activities relevant to health both voluntary and statutory. The community participation group (CPG) links with similar groups at higher levels. Adequate resources to enable CPG to undertake evaluative studies, as an autonomous unit, independent of the administrative and bureaucratic health system, but with rights of information, access and consultation. Incentives to encourage general practitioners to co-operative with community participation groups. A start be made by ensuring that one of the criteria for training practices is that they have CPG.

2. District level

Assuming that a population of a quarter to half a million be served by a district general hospital, the aim of a participative model be to identify the best interests of patients so that primary and secondary care may be co-ordinated; and that hospital/community links are maintained in order to achieve optimum care, both preventive and curative. The UK Community Health Council (CHC) is an appropriate model at this level, but CHCs have been under-resourced and some have generated antagonism.

3. Regional and central levels

The concept of an autonomous participative body separate from the NHS adminstration is crucial. This independent consumer representation ought to address itself to the decisions taken at more central levels, involving medical education, strategic planning and policies for primary health care. Apart from the RCGP Patient Liaison Group, and bodies like the National Consumer Council, this area is poorly covered in UK.

In conclusion

I quote Richardson's (1984b) address to the Annual Symposium of the Royal College of General Practitioners.

> It is probable that participation is here to stay, and it is likely to be a much more common phenomenon in 10 or 20 years than it is today. That is as true for the running of general practices as for the management of schools, or planning procedures or housing estates. The key question today is therefore not so much whether it is a good or a bad thing as how should the profession respond? What practical steps should be considered? My expectation is that many local

doctors will feel that they can see little sense in pursuing the subject further. Many others, however, will begin to experiment with new ways of running their practices and will have a great deal to learn from one another.

Those general practitioners up and down the country who begin to experiment with participation are likely to find that it has a deeper impact than they — or the patient participants — expected. It will affect *them*. The experience of participation tends to foster greater self-questioning, and therefore self-development, among professionals themselves. This, is my view, represents the crucial hidden agenda of participation. The challenge of the future, in other words, lies not simply in opening doors to patients but in opening doors to yourselves. It is probably the most difficult challenge of all, but through the process of meeting it squarely you will make yourselves, and your profession, ever more strong.

Acknowledgements

I wish to thank all those who have contributed their ideas so generously, particularly Dr Ann Richardson, Mrs Pat Turton and Dr Hannu Vuori.

REFERENCES

Arnstein S 1969 A ladder of citizen participation. American Institute of Planners Journal 53: 216–224
Byrne P Long B 1976 Doctors talking to patients. DHSS. HMSO, London
DHSS 1979 Report of Royal Commission on the National Health Service. HMSO, London
Feuerstein M-T 1978 Evaluation — by the people. International Nursing Review 25, 5, 78: 146–156
Gann R 1981 Help for health. Information for primary care. Wessex Regional Library Unit, Southampton S09 4XY
Hannay D R 1979 The symptom iceberg. A study of community health. Routledge & Kegan Paul, London
Harris T A 1970 I'm OK — you're OK. Pan books, London
Hatch S Kickbusch I (eds) 1983 Self-help and health in Europe. New approaches in health care. World Health Organization Regional Office for Europe, Copenhagen
Kaprio L A 1979 Primary health care in Europe. Euro reports and studies No 14. WHO Regional Office for Europe, Copenhagen
Levitt R 1980 The people's voice in the National Health Service. King Edward's Hospital Fund, London
Paine T 1982 A survey of patient participation groups. British Medical Journal 286: 768–772, 847–849
Pemberton J 1972 Will Pickles of Wensleydale: the life of a country doctor. Country Book Club, Newton Abbot, p 29
Pendleton D et al 1984 The consultation. An approach to learning and teaching. Oxford University Press, Oxford
Pritchard P M M (ed) 1981 Patient participation in general practice. Occasional paper No. 17. Royal College of General Practitioners, London
Pritchard P M M 1983 Patient participation in general practice. Medical Annual, John Wright, Bristol, 227–238

Pritchard P M M 1984 Professional accountability in primary health care. In: Nowotny H (ed) Social concerns in the 80s: breaks and continuities in social policy. European Centre for Social Welfare Training and Research, Vienna

Pritchard P M M, Low K, Whalen M 1984 Management in general practice. Oxford University Press, Oxford

Richardson A 1983a Participation, Routledge and Kegan Paul, London

Richardson A 1983b Patient participation in general practice. A research proposal. Policy Studies Institute; London

Richardson A 1984a Working with self-help groups. A guide for local professionals. Bedford Square Press, London

Richardson A 1984b Doctors and the receivers of care. In: Zander L (ed) Change the challenge of the future. Proceedings of the annual symposium of the Royal College of General Practitioners 1983. IRL Press/RCGP, London

Richardson A Goodman M 1983 Self-help and social care: mutual aid organizations in practice. Policy Studies Institute, London

Robinson D 1978 Patients, practitioners and medical care, 2nd edn Heinemann, London

RCGP 1983 Patients and the College. Report of a working party Journal of the Royal College of General Practitioners 33: 53–55 and editorial 33: 5–7

RCGP 1985 What sort of doctor? Report from General Practice 23. Journal of the Royal College of General Practitioners

Tannenbaum R Schmidt W H 1958 How to choose a leadership pattern Harvard Business Review 36.2: 95–101

Toynbee P 1984 The patient and the NHS. In: Teeling Smith G (ed) A new NHS act for 1996? Office of Health Economics, London

Trojan A 1983 Groupes de Sante: the user's movement in France. In: Hatch S, Kickbusch I 1983 quoted above

Vuori H 1985 Community participation in primary health care — a means or an end? In: Vuori H, Levine S (eds) Proceedings of the conference on primary health care in industrialized countries. WHO Regional Office for Europe, Copenhagen

WHO/UNICEF 1978 Primary health care Alma-Ata 1978. Report of an international conference. World Health Organization, Geneva

Wood D J, Metcalfe D 1980 Professional attitudes to patient participation groups. Journal of the Royal College of General Practitioners 30: 538–541

FURTHER READING

The following are recommended.

Fry J (ed) 1983 Patient participation — more or less? In: Common dilemmas in family medicine. MTP Lancaster (with contributions by Berg A O, Kerrigan P arguing for 'less, and Pistorius G J, Sehnert K W and Pritchard P arguing for 'more'.)

Richardson A 1983a Participation (see below)

Vuori H, Hastings J 1985 Community participation in primary health care. WHO Regional Office for Europe, Copenhagen

Collaboration

The concept of health care as requiring a graduated series of levels of increasing sophistication and complexity has been surprisingly slow to evolve. Much of the development of the various professional groups involved has proceeded with little thought being given as to how their role and tasks should relate to those of the other professions concerned or even to other members of their own profession. Thus we have the unedifying spectacle of generalist and specialist dectors competing for the same ground and doctors denying or denigrating the value of health-visitors (public health nurses) or social workers, often from a position of ignorance and blind prejudice.

The aim of this chapter is to clarify the place of primary health care within the overall system, define the role of the primary care physician and explore some of the problems of the relationship between the physician at primary care level and his generalist and specialist colleagues, the various types and grades of nurses working within the community, other professional health care workers, social workers, voluntary workers and practitioners of alternative or complementary medicine. The relationship between the primary care physician and the hospital will also be considered, as will the need for effective communication skills within a mutually supportive referral system. Finally, consideration of the problems facing us all at present should lead to a better definition of what needs must be met in the future.

PLACE OF PRIMARY HEALTH CARE

In any system of health care there is inevitably a point at which a patient or parent makes a conscious decision to take a problem beyond the informal lay referral network of family and friends and thus enter 'the system'. This decision is indeed a momentous one since it opens up for the individual the prospect of advice, investigation, treatment or referral and ultimately cure, permanent disability or even death. Simultaneously, society, either directly through a national health system or private insurance or indirectly by payment of fees and expenses by the patient, is committed to a potentially enormous expenditure of resources in an attempt to overcome the problems.

Since the nature of the problems, which are seen as appropriate to present in primary care, will vary from one society to another, and since the range of health care worker in the broadest sense to whom the patient can turn may vary widely even within a particular system, it is apparent that the nature of this interface is exceedingly complex and gives rise to the unique mixture of difficulties and opportunities which characterizes primary care. Whatever the service and whoever provides it, the essential feature is the direct contact between the consumer and the provider with no inter-mediary involved, and the frequent expectation on both sides of a continuing rather than an episodic relationship.

NATURE OF PRIMARY HEALTH CARE

Because of the exposed position of the primary health care worker, it is frequently the case that the solution to the problem presented does not necessarily lie within their particular field of competence. Thus the general practitioner, for instance, may well be faced with a somatic complaint, e.g. a headache, the roots of which may lie in anything from a brain tumour to depression engendered by the stress of life-events such as bereavement, family or marital dishar-mony, financial, employment or housing problems. Mismanage-ment of the problem at this stage by inappropriate referral has enormous implications since, down one road, may lie neurologists, brain scans and invasive investigations, whilst down another may lie marriage guidance, group therapy or a new job. Often the doctor will temporize with an analgesic or anxiolytic whilst allowing the passage of time and observing the development or regression of the symptoms. In any event an awareness of the broad range of back-ground factors which may be relevant and an understanding of how and when to mobilize appropriate alternative resources is a crucial skill which must be mastered.

Similarly, in the field of preventive medicine and health education, many different types of expertise are required, whilst the provision of family planning services, the planning and execution of immunization programmes against infectious diseases and the care and supervision of vulnerable groups within the community such as pregnant women, children and the elderly all involve a range of skills unlikely to be found within a single profession.

INTERDEPENDENCE OF LEVELS OF HEALTH CARE

Thus it is clear that the range of knowledge, skills and attitudes required by the primary care physician is very different to those required by his medical colleagues working at secondary or tertiary level. Whilst he is grappling with the broad range of physical, psychological and social problems presented by primary care, they have the much more specific and well-defined role of applying their highly specialized knowledge and skills to the diagnosis and treatment of a relatively small range of problems which have been selected for them at primary care level. The roles are complementary and interdependent and a mutual appreciation of this interdependence is crucial if the system is to function well. Whilst it is by no means universal that all primary care physicians are generalists, it is most important that specialists working in this field have a proper appreciation of the different perspectives required in primary care. Increasingly this need has been realized and specific programmes of training for doctors entering primary care have become established in many countries.

WORKING RELATIONSHIPS — DOCTORS IN PRIMARY CARE

One of the most notable features of British general practice over the past 30 years has been the increasing trend towards group practice. Indeed, it is now rare to find a young trainee even contemplating single-handed practice as a preferred lifestyle. Practical benefits include sharing the costs of practice premises and equipment and simplifying arrangements for daytime, night, weekend and holiday cover. Whilst the single-handed practitioner in most urban and suburban areas now has a commercial deputising service available these are generally seen as an inferior substitute for a well-organized rota.

However, there are other benefits of group practice, perhaps less tangible, which loom large in the thinking of those who support the concept of group practice. There is some anecdotal evidence that doctors working in group practice are more likely to enjoy their work than doctors working alone and the easy accessibility to colleagues with whom to discuss personal or clinical problems, new techniques or methods of management is an important benefit.

Since one of the most widely criticized aspects of general practice as a professional and academic discipline is the professional isolation of the practitioner, any arrangement which helps to overcome this is to be welcomed. The development of continuing education at postgraduate centres has helped to promote contact between general practitioners, but it is now clear that the way forward in continuing education is to encourage the primary care doctor to look critically at his own day-to-day work, set personal or practice standards of care in a variety of areas and then measure whether they have been achieved. The 'quality initiative' of the RCGP represents an attempt to encourage primary care doctors to develop in this way and the group practice is obviously an ideal setting in which to establish these activities.

Group practice allows the partners to develop special fields of interest, either in clinical areas or in education and research and enables these new skills to be transmitted within the practice. In addition, the organization and management skills acquired by the more senior partners can be fostered in their juniors by a gradual assumption of responsibilities. Needless to say, a legal partnership contract, regular and properly conducted meetings, goodwill and mutually supportive relationships are all necessary ingredients if the practice is to function smoothly. Unfortunately, not all group practices prove to be a success. The most common causes of dispute between partners arise from financial and organizational problems rather than major clinical disagreements. Indeed, the reason most commonly given by those practitioners who do not wish to join a group practice is the fear of loss of autonomy and independence.

Most British group practices are arranged on the basis of pooling the fees and allowances received, deducting shared expenses, and then sharing out the net proceeds in predetermined proportions. This generally works well provided that each of the partners are seen to be carrying an equivalent workload. However, with the growth of extrapractice activities, such as industrial medicine, educational appointments and committee work, there is considerable potential for disagreement. In a fee-for-service system of payment, where practice income is more closely tied to workload, the strains may become too great to bear, especially in mixed group practices, where the partners with surgical skills have a considerably greater earning capacity than their medical colleagues.

Other sources of strain relate to personality factors and dissatisfaction with the rate and direction of change within the practice. Since the universal development of vocational training for general practice in the UK many informal groups of young practitioners drawn from several practices in a locality have been formed. They discuss a variety of issues pertaining to their new role as independent professionals, but a constant theme is how to achieve change within their new practices, without alienating the more senior partners. Perhaps more emphasis should be given to this topic during vocational training!

WORKING RELATIONSHIPS — THE PRIMARY HEALTH CARE TEAM

Whilst the concept of the primary health care team is currently gaining ground in many countries and has become the administrative norm to a greater or lesser extent throughout the UK, it is nevertheless true that the term is capable of many different interpretations. However, it is manifestly the case that every community has within it many individuals working at primary care level with a variety of background, training and professional status. The details of their individual training, roles and rewards will be found in Chapter 9, but in this chapter it is pertinent to consider how these various workers relate to each other, both within and without the primary health care team.

In the United Kingdom the team always includes one or more physicians, plus, in most cases, health visitors (public health nurses) and community nurses of various grades ranging from the equivalent of hospital ward sisters to nursing auxiliaries and bath attendants. In addition, many practices employ nurses to work specifically within the practice premises and, increasingly, to undertake tasks which require skills beyond the nursing curriculum. Some of these practice nurses have developed a role similar to that of the nurse-practitioner in North America. Specialized nurses, including community midwives and community psychiatric nurses, are also commonly attached to primary health care teams.

It would seem logical to suppose that this nucleus primary health care team, consisting only of doctors and nurses with their supporting administrative and clerical staff, should find it easy to work together in order to provide a first-class service to the patient. After all, doctors and nurses are used to working with each other in hospital and co-operation should ensure that the team members are able to respond to the varying needs of the patient in the most appropriate and co-ordinated way, using their various skills and training as required. Indeed, most members of the primary health care teams do seem to function rather better than they did previously when practising as independent professionals. Nevertheless, it is all too common to hear of major problems arising and all too rare to hear of a team which has fulfilled its full potential.

Perhaps in retrospect it is surprising that primary health care teams have worked as well as they have in most cases, since little thought was apparently given to the difficulties which might arise when a group of professionals were brought together by the stroke of an administrative pen. Issues, such as the basic lack of knowledge of the other professions' training, roles and responsibilities, the effects of different employment status, remuneration, professional management structure and accountability, were rarely discussed, let alone the more subtle but probably more important issues of confidentiality, status, leadership and, above all, the need for effective communication within the team. Experience shows that where the members of a team are well motivated and of reasonably compatible personality, and when they work from the same premises and meet frequently, both informally and at more formal meetings, the arrangement can work well. Team members need to have a good understanding of, and respect for, the skills which others can contribute and also to have an appreciation of the outside pressures which may impinge upon them. Problems have arisen in the UK when community nurses and health-visitors have wished to expand their role beyond that acceptable to their nursing officers, and the increase in the number of directly employed practice nurses has partly occurred in response to these limitations. The problems which nurses have when professional accountability to a hierachy clashes with personal loyalty to a team is not always understood by the traditionally independent medical practitioner. Issues such as the need for confidentiality rarely arise within a team which is functioning well. Personal trust and mutual respect are more important than formal guidelines and, of course, there will be instances when all professionals are in receipt of a confidence which the patient forbids them to communicate to anyone or to record in the notes. The accessibility of members of the team to each others notes or, preferably, the maintenance of a unified record system is a basic requirement for effective team function.

The 'leadership' issue is a theme which constantly recurs in the literature and in discussions about the team approach. In general, it is true that the primary health care physician, because of his longer training, higher status, geographical stability and traditional role, is likely to function as a *'primus inter pares'*. However, attempts to use his position to unilaterally dictate patterns of work, decide priorities and usurp decisions which are manifestly part of the professional responsibility of the other groups will be counter productive and lead to functional, if not formal, breakdown of the team. This is particularly likely to happen if a social worker is included in the team, since he or she has quite separate statutory responsibilities which are clearly outside the health care field. Individual members of the team may well take the lead in specific areas to which their particular interests, enthusiasms and talents are best suited.

PHARMACISTS

The pharmacist is not normally thought of as part of the primary health care team but he is most certainly an important component of primary health care in any community. Progress in the direction of more enlightened self-care by members of the public depends on guidance from the pharmacist. Although this has been part of his traditional role for many years, it is only in recent times that 'clinical pharmacy' has come to be recognized as an important part of his training. The ability to manage minor symptoms appropriately and recognize potentially serious symptoms which require medical assessment is a valuable skill which should not be under-estimated. In addition, he must function as a safeguard against prescribing errors by the physician and as a source of information and education about drugs for the primary health care team. Again, there is no substitute for personal contact, mutual respect and shared experience.

SOCIAL SERVICES

The majority of social workers are not likely to see themselves as members of the PHCT in any conventional sense of the term although there are a growing number taking part in liaison schemes designed to improve communication and co-operation. Through the social services departments access is available to casework, home-care services, meals-on-wheels, aids and adaptations for the disabled, short-term care and long-term accommodation for the handicapped and elderly.

OTHER HEALTH CARE PROFESSIONALS

Clinical psychologists, physiotherapists, remedial gymnasts, occupational therapists, speech therapists, chiropodists and dieticians are usually based on hospitals in the UK, although general practitioners can often arrange direct access for the patient if required. There are no real equivalents in the UK to the 'barefoot doctors' of China and the third world, although it is possible to consider those employees who have passed basic examinations in first-aid as part-time health workers in a very limited role.

ALTERNATIVE OR COMPLEMENTARY MEDICINE

Outside of the 'official' health care system a variety of unorthodox healers flourish and there has been a considerable increase in public interest in acupuncture, homeopathy, osteopathy and other types of 'fringe medicine' during the last decade. Concurrently, the medical profession in the UK has itself developed a greater interest in these techniques and more doctors are exploring the possibility of using them in practice. Younger general practitioners especially have become involved and these topics formed the centrepiece of a recent National Trainee Conference in Cambridge in 1982. The inauguration of the British Holistic Medicine Association in 1983 and the subsequent announcement of a joint educational programme of the Association with the British Postgraduate Medical Federation in 1984 suggests that this collaboration is becoming increasingly important. The traditional antipathy between the established medical profession and other healers seems to be declining rapidly, although many general practitioners are still reluctant to make a formal referral and prefer to collude with self-referral by the patient in case they fall foul of the General Medical Council for associating with or 'covering' an 'unqualified' practitioner or traditional healer.

COUNSELLING SERVICES

There has been a similar increase in the number and variety of counselling services available in the community now that traditional counsellors such as the clergy have lost much of their influence. Thus, we now have direct access counselling services available for marriage and relationship problems, for drug or alcohol addicts, for potential suicides and for people with sexual problems or unwanted pregnancies.

SELF-HELP GROUPS

In addition, there are a multiplicity of self-help groups and organizations (see Chapter 7), which provide mutual education and support for people suffering from specific conditions such as diabetes, epilepsy or psoriasis. Many of these groups also raise considerable amounts of money with which to fund research programmes and provide educational material on their specific topics for a variety of health-care professionals. The value of this collaboration is that the professionals often become aware for the first time of the patient's view of a particular problem and its management, which in many instances changes the professional's own perspective and improves understanding between the health care worker and the patient. A recent series of articles in *Update* (1984) entitled 'Patients with Problems' has highlighted the value of this approach. At local level the primary care worker is often able to tap appropriate community resources and thus provide a type and degree of support which is beyond the range of the professional health and social services, limited as they are for time and resources. There are, of course, some potential pitfalls in this type of collaboration. The professional must be prepared to form a judgment about the quality and reliability of these local resources in order to protect the patient against harmful and disruptive influences but, in general, the voluntary associations are only too willing to engage in a dialogue with the professionals concerned and should be seen as a valuable extra resource rather than as a threat to professional integrity.

REFERRAL

In any situation where the doctor feels that some other agency or member of the primary health care team can provide a service which he is unable to provide, the doctor should make it clear to the patient that referral does not mean rejection and that the patient is at liberty to come back to the original doctor when and if he so desires. It is also most helpful if the patient is given some idea as to how the agency works and what to expect when he comes into contact with them.

RELATIONS BETWEEN PRIMARY CARE DOCTORS AND OTHER DOCTORS

This heading has been couched in general terms because the rigid separation of generalists providing primary care in the community from specialists providing secondary and tertiary care in hospital, as obtains in the UK is rarely as clearly defined in other systems of medical care. In many countries specialists provide a good deal of primary care, especially paediatricians, obstetrician-gynaecologists and specialists in internal medicine and they do not necessarily work in hospitals at all. Conversely, many generalists, especially in North America, regard access to hospital beds as an essential component of their professional practice. Notwithstanding these facts, it is quite clear that the experience of any doctor working predominantly in primary care with relatively undifferentiated problems must differ from that of the doctor dependent on referral from other doctors for his livelihood. The broadly-based skills and personal knowledge of the patient and his family possessed by the primary care doctor are complemented by the greater depth and expertise in a narrower field possessed by the specialist. If the maximum benefit is to be gained by the patient from his encounters with a range of doctors then it is most important that these doctors communicate all the necessary information to each other so that effort and resources may be applied in the most appropriate way and helpful way.

Informal consultation

Consultation between doctors about patients is an integral part of medical practice and it often occurs on an informal basis between partners in a group practice, as well as between generalists and specialists in the hospital corridors, at the postgraduate centre, over lunch or on the telephone.

Formal referral

However, formal referral of a patient for a second opinion requires considerable thought and consideration and should not be undertaken lightly. Apart from potential expense and inconvenience to the patient, the referring doctor may be setting in motion a complex series of events. Except in a case of desperate emergency, the normal form of communication should be by letter, preferably typed, with a copy kept by the referring doctor.

Ideally, the letter should be succinct, but contain all the essential information which the consultant requires. This must include the patient's name and address, date of birth and, preferably, marital state, in addition to a note of any allergic tendencies or drug idiosyncracies. A brief summary of the patient's previous medical history, followed by the history of the presenting problem, findings on physical examination and the results of any laboratory investigations or X-rays is also required. Pertinent psychological or social factors should also be incorporated at this point.

It is a good discipline for the referring doctor to commit his thoughts about the differential diagnosis or alternative management to paper before outlining what other steps he has taken or what drugs he has prescribed. In addition, it may be most important to inform the consultant about what the patient has been told and what he has been led to expect. Finally, and this is something often omitted from referral letters, the referring doctor should make it clear why he is making the referral. Does he want a second opinion about a perplexing diagnostic problem or is he asking for some technical procedure which he cannot provide himself? Does he wish to hand over the care of the patient completely in respect of this particular problem or is he quite happy to resume continuing care after receiving appropriate advice and guidance? If the patient or doctor has requested a second opinion largely for the sake of reassurance, then the referring doctor should make this clear. It may seem pedantic to labour these points but several studies have shown that it is rare for referral letters to contain all the necessary information.

The consultant's responsibility to the referring doctor is no less onerous. Firstly, he must actually read the referral letter and take note of its content! This may save considerable misunderstanding at a later date. There is no need to reiterate the patient's history, which is already well known to the referring doctor, unless significant new points come to light; similarly in respect of findings on physical examination. However, it is most valuable if he is able to summarize his clinical impressions, state clearly what action he proposes to take and what the patient has been told, and provide clear guidelines for further management as required.

If the consultant feels that the opinion of another specialist is required, then it is generally more satisfactory if this is arranged through the primary care doctor rather than directly by the consultant. In this way multiple referrals may be avoided. However, if the patient is already in hospital under the care of the consultant and the matter is urgent, then direct referral may be necessary. When the patient is discharged, a brief summary detailing diagnosis and drug therapy should accompany him, plus a telephone call to the primary care doctor if there is some particular problem outstanding. The discharge summary, which should be typed and delivered to the primary care physician as soon as practicable, should contain all the relevant information arising from the patient's stay in hospital in a form which is relevant to, and easily assimilable by the referring doctor.

Some of the discharge summaries, especially from highly specialized units are so technical as to be unintelligible and are clearly written for the purpose of providing an inpatient summary rather than communicating information to the primary care doctor.

COMMUNICATION

Generally speaking, the quality of communication between doctors varies inversely with the distance between them, both geographically and professionally, although there are notable exceptions. Where the relationship is close and personal there is more likely to be mutual respect and close co-operation. The traditional bedside domiciliary or hospital consultation with both parties present is seen less often nowadays but the increasing tendency for consultants to hold outpatient clinics in health-centres and community hospitals is an excellent and cost-effective substitute. However, even in a district general or teaching hospital the primary care physician who takes the trouble to visit his patient in hospital and meet the specialists on the wards, in the dining-room and at the postgraduate centre wll reap rich rewards in terms of professional satisfaction and an improved quality of service for his patients. Some primary care doctors enjoy working as part-time members of specialist teams, whilst others develop links with consultants whilst planning education programmes or taking part in committee work.

PRESENT PROBLEMS

When we consider the difficulties and obstacles which at present serve to hinder effective collaboration between all those involved in primary care, it appears that the basic problem is one of professional isolation, exemplified perhaps by the single-handed general practitioner who knew what his patient needed and was quite capable of providing it! I doubt whether this was ever really possible and I am quite sure that in a complex modern society it is certainly not feasible or even desirable. Nevertheless, there are still members of all the relevant professions who, quite rightly, see themselves as independent professionals but, wrongly, interpret this to mean that collaboration with others is either a sign of professional inadequacy or an admission of defeat! Ignorance of the education, training, ethos, role and work-patterns of the other professions is still widespread, as is a lack of understanding of the place of primary care within the overall network of health and social security provision in society. Relatively little consideration is given to the existence of unorthodox healers or counselling agencies, even though the orthodox professionals might benefit by giving thought as to why these alternative sources of help seem to be gaining ground amongst consumers. It is perhaps because they are offering the patient or client something which the orthodox health professionals, for all their skills and training, have lost sight of or choose to dismiss as unimportant?

Even within the primary health care team itself, there are still many problems interfering with effective collaboration. A lack of care in choosing individuals who may be working together for many years can seriously disrupt a team. Personal and professional compatability are essential if the team is to function well. Whilst a basic knowledge of the other members' training and responsibilities is more often found amongst younger members, emphasis has rarely been given in their training to the problems and difficulties of working in groups even with their peers, and thus they are rarely properly prepared to function as part of a group practice and, even less, as part of a primary health care team. On occasion, their experiences of teams to which they have been attached during their training has been a negative one. Basic training in communication skills relating to interactions between doctor and patient have now been introduced into the undergraduate medical curriculum, but little attention is paid to communication between doctors or communication with other health professionals. Some postgraduate training programmes for general practice are exploring this field and making a valuable contribution to the development of appropriate skills There is little evidence, however, that those responsible for continuing education for established professionals see the need for improvement of communication skills as a high priority and, similarly, there is little emphasis on management skills and the achievement of change within an organization.

FUTURE NEEDS FOR EFFECTIVE COLLABORATION

Consideration of the present problems which inhibit effective collaboration in primary care lead one to the conclusion that it is a change in educational emphasis which is required. Action is required in the three areas of knowledge, skills and attitudes. As always, the acquisition of knowledge is the easiest task, the development of skills more difficult and the changing of attitudes can at times seem an almost insuperable problem. It seems probable that the earlier in the educational process these issues are tackled, the more likely they are to be successfully resolved.

Undergraduates

At undergraduate level, the acquisition of technical knowledge and skills should take place against a broad background of how society functions, especially in regard to the provision of health and social care in the widest sense. The presence and functions of other professions and helping agencies should be acknowledged and some attempt made to place them in context. Opportunities for joint educational initiatives, bringing together students of the various disciplines for educational and social purposes could be explored, although the practical difficulties of aligning different curriculae from different institutions often appear insuperable. However, educational input from teachers of other disciplines is less of a problem to arrange. During their undergraduate training, all of the caring professions have some exposure to fieldwork and it is important that, whenever possible, they should experience effective collaboration and teamwork in action and learn to understand the beneficial effects which accrue to the patient or client.

In particular, medical students should have the benefit of seeing high-quality primary medical care in action and understanding how it relates to the secondary and tertiary levels of care which still constitute the bulk of their learning material. This experience is particularly important for those who are destined to be specialists, since few of them will have the opportunity to practice primary care at postgraduate level. However, a few specialist training programmes, especially in paediatrics and psychiatry, have acknowledged the benefits of experience in primary care for their postgraduate trainees.

Postgraduates

Some of the difficulties of interprofessional learning at postgraduate level in the UK were explored at a symposium held at the University of Nottingham in July 1979 (England 1979). England emphasizes the need for a primarily informal educational approach relying on simulation exercises, joint problem-solving activities and relatively unstructured discussion, rather than the different professions merely learning about a clinical topic together, with the assumption that this will somehow improve their relationships and understanding. The skills of communication and joint decision-making must be practised if they are to be improved, and exercises such as simulated case-conferences, patient-management problems and the role-playing of difficult situations, have proved helpful. If these educational exercises are to be successful they require a good deal of planning and thought beforehand, and this implies successful co-operation between the tutors from the various disciplines, a model of collaboration which is in itself valuable for the students to observe. It is salutary to note that these educational efforts do not necessarily focus on 'the primary health care team' as the only model for collaboration and it is important to enable people to communicate better across whatever organizational boundaries may exist in a given situation. Those responsible for the vocational training of general practitioners or their equivalent will need to take steps to ensure that the trainees are exposed to a wide range of other providers of primary care as well as representatives of self-help groups and counselling services in the course of their postgraduate training. In addition, discussions focussing on the referral process and relationships with other doctors, both inside and outside the hospital, will help to draw attention to the skills of communication and referral. In particular, the need for the referring doctor to choose a specialist, who will meet not only the patient's technical needs but also, if possible, his personal needs, may be emphasized.

Established practitioners

Whilst changes of emphasis in undergraduate and postgraduate training should improve collaboration in the future, most of the practitioners of all professions at present working in the community will have had little or no specific training in this area. Those who are well-motivated, or have been fortunate enough to establish a close liaison with members of other disciplines, will have learnt gradually how to co-operate in the best interests of their patients and clients by working together on a variety of problems. Others, however, less well-motivated, or having experienced unsatisfactory co-operation from other disciplines, are likely to discount their value and pursue an independent line. The evidence is that attempts to develop interprofessional liaison groups at local level have usually managed to attract only the converted. Nevertheless, more could be done in the field of continuing education to encourage a multidisciplinary approach to primary care problems and this is much more likely to occur when educational priorities are decided and educational efforts directed by general practitioners themselves, working together with their colleagues in the community.

FURTHER READING

Barber J H, Kratz C R, 1980 Towards team care. Churchill Livingstone, Edinburgh, London, New York

Brooks M B 1973 Management of the team in general practice. Journal of the Royal College of General Practitioners 23:239

Cartwright A, Anderson R 1981 General practice revisited. Tavistock Publications, London

Cormack J, Marinker M, Morrell D 1981 Teaching general practice. Kluwer Medical, London

Dowie R 1983 General practitioners and consultants. Kings Fund Publishing Office, London

Edwards C, Stillman P 1982 Major illness and minor diseases — A guide to prescribing in the pharmacy. Pharmaceutical Press, London

England H (ed) 1979 Education for co-operation in health and social work, occasional paper 14. Royal College of General Practitioners, London

Fry J (ed) 1980 Primary care. Heinemann, London

Fry J (ed) 1983 Present state and future needs of general practice. MTP Press, Lancaster

Goldberg E M, Neill J E 1972 Social work in general practice. George Allen & Unwin Ltd, London

Hicks D 1976 Primary health care. HMSO, London

Horder J P 1977 Physicians and family doctors: a new relationship. Journal of the Royal College of General Practitioners 27: 391–399

Jefferys M, Sachs H 1983 Rethinking general practice. Tavistock Publications, London, New York

McWhinney I R 1981 An introduction to family medicine. Oxford University Press, Oxford

Marsh G, Kaim-Caudle P 1976 Team care in general practice. Croom Helm, London

WHO 1984 The role of WHO participating centres in continuing education. Specialty training and educational research. WHO Regional Office for Europe, Copenhagen

Workers

In the small village in Papua New Guinea, the aid post orderly is dressing a foot. In his rural community, he is the first point of contact with the health services and the nearest doctor is many miles away. But he knows the villagers well and, although his knowledge of medicine is relatively small, he is trusted by the rural community he serves.

Many thousand miles away, on the other side of the Pacific Ocean, one of the family practice nurses in a well known American city is showing a lady into the examination room for her regular Pap Smear. It is the last of several gynaecological examinations that day and on many previous days.

Another four thousand miles to the east again, it is night time and, in a farmhouse in the Pennine mountains of Northern England, the old farmer is dying. The district nursing sister is preparing to give him another pain killing injection, which will see him through until morning. Although, in theory, she went off duty several hours ago, she has known the family for over 20 years and has willingly come back to do what needs to be done.

Three very different examples of primary care teamwork in three places separated by time, distance, culture and provision of health care. And there are many other such examples of equal diversity. Yet in spite of such variation, the basic needs of the population of the world are perhaps not so very different.

WHO ARE THE WORKERS?

In Chapter 8, the members of the nucleus primary health team in the United Kingdom were listed as physicians, health visitors (public health nurses) community and practice nurses, nursing auxiliaries and bath attendants. The list applies to many other countries, but with two provisos. The ratio of the different workers to each other varies widely from country to country and to many the list will seem unduly restricted.

First, it is necessary to be clear at what point people enter the health care system and seek advice. In most developed countries this will be at the time they consult a physician. Already they have consulted relations and friends and they may have also discussed their problem with a pharmacist, since many medicines are sold over the counter. In more remote areas, patients first may go to nurses, such as health visitors or district nurses in the United Kingdom, or physician's assistants in the United States.

In many less developed countries, the first and frequently only health advice will come from a relatively untrained worker, such as an aid post orderly, barefoot doctor or health technician. Here, the doctors and nurses are operating one degree removed from the patient and their role has a much greater proportion of management education and supervision, than the work of their counterparts in more developed countries. However, the fact that a higher percentage of primary health care is given in this way in the less developed parts of the world should not be taken as necessarily indicating that the populations in these countries are receiving a significantly lower standard of care. The problems are frequently different to those of more developed countries and the local village worker's advice and treatment may very well be followed, whereas the doctor's advice may not.

Second, even in the more developed countries, there is an increasing interest in health care provided by workers other than physicians, nurses and supporting professionals, such as physiotherapists and occupational therapists. In the United Kingdom there is a growing number of people, previously described as being in the realm of fringe medicine, who are providing some primary health care, particularly for problems such as musculoskeletal disorders and stress. These are osteopaths, chiropractors, acupuncturists, hypnotherapists and others who aim to fill gaps where it appears the more conventional health workers are less effective. This may be due partly to medical science having relatively little to offer people with backache and stress and partly because increasing medical technology and pharmacology may have reduced the importance of dealing with the whole person. An increasing number of general practitioners in the United Kingdom are incorporating some of these techniques into their everyday medical practice.

Nevertheless, the workers in these various fields cannot be regarded as central figures in primary health care, since they do not offer a comprehensive assessment and diagnostic service which can deal with any problem, however superficially, in the first instance. So we might regard our central primary health workers as:

1. Physicians (family physicians or general practitioners)
2. Nurses
   a. Nurse practitioners (physician's assistants)
   b. Preventive nurses (health visitors, public health nurses, occupational health nurses)
   c. Community nurses (district nurses)
   d. Office nurses (practice nurses)
   e. Midwives
3. Auxiliaries (health technicians, nursing auxiliaries, aid post orderlies, bath attendants)

It should not be forgotten that, with the increasing sophistication of primary health teams, an increasingly complicated administrative support system is required. Indeed, it has become clear in the United Kingdom that many of the deficiencies in prevention and in the monitoring of chronic disease are related more to deficiencies in management than to deficiencies in the clinical expertise of the doctors and nurses.

Physicians

In a number of countries, including the United Kingdom, Australia, and Canada, general practitioners occupy a central role in the health service, since (with a few exceptions) patients have to consult their general practitioner before they can consult specialists. In other countries this is not the case.

As medicine has become more specialized, so it has become clear that the doctor who works at the primary care level has to have certain skills and expertise, which are not just the superficial ends of each specialty put together. In North America, there has been great emphasis on the family and on behavioural sciences and the important effects different members of the family have on the individual's illness. United Kingdom general practitioners have a significant theoretical advantage over most other primary care doctors in the world, they have registered lists of patients, whom they can identify clearly and for whom they are responsible, although many of them have been slow to exploit this. But doctors from many countries have not only accepted the need for family medicine, but, increasingly, are realizing the need for management and epidemiology so that they can demonstrate their effectiveness of prevention and chronic disease surveillance for their patients.

By comparison, in the developing countries, the physician provides the point of the first contact for a smaller percentage of the population. His work will consist not only of attending patients, but of supervision, education and guidance of other members of the health team, some of whom may have only a very short training.

Nurses

The range of activities and responsibilities of primary health care nurses is now very wide. At one end of the spectrum they have been trained to function as practitioners in their own right, taking over much of the work traditionally regarded as that of the doctor. The nurse practitioner educational programmes in Canada grew from the necessity to provide health care to the comparatively deserted northern parts of that country. Elsewhere, physician's assistants usually work alongside the physician, taking medical histories and performing routine physical examinations. Their introduction has raised some difficult questions about the borderline between doctors and nurses and the best physician's assistants may appear to their patients to be replacing the physician himself. In developed countries, they have remained a small minority and it may be that their most important role in the end will be to challenge the relevance and balance of existing undergraduate education for the doctor.

Nurses involved in prevention occupy a much more secure place in primary care. In the United Kingdom they are known as health visitors and have a quite separate role from the nurses involved in treatment. They are trained to deal with family and social problems and in health education and although a large amount of their time has been traditionally with young children and their mothers, they are moving now into a greater involvement with other age groups, especially the elderly. By contrast, in other countries such as India, the health visitor, like the physician, spends a significant amount of time supervizing her auxiliary colleagues, although, once again, her work has been largely in maternal and child welfare.

Whilst nursing in the patient's home has been a feature of primary health care in many countries for a long time, the introduction of office, or practice, nurses has been a more recent development. In North America their work is, to a large extent, dictated by those kinds that health insurance will pay for and this may mean that their full range of skills are not deployed. In other countries, such as the United Kingdom, there are no financial constraints imposed by the health service on nurses' work. Those nurses employed directly by the doctor have most of their salary reimbursed, and the amount and diversity of practice nurse work has increased over the years. It includes not only routine dressings and injections, but suturing, ear syringing, electrocardiography, venepuncture and simple advice.

In the less developed countries the nurse often occupies a different position in relation to the doctor. Whereas her role in developed countries is usually acting as an assistant to the doctor once the patient has been seen, in some less developed countries she will act as a filter, passing on to the doctor only those people who are going to need his skills.

The midwife (now rarely seen in North America) has a fairly clearly defined role although in developed countries her role in primary care in the community has become progressively more to do with ante and postnatal care than with the actual supervision of deliveries.

What has happened over the years is that many nurses, having started first as subordinate to the doctor, have now become increasingly autonomous in their own right. The challenge of the nurse practitioner movement has forced doctors, not only to look at the relationship between themselves and nurses, but also to where the real needs of patients lie.

Auxiliaries

In the developed countries, auxiliaries are used mainly to assist fully trained nurses in the less technical work such as bed bathing. But in the underdeveloped countries, there has been increasing effort to train auxiliaries to bring basic health care to populations that would otherwise not receive it. Just as the nurse's role has changed in relation to the doctor, so the auxiliary's role has changed in relation to the nurse: the auxiliary is not so much assisting the nurse, but deciding to whom he or she needs to refer, and what she can do for herself. There is a danger that the title 'auxiliary' may be seen as pejorative and yet there is no way that health care in the less developed countries could be provided without them. In China, more than 1 million 'barefoot' doctors have been trained: other training programmes have been started in Bangladesh and Bhutan.

The training varies considerably in sophistication and length; in some countries health aides may receive only a few weeks of instruction.

The importance of the auxiliary in many less well developed countries cannot be overemphasized. It is crucial that these workers remain in close contact with their communities and are not pressed into more sophisticated health care.

Thus, although doctors, nurses and auxiliaries form the nucleus of the primary health team, their roles and relationship vary widely from one country to another and which of them deals with the presenting complaints will depend on the nature of the health service and the numbers of different workers per head of population.

WHAT GENERAL PRINCIPLES APPLY?

Given this great variety in the way primary care workers operate and given the widely differing needs of populations, there are certain general principles for better care:
1. Goals and roles
2. Relationships with patients and communities
3. Relationships between workers
4. Management and effectiveness
5. Manpower

Goals and roles

For any team to work effectively, certain characteristics are necessary, one of which is that each member has a clear understanding of his own function, appreciates and understands the contributions of other professions, and recognizes common interests (Gilmore et al 1974). Although this may sound like common sense, unfortunately it seems to be somewhat difficult. Why should this be?

First, there may be problems in training. Medical students' education is largely hospital based and, until the widespread introduction of university departments of general practice and vocational training in the United Kingdom, many doctors entering general practice had never met health visitors or community nurses. Equally, nurses and auxiliaries may be quite unaware of the modern training of family physicians and general practitioners as it now occurs in many developed countries.

Second, roles are less clearcut than in secondary care and overlap much more. A surgeon, his operating theatre sister and technician will be quite clear what is expected of them and who does what. But in primary care matters are different, especially in the family and social aspects of health and illness. An identical problem may be dealt with by the general practitioner in one family, by the health visitor in another and by the district nurse in a third, depending on the individual skills and the particular relationship between health worker and patient. With the advent of more active prevention in primary care, there is further scope for confusion: for example, blood pressures may be measured by doctors, health visitors, nurses, midwives or even receptionists.

People do not behave in isolation or in a random manner and their behaviour is influenced partly by the expectations of others. So, the role that individual team members adopt is partly determined by the other team members. Furthermore, if individual workers and teams are not clear about their individual and collective roles there will be no means of measuring the effectiveness of the care they are trying to provide.

Relationships with patients and communities

There is increasing interest in what has come to be known as consumerism. One example of this in primary health care in the United Kingdom has been the introduction of patient participation groups. These groups of people served by an individual primary health team meet regularly for the purpose of influencing the health care being provided. (see also Chapter 7.)

By its nature, primary health care has a much closer relationship with the community it serves than does the hospital and specialist services. Primary health care operates in the community, including patients' homes, and is influenced heavily by social and environmental factors, such as housing, industry, nutrition, water supply, drainage and poverty. It is essential, therefore, that primary health care takes account of these factors and understands how they influence health care.

In many parts of the world, general practitioners still need to be encouraged to become responsible for local communities and identify the needs of those communities. This is one of the arguments for having some kind of state involvement in primary care.

But there is a more fundamental reason why primary health care workers need to have a close relationship with the people they serve. One of the conclusions reached by those who have attempted to evaluate primary health care in underdeveloped countries is that the village worker, auxiliary or aid post orderly, or volunteer is the key to success because they are accepted as part of the community and because they are there when needed. They are not only available, but subscribe to the common beliefs and philosophies of their own people.

Equally, in the more developed world, it is becoming clear that primary health workers, especially doctors, need to have a more equal and less heirarchical relationship with patients. That relationship needs to be manifested in two ways. First the doctor needs to understand and discuss not just the medical symptoms and aetiology, but also patients' ideas, concerns and expectations. Second, he needs to involve patients in the decision making and management.

Relationships between workers

The need for workers to have clear goals and perception of roles has already been stressed. For a team to work effectively, its members must relate well to each other. For them to do this they must share a common purpose. It is essential that they make time to communicate with each other and provide each other with support.

There is an inverse relationship between the size of the team and how often the members are able to communicate with each other face to face. So this is obviously a problem in those countries where primary health workers are widely dispersed, which is likely in the underdeveloped world.

Ironically, however, communication may be less effective between health workers when they are geographically close together. At least those workers who are widely scattered recognize there is a problem and their relationships may be clearer than those of the primary health care team who work in developed countries under one roof. Here, status problems may well be more acute. Doctors and nurses in the developed world train largely in hospitals which are very heirarchical by nature and these heirarchical relationships often persist into later life. Roles and role boundaries may be blurred, the patient does not proceed in an orderly fashion through less trained to more highly trained worker but may present to any member of the team.

In some countries, there are further potential problems related to accountability. Doctors and nurses may be either self-employed or employed by the health service: there may be a mixture of the two and doctors may be directly employing staff as well. In the United Kingdom, the general practitioners are self-employed, although the vast majority are in contract with the National Health Service; the health visitors and many of the nurses will be directly employed by the health authority and accountable to a nursing manager, while practice nurses and administrative staff are usually employed by and accountable to the doctors. A more complicated potential for difficulties could not have been devised.

A primary health team can only be regarded as a team if all the members are clear about the roles of themselves and other members, and if they also communicate, and co-operate with each other, and respect each others' contribution.

Management and effectiveness

Management, except in the strictly clinical sense, is not part of most doctors' and nurses' curriculum. We have already seen some of the factors that need to be considered in primary health teams, such as goals, roles and relationships, and the need to have a common purpose. But how can the effectiveness of a primary health team be measured? We need some unit of measurement or indicators of performance.

Some of the questions a team needs to ask itself have been listed by Pritchard (1981) and are set out in Table 9.1.

Increasingly, however, primary health workers should be starting to ask themselves questions about outcome in addition to operation. Thus, it should be possible to produce data on immunization, contraception, cervical cytology, blood pressure recordings, and antenatal care and so on, so that each team can see how well it is doing. Equally, it should be possible to look at criteria of good chronic disease management, such as hypertension, asthma or diabetic control (Hasler & Schofield 1984).

Manpower

Management of manpower is a major problem. Yet, without it, health workers are often utilized uneconomically, they are likely to be in imbalance in relation to their skills and may well be distributed inadequately.

Some countries have started to attempt to rationalize the numbers

Table 9.1 Questions about team working

Aims, tasks
1. Are we all here for a common purpose?
2. What is that purpose?
3. Do we agree about the tasks we set ourselves?
4. Do we define them adequately?
5. Can they be measured, so that we know if task has been completed?

Roles
6. Are we clear about our own role in the team?
7. Are we clear about the roles of others in the team?
8. Are these roles in conflict, and if so where?
9. Are we unable to fulfil our role (e.g. due to overwork)
10. Is our ability to carry out our role hampered by outside constraints (e.g. not being allowed to make decisions, fear of litigation, etc.)

Procedures
11. In making decisions do we take adequate notice of:
    (a) who has the relevant information?
    (b) who has to carry out the decision?
12. Are decisions usually made:
(a) unanimously? (b) by majority? (c) by team leader? (d) by default?
13. When a decision is made, is it carried out, or forgotten?
14. Does the team follow up its decisions, question the outcome, and learn by its mistakes and successes?
15. When a conflict arises do we:
(a) ignore it? (b) allow one person to force a decision? (c) compromise? (d) look for alternative solutions?
16. Do we let everyone have a chance to speak, or let one or two members do all the talking?
17. Does everyone feel free to challenge any statements made in the group?
18. Do we waste time, or allot it according to the priority of the task?
19. Does the team meet often enough and in the right circumstances, and is the size of the group right?
20. Do team members concentrate on the task or waste time trying to impress, or raising irrelevant issues?

Interpersonal relationships
21. Are team members sensitive to how others in the group feel abour discussion?
22. Can the team tolerate failure, and give mutual support rather than blame?
23. Is team morale high? If not, why not?
24. Can any member suggest any way in which team working could be improved?

Reprinted from: Pritchard P 1981 Manual of primary health care, 2nd edn. Oxford University Press, Oxford, p 63–64.

of their health workers, but at the moment the variation between countries is considerable. In Canada, for example, there is a physician per population ratio of 17: 10 000 compared to Haiti with 1.4: 10 000. Nurse to physician ratios vary equally widely with 4:1 in Canada and 6:1 in Finland compared to Bolivia with 0.6:1 and India with 0.65:1.

If primary health care is to become generally available by the year

2000, it will be essential to have enough appropriately trained workers in every country. Few countries seem yet to have produced health manpower plans and policies. These policies need to take account of how primary health workers are needed and the ratio of one kind to another.

WHAT EDUCATION AND TRAINING IS NEEDED?

Physicians and nurses have traditionally been educated and trained mainly in large teaching hospitals. As technology and superspecialization has advanced, the knowledge and skills of the teachers and the type of patient seen become less relevant to the everyday basic health needs of communities, whether they be in the more or less developed countries. The need for reorientation is world wide. In Chapter 8, the needs of the medical undergraduate have been identified and the need for doctors in training to understand the broad concepts of health care and the behavioural sciences. The same is true for nurses.

These changes can only come about if a larger proportion of education and training is based in the community away from the hospital ward and laboratory. The growth of university departments of family medicine and general practice in North America, Europe, the Middle East, Australasia and elsewhere has had some effect on medical undergraduate curricula, but not nearly enough. They have had to compete for resources with powerful specialist departments, and primary care has been seen purely as an additional specialty rather than something much more fundamental.

Not only are moves into the community important for the content of what doctors and nurses learn, they are important, too, for helping to solve relationship problems. In hospitals and universities, relationships between physician, nurse, auxiliary and patient is clearly influenced by status. This means that the early training of budding family physicians and community nurses after qualification has to be in some way remedial, so that each group can start to regard the other as an equal and can relate to patients in a way that does not remove their autonomy. This can best be achieved by shared learning and problem-solving, where different professionals work together before their attitudes become too difficult to alter.

New initiatives are needed in continuing education where segregation between different professions often persists. The need for goals in the management of prevention and chronic disease means that, for the more highly trained professionals, what is needed is not more detailed clinical facts, but help, for example, in reviewing ways of achieving high immunization and cytology rates, how to help people to stop smoking and use contraception and, equally important, to devise ways of monitoring these activities.

A number of new initiatives in various developing countries have been described by the World Health Organization. These have not only been in education for physicians and nurses but also for auxiliary personnel, now that the important need for the front line workers has been recognized.

NEEDS FOR THE FUTURE?

Although the immediate needs of countries vary considerably across the globe, there are some general lessons we can learn for the future. Nor should those responsible for providing health care in the more developed countries feel in any way satisfied since, although the detailed problems will vary in emphasis from those in underdeveloped countries, the principles are the same.

The *primary health team* seems to be an efficient and effective system for delivering care to individuals and populations, both for prevention and for the point at which individuals seek advice and treatment. There are questions, however, which each country and each individual team must ask.

Which member is the point for first contact?

Is it the most or least highly trained?
If it is the latter, then the nurses and doctors will have to assume a greater management and supervisory role than if they see the patients first. The answers must be influenced by cultural and social factors, the numbers of health workers available and whose advice patients are most likely to follow.

How can teams become more democratic?

If auxiliaries and comparatively untrained workers are to be properly integrated and accepted into the system, can they have more involvement with the decision making? The professionally qualified must take the lead in answering this question and accepting that their own attitudes are a major factor in whether team members work co-operatively together. Physicians can no longer assume that many primary health needs should always be met by themselves.

How can teams become more effective?

The need for clear goals and roles has been emphasized, as has the need for good communication. Team members need to be more aware of management as a discipline in its own right and for valid criteria of effectiveness to be developed and monitored.

How can teams become more accountable?

Whilst many teams have been functioning progressively well in recent years, others have not. Some form of accountability may be needed both for local communities and for health services as a whole. Each team should consider producing annual reports to demonstrate its effectiveness.

The *balance* between high technology specialist health care and low technology primary care needs altering in the favour of the latter and the necessary *resources* need to be available from governments. The needs for different workers and their support will vary from country to country. For example, in the United Kingdom, with an increasing proportion of the very old and a shift to community care, what will be needed most will be more community nurses and auxiliaries.

Policies for manpower need to be developed in each country. These have to take into account how many professionals each country needs in order to achieve the targets of the year 2000, and what the ratio of different workers should be.

There has to be a *change in emphasis in the basic education* of doctors and nurses, with a greater emphasis on population needs, care in the community, behavioural skills in communication and management and multidisciplinary learning.

CONCLUSION

Health service workers are the most important asset each country possesses in its quest for better health care for its people. They will need more attention and support between now and the end of the decade if the declaration of Alma Ata is to be achieved.

REFERENCES AND FURTHER READING

Andrus L H et al 1978 The health care team. In: Taylor R (ed) Family medicine, principles and practice. Springer Verlag, New York

Burrell C D, Sheps C G (eds) 1978 Primary health care in industrial nations. New York Academy of Sciences, vol 310

Gilmore M, Bruce N, Hunt M 1974 The work of the nursing team in general practice. Council for the Education and Training of Health Visitors, London

Hasler J C, Schofield T P C (eds) 1984 Continuing care — the management of chronic disease. Oxford University Press, Oxford

Hetzel B S (ed) 1978 Basic health care in developing countries. Oxford Medical Publications, Oxford

Jeffrey M 1984 General practice as a setting for primary health care development. In: Nowotny H (ed) Social concerns for the 1980s. European Centre for Social Welfare Training and Research,

Newell K W (ed) 1975 Health by the people. WHO, Geneva

Pendleton D A, Hasler J C (ed) 1983 Doctor–patient communication. Academic Press, London

Pritchard P M M 1981 Manual of primary health care, 2nd edn. Oxford University Press, Oxford

Pritchard P M M, Low K, Whalen M 1984 Management in general practice. Oxford General Practice Series, no 8. Oxford University Press, Oxford

WHO 1982 Review of primary health care development. WHO, Geneva

Looking ahead to a child survival revolution

MORTALITY

Each year in the 1980s 15 million children under 5 will die on our planet. At least 95% and probably 97% of these deaths will take place in the less developed countries of the south.

From conception onwards, for every human being, there is one certainty and that is death. However, there may be a great variation in when this death will take place. For many in our world death can be relegated to the years of retirement, thanks to developments in many fields of human endeavour.

In Figure 10.1 we see that whereas 80% of coffins in the more developed countries of the world are only required after retirement, the situation is very different in the less developed countries. Here three-quarters of coffins are required before the age of 65 and, in many countries, half of these may be the coffins of children. Except for those due to malaria, few of these children's coffins are the result of tropical disease. These deaths are due to an interaction of poor nutrition, infectious diseases and a lack of basic resources in the living environment.

WHEN DEATH OCCURS ?

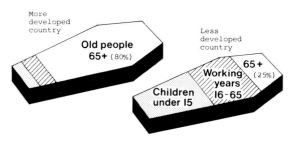

Fig. 10.1 Deaths by age group as percentage of all deaths (data from Taylor, 1984)

This chapter will briefly attempt to summarize some of the problems that face mothers and children in the less developed countries of the world and suggest some new approaches to overcoming these problems.

RESOURCES

The greatest problem is the maldistribution of resources. Although three-quarters of the world's people live in the less developed countries, they can avail themselves of less than a third of the world's resources and in many cases very much less even than this (Figure 10.2).

THE DEVELOPING WORLD HAS . .

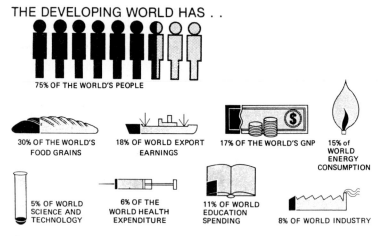

75% OF THE WORLD'S PEOPLE

30% OF THE WORLD'S FOOD GRAINS

18% OF WORLD EXPORT EARNINGS

17% OF THE WORLD'S GNP

15% of WORLD ENERGY CONSUMPTION

5% OF WORLD SCIENCE AND TECHNOLOGY

6% OF THE WORLD HEALTH EXPENDITURE

11% OF WORLD EDUCATION SPENDING

8% OF WORLD INDUSTRY

Fig. 10.2 Proportion of resources available to the developing world

Although there is this maldistribution between north and south, there is, equally, a maldistribution within less developed countries between the elite, largely urban, population and the poor who live in the rural areas or shanty towns. Not only is there this maldistribution of resources but the evidence suggests that the total resources available per capita in our world has declined. As the amount used in the north is increasing, or stabilizing, the proportion available to those in the less developed countries is decreasing. Perhaps one of the most serious to decline is the availability of wood. Two-thirds of the world's population cook on wood or charcoal and, as the quantity of these available diminishes, mothers tend to cook less frequently and the child with his small stomach is likely to receive fewer meals and more highly contaminated food. Bacteria multiply rapidly in hot climates in food not eaten soon after cooking.

POPULATION

The number of children in the more developed countries is now almost constant at just under 300 million. The same is not true in the less developed countries where in 1980 there were around 1300 million. This number will increase by 200 million each decade until the end of the century (Fig. 10.3). By that time the speed of increase will be slackening off and a stable figure of 1800 to 1900 million children will be reached by the year 2100. This increase in the child population gives a particular responsibility to those concerned with children during the last two decades of this century. In this period we are working to improve the lot of children with limited or declining resources, and yet the number of children is increasing rapidly. For this reason the appropriate use of these resources must be a priority in planning.

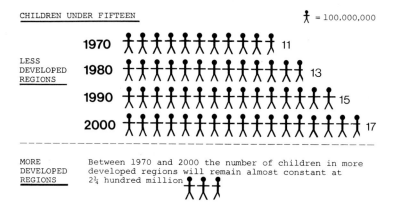

Fig. 10.3 Estimated child population 1970–2000

MORBIDITY

Few studies exist in which the frequency of illness in children in the north and south has been compared. However, all show that during the first 3 years, and particularly in the second year of life, the child has frequent infections in the south (Fig. 10.4). The child

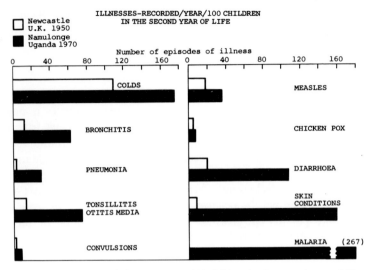

Fig. 10.4 Illnesses recorded per year per 100 children in the second year of life (data from Parkin M, The Child in the African Environment)

living in the less developed countries of our world is likely to have 5–10 times as many infections and many of these will be more severe than those experienced by the child in the industrialized north. In the south each child is likely to have 10 days each month when it is unwell. This compression of so much illness into the first 3 years of life is one of the outstanding disadvantages for children in less developed countries. It is not surprising that these children cannot eat sufficient of their bulky diet to meet their food requirements. As a result, in most countries at least three-quarters of the children fail to grow as they should.

Cycle of malnutrition

This failure of growth in the small child under 3 years is just one, but an important, step in the cycle of malnutrition in women shown in figure 10.5. Children who have been stunted in the early years are unlikely to catch up in their growth and are likely to result in short women. Such women will themselves have frequent infections during pregnancy and are likely to deliver children of whom perhaps a quarter may be considered low birth weight. These low birth weight children are more liable to poor growth and early death and perhaps also poor intellectual development (Fig. 10.5).

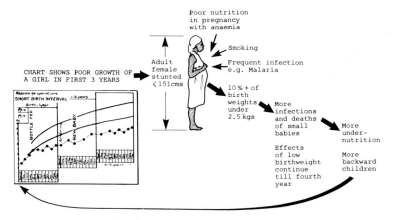

Fig. 10.5 The cycle of undernutrition

A similar cycle can be defined amongst men. Here the shorter man will be less productive in his physical work, receive lower wages, be more likely to be unemployed and, as a result, have a less able wife. Such parents have a higher chance of deprivation for their children.

Birthweight

The effects of birth weight are dramatic (Fig. 10.6). This study in

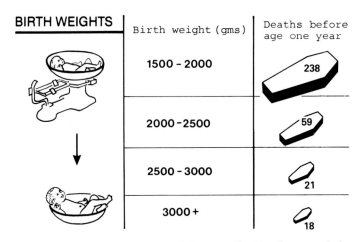

Fig. 10.6 The effect of birth weight on infant mortality (data from a study in New Delhi, India, by Ghosh, 1978)

New Delhi showed that infants born at a birth weight greater than 3 kilograms are likely to suffer no higher mortality than the average infant in many of the developed countries of the north. However, those of a low birth weight are likely to succumb in the first year of life and other studies have shown that this increased risk of mortality of low birth weight babies is likely to continue until the fourth birthday in less developed countries.

Measures in the antenatal period to reduce the incidence of low birth weight, such as providing antimalaria in a malarian area, are of great importance in decreasing the cycle of malnutrition.

HEALTH EXPENDITURE

The next problem is the low level of health expenditure in the south. The median figure for countries in the north in 1980 was $220. Half the countries were spending more than this and, in some, several times this amount.

In the south the median figure was $4 and many of the large countries were still spending only about $1–$2 per head for all health care during a year (Fig. 10.7).

Health services have to be created and run for about 2% of the per capita sum spent in Europe or North America. Unfortunately, many countries in the south have modelled health services on those in the north. As a result the services are curative, doctor and

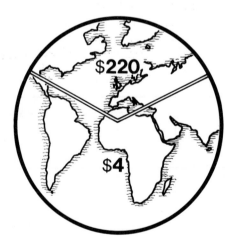

Fig. 10.7 National expenditure on health per person per year: median figures for 32 more developed and 92 less developed countries (Health Sector Policy Paper, World Bank, 1980)

IN INDIA 13 MILLION PEOPLE ARE ADDED EACH YEAR

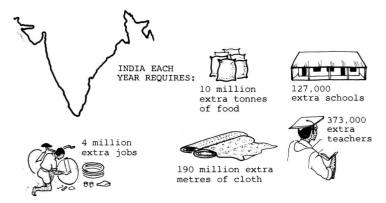

Fig. 10.8 Extra resources required in India relative to population growth (Bull UNESCO Reg. Asia Office, 22 June 1981)

hospital orientated and frequently restricted to those better off living in the cities.

With the pressure of population increase, the amount to spend on health care is unlikely to increase. To India each year is added a population equivalent to that of Australia, that is 13 million additional individuals to be cared for. Each year the Indian people have to build 127 000 extra schools so that education can be no worse in December than it was in January (Fig. 10.8). Analysis of health expenditure in India, however, shows that, in common with most countries, it spends more than 90% on large specialized hospitals and other services confined to urban areas. The Mangudkar commission in Maharashtra State in 1976 found that 80% of the $1.60 per head of population was spent in Bombay and other cities and just US $0.02 per head spent in rural areas. Few countries produce such figures, but, where estimates of expenditure can be found, it is rare to find more than 10% allocated to the health care of a large rural population.

About 1% of health expenditure in Britain is devoted to the prevention of disease and one third of 1% in the USA. Unfortunately, this pattern of health care has been exported to the less developed countries of the world. They too have invested in large specialist hospitals and curatively orientated medical schools (Fig. 10.9).

Unfortunately, investment of resources in prestigious 'disease

Imbalance in present investments in health
CONCEPT: Cost increases with specialisation

Primary •Low cost
health •Difficult to introduce
care •Great effect on
    common health problems

Specialised •Expensive
health care •Easy to introduce
•Prestigious
•Little effect on
    health problems

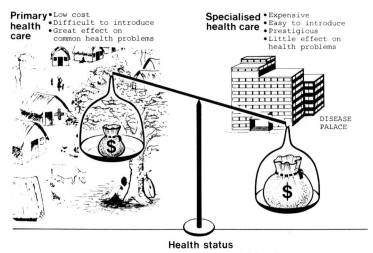

DISEASE
PALACE

Health status

Fig. 10.9 Imbalance in present investments in health in less developed countries

palaces' is easy and politically satisfying. Investment in primary health care is difficult and can run into social and political problems. Perhaps it is not surprising to find some of the best primary health care services in small countries such as Lesotho, Botswana, Malawi and The Gambia, none of which have expensive medical schools. Much of primary health care is concerned with mothers and children and it is largely they who go without when resources are taken up by large 'disease palaces'. In this situation, of very large numbers of children with limited and even declining resources, there is a great need to try to identify priorities.

PRIORITY HEALTH MEASURES

Over the last 3 years, UNICEF particularly, through its publication *The State of the World's Children*, has been attempting to sharpen and refine priorities. These are now memorized by the acronym GOBI-FFF (Fig. 10.10). These are:

1. Oral rehydration.
2. Immunization.
3. Breast feeding and birth spacing. (This is the first 'F' for family planning.)

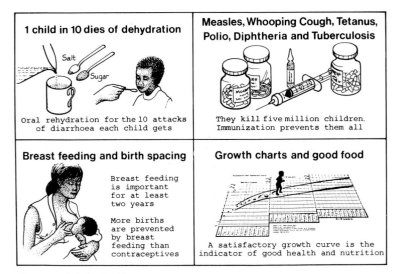

Fig. 10.10 Priority health measures in third world countries (GOBI–FFF)

4. Growth charts and food supplementation of the small child. (This is the second 'F' for food.)

The third 'F' relates to all the above and stands for female literacy. Here again, studies in many countries have shown a strong correlation between infant mortality levels, nutrition of the children and success in family planning, with the education of the mothers.

Oral rehydration

Wide variations in the frequency of diarrhoea exist. In Bangladesh a child may have 7 episodes a year and have diarrhoea 55 days or 15% of the whole year. In general, we can expect every child to have 10 episodes of diarrhoea before the age of 5. Of every 100 episodes 10 are likely to lead to significant dehydration and 1 of these to the death of the child (Fig. 10.11). To prevent this death we must expect to provide oral rehydration therapy for 100 episodes of diarrhoea. Through management of dehydration we can also hope to prevent much malnutrition, which frequently follows on repeated attacks of diarrhoea.

Preventing the 5 million estimated deaths from diarrhoea on our planet with simple salt and sugar solutions that can be made up in the home must be our priority in primary health care.

Diarrhoea EACH CHILD IN LESS DEVELOPED COUNTRIES HAS 10 ATTACKS

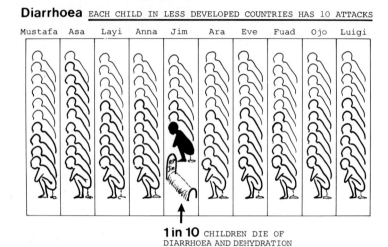

Mustafa Asa Layi Anna Jim Ara Eve Fuad Ojo Luigi

1 in 10 CHILDREN DIE OF
DIARRHOEA AND DEHYDRATION

Fig. 10.11 Representation of morbidity and mortality rates as a result of diarrhoea in less developed countries

Around the world, it is now appreciated that diarrhoea causes death through loss of salt and water from the body. In its management medicines have a very small part to play. Instead the child must be fed solutions containing common salt, together with either glucose or a substance such as starch or sucrose which will break down to glucose. The medical approach to this has been the distribution of packages of oral rehydration salts, the production of which achieved 300 million in 1983. A more practical and appropriate method is through teaching and demonstrating to the mothers, through every means possible, how they can make up their own solution of salt and sugar, so that the child can be treated in the very earliest stage of diarrhoea (Fig. 10.12). Just as we accept that calorie-protein malnutrition should be prevented and treated in the home, so also the more acute water-electrolyte malnutrition is better prevented and treated there.

Immunization

Around 5 million children die each year from diseases that could be prevented by immunization. A similar number survive but have a severe disability. Of every 1000 children born:
    5 are likely to develop severe paralysis from poliomyelitis
    10 will die in the spasms of tetanus

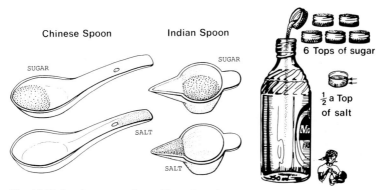

Fig. 10.12 Local measures for making salt and sugar rehydration solution

20 will die in the prolonged spells of coughing from whooping cough in infancy,

30 at least in most less developed countries will succumb to measles and its after effects.

Already in South America and in some other countries we are seeing a mass movement headed by political leaders who, through compaigns, aim in 1 or 2 days every year to achieve a very high level of immunization amongst children (Fig. 10.13). This started with just poliomyelitis, but now, with adequate logistic and mass media support, a range of vaccines is being offered, and the results entered onto the child's growth chart.

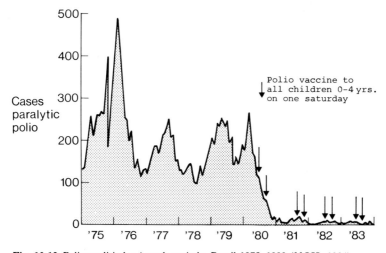

Fig. 10.13 Poliomyelitis by 4-week periods, Brazil 1975–1983 (MOH, 1984)

Breast feeding

The International Confederation of Midwives in late 1984 affirmed;

> . . . the right of all babies to be breast fed, the right of all mothers to proper advice, encouragement and counselling; and the right of all families to accurate information.

Already the right of every child to be breast fed is widely accepted by the mothers and health professionals of the north, as well as the advantages to the mother of suckling her child (Fig. 10.14). Unfortunately the same cannot yet be said for babies born in less developed countries of the world. Inappropriate advice from health professionals and incursions of international milk marketing conglomerates leads to the feeding of dangerous cows' milk substitutes for breast milk. So often the baby is given this in an over-diluted and highly infected condition.

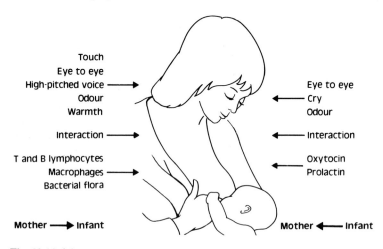

Fig. 10.14 Advantages to mother and infant of breast feeding

Weaning

Where possible, breast feeding should be continued for at least 2 years, so that a birth interval of between 3 and 4 years can be created. However, other foods must be introduced. The paps and porridges fed to so many children are so bulky that the child may be unable to eat enough to achieve its energy requirement (Fig. 10.15). For this reason much more emphasis is now placed on high-energy dense foods than protein foods. Those containing

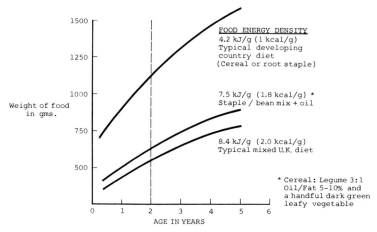

Fig. 10.15 Food intakes in relation to energy density

oils and fats are needed as they reduce the water content and, there-fore, the bulk of the food.

The concentrated calorie content of foods fed to children in the north results in their receiving an adequate calorie intake at all times. The improved nutrition that results from this may be the important factor in the high level of health experienced by those more fortunate children compared with children from the south.

Growth charts

Research from many countries shows that mothers with stunted and even malnourished children do not recognize that their children are not as they should be. For this reason simple growth charts have now been universally accepted (Fig. 10.16), although there are still great problems in their use. The charts are held by the mothers and wherever she makes contact with health services her child will be weighed and the weight recorded. A new concept, which is likely to spread with the introduction of low cost scales, is that mothers in groups weigh their children and support each other where the growth of some children is inadequate. As politicians begin to appreciate the link between adequate growth of the child and adequate growth of the brain, more emphasis will be placed on growth in the first 2–3 years.

The growth chart is a problem-oriented record system. Through

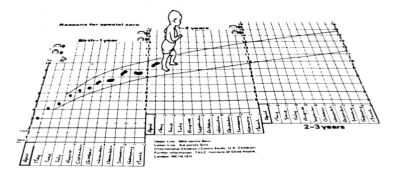

Fig. 10.16 Simple growth charts

its use the various elements of GOBI-FFF can be integrated together with management of nutrition and frequent infections.

LONG-TERM MEASURES

Primary health care teams

Success in developing primary health care with the people will depend on an army of new health workers. The present training of the doctor makes him inappropriate as the provider of primary health care (Fig. 10.17). However, given adequate orientation and new training, a proportion can become the leaders of primary health care teams. Nurses and medical assistants with appropriate training will work with an army of part-time community-based health workers. Because they remain involved in farming, or the work of the community, these part-time health workers have an ability to bring about health education and behavioural change in a way that is difficult or impossible for the full-time worker.

Unfortunately the whole structure of health services in most less developed countries is inappropriate to the development of primary health care programmes (Fig. 10.18). Ministries of Health require economists, sociologists and many other disciplines if they are to plan appropriate new services. Similarly, great changes are required at district level if those providing primary health care are to be recognized as the priority workers.

Private practice is difficult to control because of the implications for doctors' incomes. They remain one of the more powerful political groups in every state: they have an access to and power over the politicians and their families which is difficult to control.

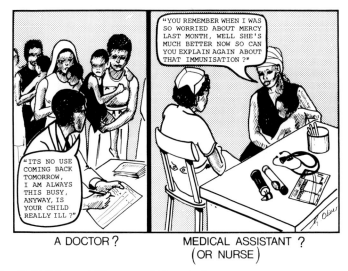

Fig. 10.17 Primary child care — which option?

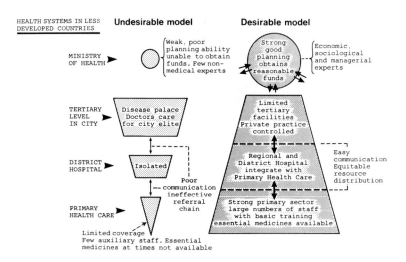

Fig. 10.18 Health systems in less developed countries

Unfortunately, educational investment is almost entirely in the initial training of health workers. Expenditure in ongoing education is limited, and a change away from curative doctor and hospital orientated training can be difficult.

Redistribution of resources

While new emphasis on priorities in health care will play its part in reducing mortality and improving the health of the underprivileged, the real change will only come with a better distribution of resources. As this study (Fig. 10.19) showed, a 10-fold increase in resources in New Delhi could be correlated with a 10-fold decline in child mortality.

Unfortunately socioepidemiological studies of this nature are relatively new in the more developed countries of the north. In the south such studies are uncommon, but those that exist suggest the economic position of the family and the schooling of the mother are far more important in reducing child mortality than health services as they exist at the present time.

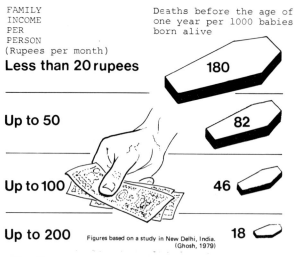

FAMILY INCOME PER PERSON (Rupees per month)

Deaths before the age of one year per 1000 babies born alive

Less than 20 rupees 180

Up to 50 82

Up to 100 46

Up to 200 18

Figures based on a study in New Delhi, India. (Ghosh, 1979)

Fig. 10.19 The relationship between family income and infant deaths (data from a study in New Delhi, India, by Ghosh, 1979)

Political change

In many countries success will need some degree of political change. Only with redistribution of wealth can we expect the death rate to fall, and only in countries where children survive has it been possible to bring down the birth rate (Fig. 10.20).

Unfortunately, true development in so many countries is impossible while so much of the resources available are absorbed by the population increase.

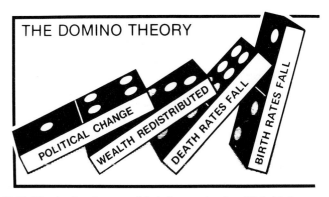

Fig. 10.20 The domino theory: political change related to fall in birth rate

Acknowledgement

The illustrations in this chapter are taken from a book, *Her Name is Today*, being prepared by David Morley.

FURTHER READING

Morley D, Rohde J, Williams G 1983 Practising health for all. Oxford University Press, Oxford
Grant J P 1984 State of the world's children. Oxford University Press, Oxford.

PART TWO

National perspectives

Australia

NATIONAL FEATURES

History

The original Australians — the Aborigines — can be traced back well over 30 000 years. Probably the oldest race on earth, their numbers now amount to only 160 000, half of which still live in tribal areas. The new Australians — mostly of European origin — began arriving about 200 years ago when a British colony was established at Botany Bay in Sydney. The population is now 15 million.

Cultural and social features

Although a young country, Australia's culture is enriched by its diverse ethnic composition. 20% of Australians are immigrants, 8% from the United Kingdom, 8% from Greece, Italy, Yugoslavia and other European countries and, more recently, increasing numbers have come from countries in the Asia-Pacific region (Australian Bureau of Statistics 1980a).

Geographical features

Much of Australia is desert. A narrow but fertile coastal belt extends from the tropical north of Queensland to temperate southern Victoria and South Australia. Tasmania and the south west of Western Australia, too, are fertile and productive. Central Queensland and New South Wales are drier, subject to drought and at time floods, and less productive.

The geography determines the distribution of the population: 86% are urban dwellers; only 14% live in rural towns of less than 1000 people (Australian Bureau of Statistics 1980b). About 3 million people live in Sydney and in Melbourne and about 1 million in Brisbane, Adelaide and Perth. The population shows a high degree of mobility.

Economic features

Its vast natural resources, particularly minerals, and its highly developed manufacturing industries contribute to Australia's high GDP. Per head of population, it matches many larger nations. Typified as a rural country, only 5% of GDP is now derived from agriculture.

HEALTH SYSTEM — EVOLUTION AND FORMAT

Hospitals have been a central element of Australia's health care system since colonial days, but private practice and public health services have developed strongly alongside the hospital system. Private practitioners, who charge on a fee-for-service basis, comprise 23 600, and salaried (mostly hospital) doctors 8100 of Australia's 30 700 medical practitioners. Of the private doctors, 13 800 are general practitioners (family physicians) and 9800 specialists (Permail Pty Ltd 1984). A 1980 survey showed that 70% of all consultations occur in private consulting rooms, and 11% in the home. The general practitioner provides 78% of all doctor consultations, specialists 12% and hospital doctors 10% (Australian Bureau of Statistics 1980c).

In 1981–1982, Australians spent A$11 billion on health care: 7.4% of GDP. Of this, Governments spent A$7 billion (Commonwealth Department of Health 1984). A taxation levy is used to finance Medicare, Australia's compulsory health insurance system, which provides cover for most medical expenses, some pharmaceutical expenses, free public hospital care and subsidized private hospital care. Additional insurance against private hospital costs is available and taken out by about 50% of the population. Health care expenditure is disproportionately high in some age groups: the very young, women aged 20–44 and the over 65-year-olds. 10% of the population are over 65 (Australian Bureau of Statistics 1983), yet account for about 40% of expenditure on health care (Commonwealth Department of Health 1984). Hospital care accounts for 40% of health care expenditure, general medical services 15%, pharmaceuticals 8.5% and nursing homes 6.5% (Commonwealth Department of Health, 1979).

THE PLACE OF PRIMARY HEALTH CARE

Organization

In Australia, primary health care is provided principally by the 13 800 general practitioners who, each year, provide over 60 million consultations, an average of 4.5 per head of population. Estimates of the number of consultations provided by practitioners of alternative health care vary from 1 to 2 million per year, but the figure may be much higher. Nobody really knows how many times the chiropractor, osteopath, naturopath, homeopath, acupuncturist, herbalist, iridologist or other alternative practitioner is consulted. The strong impression is that it is not only high, but rising.

With a few exceptions, allied health professionals provide little primary care; however, they do provide valuable supportive ancillary services. Community-based nurses, physiotherapists, occupational and speech therapists, dietitians, social workers, psychologists, counsellors, family therapists, podiatrists and several others supplement medical services, mostly on referral from doctors. Practice nurses and receptionists assist general practitioners in their practices and occasionally a social worker or physiotherapist is employed by the practice.

The exceptions are dentists and optometrists who do provide primary care; most of their patients are unreferred. Pharmaceutical chemists, too, provide a large amount of primary care, especially for uncomplicated problems. It is recognized that only 1 in 5 people with a symptom consult a doctor (Fry et al, 1984). Family, friends, neighbours, the nurse down the street, the chemist and others provide the needed advice.

The 9800 specialists in private practice and the 7000 hospital doctors provide secondary and tertiary care, usually on referral from general practitioners. With the exception of those staffing hospital emergency rooms, very little primary care has been provided by these doctors in the past; Australia's health insurance system discourages direct access to specialists. However, a recent trend has become apparent — the increasing number of outpatient services provided by hospitals. By contrast, inpatient services and surgical procedures have remained static.

Another recent trend is the advent of the 'shop front' practitioner who provides a very limited range of services (treatment for minor complaints, prescriptions, certificates and referrals), on a short consultation basis, which is lucrative, leaving the more difficult and time-consuming problems, which are less well remunerated, to his more thorough colleagues.

How independent is the general practitioner?

Almost all general practitioners practise in private consulting rooms. They operate a small, and sometimes not so small business. Most are in partnership or group practice, but perhaps as many as 4 out of 10 still work in solo practice. Group practices are generally small, consisting of 4 to 8 doctors; seldom are larger groups encountered.

Whilst fees charged are at the discretion of the doctor, most charge a fee based on a schedule of rebates set down by the Commonwealth Department of Health. Patients are entitled to an 85% rebate of the scheduled fee for general practitioner consultations, and a higher proportion of specialist fees. The doctor usually accepts a discounted fee equal to the rebate for pensioners or socially disadvantaged patients, and he may do so for all patients and elect to bill the Department of Health directly (bulk billing).

So, although the private general practitioner is quite independent in a legal sense, he has allowed his fees to be regulated by the current schedule of rebates. Few general practitioners charge a fee outside of the schedule, although they know that many of their services are worthy of a higher fee. Most of the services rebated are for curative care. Although prevention is promoted strongly by the Department of Health, the current schedule of fees offers little financial incentive to provide such care.

Remuneration

Although the fee schedule is revised regularly, with double digit inflation the real value of the general practitioner's consultation fees has slipped in recent years to the point where the quality of the services he provides is in jeopardy. A falling patient load, resulting mainly from an increasing number of general practitioners (the number has almost doubled in 10 years), has reduced his income further. The number of consultations per general practitioner per week has dropped from 160 in 1974 (Bridges-Webb 1981) to a contemporary 120. The median net annual income of general practitioners in Australia is estimated to be close to A\$44 000, with the lower 33% earning under A\$30 000 and the upper 33% over A\$50 000 (Royal Australian College of General Practitioners 1985). Many young doctors are finding it difficult to establish themselves in a financially viable practice.

Some consider there are too many general practitioners and that medical school intakes should be reduced substantially; others believe that all could be gainfully employed if greater emphasis was given to preventive care and health promotion and if financial incentives were provided to supply such services.

The average suburban general practitioner now cares for little more than 1000 patients and even in remote rural areas he seldom cares for more than 2000. Urban general practitioners work on average 50 hours a week (including 7 hours administration and 3 hours travelling) and rural doctors somewhat longer (Bridges-Webb 1981). In the larger cities, deputizing services provide out-of-hours cover for a significant but diminishing number of doctors. With the steady increase in the numbers of general practitioners, more and more are reverting to providing their own out-of-hours care.

One-third of general practitioners are female (Rowe & Carson 1982). However, this proportion will increase, as 46% of general practitioners currently in training are female (Family Medicine Programme 1984).

EDUCATION AND STANDARDS

Undergraduate

10 medical schools graduate 1300 doctors annually. In all except New South Wales the medical course lasts 6 years; in New South Wales, 5 years. All medical schools have departments of community medicine/practice/health, which provide undergraduates with exposure to the principles and practice of primary health care as provided in general practice. Following graduation, all undertake a compulsory intern year in a teaching hospital.

Vocational training

Currently 8 out of 10 doctors seeking training for general practice are provided with 4 years of training through the Family Medicine Programme (FMP), conducted by The Royal Australian College of General Practitioners (RACGP) with the support of an annual Federal Government Grant of over A$7 million. 2 years of hospital training beginning after the intern year and 2 years of general practice experience, including 6 months of intensely supervized training in an accredited teaching practice, comprise the inservice elements of training.

A comprehensive 2-year cyclical educational programme accompanies this training, and a wide variety of educational material is available to augment this programme. A large National Resource Centre and Video Studio houses and produces educational resources, especially audiovisuals, and smaller Resource Centres supplement this in each State.

The Programme aims to train family doctors to serve the diverse and widely scattered population. Different training is provided for those intending to practise in the cities, the suburbs, rural areas and in the tropical north. The curriculum places great emphasis on the *process* of providing care as well as the problems to be managed. The basic concepts and principles of the discipline of family medicine are an essential part of the trainee's learning.

During the four years, regular assessments of the trainee are made, leading to a certificate of satisfactory completion of training. The Programme espouses a self-directed learning philosophy and encourages each trainee to assume responsibility for his own education. A learning plan, called a 'contract', is drawn up by each trainee with the assistance of a training adviser. The contract describes the trainee's learning goals, the resources which are to be deployed to achieve these goals, and the nature of the evidence which will signal their achievement. The contract is a commitment by both parties, trainee and Programme, to achieve the goals set. It can be renegotiated as circumstances change.

Most trainees elect to undertake the Fellowship examination of the RACGP during or at the end of the training period.

Satisfactory completion of a training programme is not yet a prerequisite for independent practice in Australia (as it is in the UK), but moves towards this are afoot. Vocational registration would give the leverage necessary to ensure that all entering unsupervised practice were properly trained.

The FMP is a nation-wide programme involving almost 2000 trainees, situated in over 150 hospital programmes and almost 700 general practices accredited for training, throughout 80 training areas scattered from the north of Queensland to the remote west of Western Australia. The Programme is co-ordinated through area co-ordinators, State offices and a National office in Melbourne. It combines peripheral autonomy with central co-ordination and support, and uniform standards of training. Policy making involves all sections of the Programme, including the trainee body, through State and National Trainee Associations.

The large size of the Programme, its decentralization, its national co-ordination and standards, its use of regular general practices as teaching practices, its philosophy of self-direction and contract learning, and the intimate involvement of the trainee group in management decisions are amongst its unique features.

Over 5000 have already undertaken training with FMP, and in the next 10 years a further 6000 will do so. By 1991 two-thirds of the general practitioner workforce in Australia will have been trained through FMP.

Continuing medical education

The RACGP provides continuing education through its monthly journal *Australian Family Physician*, its monthly *CHECK programme of self-assessment* and other publications, and through its six faculties, which conduct hundreds of regular and intermittent courses, workshops, seminars and conventions varying in duration from an hour or two, through weekends to week-long courses, to continuing courses over months and years. Almost everything one could hope for is provided. The College conducts an annual examination for Fellowship which embodies modern techniques tested for reliability and validity.

COMMON DISEASE PROBLEMS AND PREVENTION

The disease pattern seen in Australia is similar to that in other Western countries, as is demonstrated in Table 11.1 from the 'Australian general practitioner morbidity and prescribing survey. 1969–74' (Bridges-Webb, 1976). It showed that 1 in 5 consultations were for respiratory illness, 1 in 9 for cardiovascular illness and 1 in 11 for mental disorders. 12% of consultations were for preventive care, many of which were for antenatal care. The incidence of chronic conditions is high. 45% of the population are so afflicted (Australian Bureau of Statistics 1980d) and are high users of medical services.

Prevention

The time devoted to preventive care is less than it needs to be if we are to build a healthier nation. Much of the illness in Australian society today is due to lifestyle — excessive drinking, smoking, poor nutrition, inadequate exercise, and stress in the home and workplace leading to abnormal behaviour, family disruption and social disorders. High unemployment, especially amongst young

Table 11.1 All disease contacts by class as a percentage of total disease contacts and male:female ratios, 1969–1974

Disease class	% of all disease contacts	Male:female ratio
Infective and parasitic diseases	4.4	42:56
Neoplasms	0.8	42:56
Endocrine, nutritional, and metabolic diseases	2.9	38:60
Diseases of blood and blood-forming organs	0.9	20:79
Mental disorders (and psychologic conditions)	9.1	30:70
Diseases of the nervous system and sense organs	6.0	44:54
Diseases of the circulatory system	11.6	38:60
Diseases of the respiratory system	20.5	47:51
Diseases of the digestive system	4.0	44:54
Diseases of the genitourinary system	4.2	18:80
Complications of pregnancy, childbirth, and the puerperium	0.6	0:100
Diseases of the skin and subcutaneous tissue	5.7	44:54
Diseases of musculoskeletal system and connective tissue	6.5	38:61
Congenital anomalies	0.1	42:57
Certain causes of perinatal morbidity and mortality	0.0	55:34
Symptoms, signs, and ill-defined conditions	5.4	37:61
Accidents, poisonings, and violence	4.9	60:39
Supplementary classifications (preventive medicine, care of normal pregnancy, family planning, social problems)	12.0	22:77

Source: *Adapted from Bridges-Webb C (ed): The Australian general practice morbidity and prescribing survey, 1969 to 1974. The Royal Australian College of General Practitioners. Medical Journal of Australia (Suppl) 2:9, 1976, with permission.*

people, brings with it unique social, psychological and even physical problems. Much of this illness could be prevented if enough time and skill were brought to bear on these problems. The general practitioner is well situated to be an agent for change in his patient's lifestyle if he is trained in behaviour modification and properly remunerated for the time such activity takes.

The heaviest users of medical services are infants — 10 consultations per year with the general practitioner. Usage drops to 7 in preschool children and 3 in children and adult males, but rises in adult females to 6 per year and in the over 65 group to 7 per year, giving an average over the whole population of 4.5 general practitioner consultations per year (Bridges-Webb 1973, 1974). 80% of the population will see the general practitioner each year and about 90% of children under 5 and the elderly will do so. The implications for preventive care are clear.

The over-65-year-olds, which now comprise 10% of the population, will continue to increase to 12% by 2000, (Australian Bureau of Statistics 1980e) and use an increasing proportion of health care resources. One way of off-setting this is through the provision of community-based support and preventive care, which avoids, delays or minimizes institutional care.

PRESENT PROBLEMS AND ISSUES

Australia's health problems are set against a background of social problems common to industrialized nations: urbanization, environmental pollution, high unemployment, substantial but often hidden poverty, a growing number of aged and disabled, a number of ethnic minority groups, changing family structure and social values, and increasing alcoholism, drug dependency, violence and crime. Of the many current problems and issues in health care in Australia, the most important, as far as general practitioners are concerned, include:

1. The rising cost of health care
2. The changing needs and expectations of the community
3. The increasing complexity of the health care system
4. The low morale of the medical profession
5. Technology in general practice
6. Quality assurance
7. The need for an Australian health policy.

The rising cost of health care

The most pressing problem for governments is the rising cost of health care and how to contain it. There would be less concern if the increasing expenditure was paying reasonable dividends. Such is not the case. Using infant mortality, longevity and the incidence of cardiovascular disease as criteria, increasing per capita expenditure does not concomitantly improve these health outcomes; indeed some are worse (Commonwealth Department of Health 1984). We are in a state of diminishing, static or even negative returns for increasing expenditure.

There are many reasons: the nature of the illnesses which predominate, especially chronic degenerative and lifestyle illness; the unnecessary use of investigations, medications and referral to specialists and hospitals; the high and increasing cost of medical technology; and the attitude and approach of some of the medical profession which elects not to ask the critical questions, 'In what way will the results of this investigation alter my management?' and, 'Will my management significantly alter the illness?'. Medical decision making, which almost always generates costs, is hampered by insufficient information about the predictive value of medical information and the outcomes of interventions. So it is hard for the doctor to be sure he is using cost effectively the resources he has at his disposal.

One approach to the cost problem is to shift the burden of care towards the providers which give the best value for money in terms of health outcomes and patient satisfaction. The cost of general practitioner services is about 25% of the cost of the same services provided by hospital outpatient departments. The cost of home care or nursing home care is a fraction of that in hospitals. Aware of this, governments are beginning to shift the focus of health care from hospitals to the community. Hospital beds, even whole hospitals, are being closed. Anticipating such a shift, hospitals have responded by increasing outpatient services as a hedge against static or contracting inpatient services. A 1984 study in the USA predicts a 12% reduction in inpatient admissions and a corresponding increase in outpatient services, which it is predicted will provide 25% of hospital revenue by 1995 (Arthur Andersen & Co & ACHA 1984). Aggressive marketing of these services is predicted. Already this trend is apparent in Australia. If general practitioner services are to compete with this trend, they will need to be relevant, efficient, economic, cost effective and competently marketed.

The changing needs and expectations of the community

Interest in health has surged in recent years. The public is increasingly concerned with nutrition, exercise and health maintenance. Dietary regimes abound, health food stores are proliferating, fitness centres are springing up and joggers and cyclists are everywhere. And the people are not just taking more care of their health, they are insisting on more say in the management of their illnesses. They want doctors who will give them time, who will listen to them, explain things to them, and counsel them about their health and how they can maintain it. Often all they want is advice and reassurance. They do not want them to reach reflexly for their prescription pad.

For his part, the general practitioner, if he is able and willing, has a unique opportunity to meet these needs and to accept the challenge of combating the high incidence of lifestyle illness. To do so, he needs a preventive attitude to health care, and specific knowledge and skills in preventive care, health promotion and health education.

Until now, illness prevention has been focussed largely on the individual, but the involvement of governments, commerce, industry and the public generally in making the workplace and community environment less hazardous to health, is beginning. The importance to health of congenial work is being recognized. General practitioners will need to work in concert with these community developments.

More comprehensive care for the increasing proportion of aged and disabled is another changing health care need to which general practitioners are responding. The Federal Government, as part of its health policy, has given community-based care of the aged top priority. Occupational health is another high priority area for the Government, and general practitioners are providing much of it. The health problems of the unemployed, the poor, and ethnic groups are also receiving special attention.

So what Australia needs is community-oriented doctors who are able to assess health needs and respond to them. Research into community health needs and how to deploy available resources to satisfy them, is the most important research to be done in general practice.

Given the health problems that exist, the properly trained general practitioner is the most appropriately placed health care provider in Australia to meet the community's current and emerging primary and continuing health care needs, preventive and promotive, as well as curative and rehabilitative. People still prefer to consult first their family doctor in illness, or for advice. But that advantaged position needs to be maintained and enhanced. Other providers abound and are expanding. Almost daily, some new service or agency is established in the larger cities. The general practitioner can confirm his position only if he is readily accessible, competent and caring, and only if he provides the services the community needs and wants.

The increasing complexity of the health care system

A major problem for consumers and providers alike is the rapidly increasing complexity of the health-care system. Apart from the 30 700 doctors with their numerous subspecialties, there are thousands of allied health professionals and a large but unknown number of practitioners of alternative medicine. There are hundreds of hospitals, public and private. In addition, there are thousands of other health services, agencies and foundations set up to provide support for particular age groups or problems. Examples include infant welfare centres and aged care facilities, family planning clinics, agencies for the care of alcoholics, asthmatics, epileptics, the mentally retarded, those with family problems or drug dependency, those with multiple sclerosis, and so on. Sometimes multiple agencies exist for one problem, for example, alcoholism. Often there is inadequate communication between similiar agencies, they sometimes arise and disappear without notice, and they often change their address and telephone numbers.

The difficulty the general practitioner has in keeping up with all of these services can be imagined; the patients must find it bewildering.

More than ever, patients need an adviser to guide them through this health care maze. The general practitioner is the most appropriate one to do this. His role is to *co-ordinate* the contribution of other health professionals and services to the health of his patient, and to *integrate* the information they provide with his own data to construct a comprehensive profile of the patient and his health problems.

The general practitioner therefore needs to have up-to-date information on all health services. This is presently available in many cities in the form of a directory, but updating is a problem. This information needs to be on a central computer file accessible to the doctor through his own computer.

This so called 'gate keeper' role of the general practitioner is not well understood. Yet the way in which he is aware of, understands and evaluates these services, the way he opens gates to effective ones, and the extent to which he monitors their contribution to the care of his patients has a critical influence on the outcome of many of the conditions he is called upon to manage. It necessitates him working as a member of the health care team and often acting as the manager of the team — 'the conductor of the health care orchestra'. At all times he is the patient's adviser, advocate and, if the patient elects, the manager of the patient's illness.

The low morale of the medical profession

Beset by Federal Government accusations of fraud and overservicing on a major scale, by an unsympathetic, and at times hostile media, which paints doctors as avaricious rogues, by mushrooming alternative health care providers to which the public are flocking, and facing falling incomes and rising expenses, it is not surprisng that the morale of the medical profession in Australia is low. Doctors no longer feel the pride they once felt in belonging to this noble profession.

The problem for the profession is how to reverse that image. The Australian Medical Association (AMA), which now represents a declining number of doctors, has not improved the image, despite its best attempts to do so. It comes across as being overly concerned with the doctors' fees and not so much with the health care of the people. Its inability to represent the profession adequately has become even more obvious lately as one section vies with the other for a bigger slice of the health care cake.

So where is the answer? For general practitioners, the answer is to go it alone. The RACGP which represent 4000 general practitioners who are its members, and the National Association of General Practitioners of Australia (NAGPA) which acts on behalf of some 7000 general practitioner members of the AMA, are bodies which can speak for general practice. The College, particularly, with its emphasis on education and research and its concern with standards of care, is particularly well placed to provide the leadership general practice now needs.

RACGP survey of standards and fees

In 1985 the College conducted a nation-wide determination of the standards required of general practitioners using a Delphi technique to survey a wide range of consumer and provider groups (RACGP & Arthur Andersen & Co 1984). At present, it is conducting a relative work value study to reassess the relative value of the services provided by the general practitioner and to compare these with the services of other medical providers (RACGP 1984). For years, many general practitioner services have been undervalued, and inflation has eroded their value still further. In contrast, remuneration for surgical procedures has been overvalued.

The relative work value study will reset the values of medical services. Hopefully, it will be accepted by the Federal Government which sets the level of rebate for medical services. Government subsidy of medical services, a blessing when introduced, has now become a millstone around the general practitioner's neck as he struggles to maintain his economic situation in the face of a diminishing return for his services brought about by pegging of the rebate at an unrealistically low level. Until and unless the general practitioner places a realistic value on his services, irrespective of the rebate, he will remain fettered by the system, and the quality of care he provides will fall. Hopefully, the work value study will restore his economic status and enable him to enhance the quality of the care he gives.

However, some fear that if fees are set at a level which is equitable for the practitioner, he may price himself out of the market. Fee structures are governed to a considerable extent by what practitioners believe their income should be, giving the skill, responsibility and time involved. Some consider that high medical incomes are a thing of the past and that doctors will need to accept more modest incomes. Others feel that the fee-for-service system will become unworkable and will soon be replaced by salaried or prepayment systems. Whatever the outcome, it is essential that the general practitioner's pride in his vocation is enhanced and that he is equitably rewarded for his contribution to the health of the nation. It is the College's task to see that this is so and that his morale is restored.

Technology in general practice

General practice in Australia could still be regarded as a cottage industry. Although the use of electrocardiography, spirometry and a limited range of pathology tests is long established, few practices have sophisticated equipment for performing blood examinations, biochemistry and radiology. However, it seems likely, with the recent development of new biochemical methods — so-called 'dry chemistry' — that accurate biochemical tests will be performed in the doctor's office. As technology is simplified and the cost falls, the general practitioner needs to assess its value to his practice and adopt it accordingly. General practice needs to move from being a cottage industry to becoming a technologically sophisticated one, using the best that technology can offer in a rational and cost effective way.

One technology which will burgeon in the remainder of this century will be the computer. Although used now by many practices for accounting, basic patient information and recall procedures for routine screening or immunization, and occasionally for medical record keeping, its value will grow as medical information becomes more readily available. It will be an electronic encyclopaedia of medical information which will be more accessible and up-to-date than any book could ever be. It will be invaluable in continuing education as the number of programmes expands. It can provide questions and problems for the user to solve, give him feedback on his performance, and update him when deficiencies are identified.

Whilst programmes will be developed to assist the doctor in diagnosis, perhaps in the form of algorithms, decision trees or simply information about the predictive value of medical information, especially investigations, it is unlikely that the general practitioner will use his computer to solve patient problems by processing patient data. That would require a highly sophisticated programme and much time to enter the data. The human computer is much superior, provided up-to-date information is available.

Central data banks will become accessible through landlines, giving the practitioner a volume of information which would be impossible for him to store on his in-house computer. The importance of medical records will increase and computers will be used more and more to assist with the storage and transmission of patient information. The potential of the computer for improving communication is enormous, yet currently most of this potential is unrealized. Major developments will occur in this area as we approach 2000.

Quality assurance

The public and governments are showing increasing concern about the quality of health care and are pressing for some form of quality control. This requires assessment of the quality of care (quality assessment) and action to remedy the deficiencies disclosed (quality assurance). In 1978, the Federal Government warned the profession that unless it implemented peer review, the Government itself would consider doing so. The AMA responded by establishing a resource centre and has assisted academic colleges and institutions to establish experimental peer review.

The RACGP is responding to this challenge by conducting studies to demonstrate the most appropriate methods for general practitioners and by introducing the concepts of quality assurance and cost effectiveness during training. The Family Medicine Programme's philosophy of self-direction encourages life-long surveillance of standards of care and the correction of deficiencies by continuing education. The RACGP, through the setting of standards of care in general practice, will be providing the guidelines the practising doctor needs to maintain and enhance the quality of the care he provides.

Beyond quality assurance is the question of ethical behaviour. Alarmed by accusations of fraud and overservicing by medical practitioners, governments and the public are questioning the ethics of the profession. The demand is for more ethical behaviour and for a greater sense of responsibility to the public and those who fund health care. Again, the RACGP has responded by re-emphasizing ethics in its courses and by providing better information to its trainee doctors on their responsibilities to government.

The need for an Australian health policy

The Federal Government's health policy focusses on the introduction of an equitable health insurance programme for all Australians (Medicare), community-based care of the aged, a preventive health programme, Aboriginal health, occupational health, and an upgraded community health programme.

It also has a policy on a number of other issues, for example, manpower and medical immigration. State governments, too, have their policies. However, there is no integrated national health policy which guides and governs the development and deployment of health services in Australia. Until this is a reality, health care will remain fragmented, unco-ordinated and to some extent wasteful of resources.

A comprehensive enquiry is needed into the current and future health needs of the community and how the limited resources can be used most effectively. It is encouraging to see that the Federal Government is currently developing a preventive health strategy for Australia.

FUTURE NEEDS FOR 2000

Several have been mentioned in the previous section and will not be detailed further here. Instead this section summarizes the anticipated changes in the next 15 years, and the needs arising therefrom.

The unchanging

Not everything will change. General practitioners will still need to provide whole-person continuing care to individuals and families in their community setting, something which they and they alone uniquely provide. They will continue to recognize the central importance of the family in health and illness and the need to assess individuals in physical, psychological and social terms in the context of the family and community environment. They will still need to be readily available and make adequate provision for round-the-clock cover for emergencies. They will still need to be highly competent clinically, and caring and committed to the health and welfare of their patients.

The changes

But many things will change, and unless general practitioners can accommodate to these changes, they will fossilize. However, reacting to change will not alone create the future they desire. They will need to grasp every opportunity to contribute assertively to the shaping of better quality health care for all.

The most significant changes and challenges general practitioners will face are:

1. An escalating requirement for care of the aged and disabled and those with chronic conditions.

2. More demand for the effective management of lifestyle illness and abnormal behaviour.

3. An increasing demand for preventive care, health promotion and health education, both on a personal and community level.

4. More insistence by patients on self care and a greater say in the management of their illnesses.

5. Increasing pressure on the general practitioner to offer an enhanced range of services and a higher level of availability to provide continuing care.

6. The demand for a higher level of co-operation with, and co-ordination of, health care resources by the general practitioner, and for him to work in a health team.

7. Increasing competition from other health providers, especially alternative health practitioners and hospitals.

8. An increasing emphasis by governments, the public and the profession on quality assurance and ethical behaviour.

9. Increasing community involvement in decisions about health care services.

10. An increasing demand for the cost effective use of health care resources.

11. A steady shift from high cost institutional to lower cost community-based care.

12. A shift of some technology from institutions to general practice.

13. A revaluing of general practitioner services relative to other medical services.

14. A more effective marketing of general practitioner services.

15. The advent and extension of alternative methods of remunerating practitioners.

The general practitioner who is able to accommodate to these changes will derive great satisfaction from the application of his expanded knowledge and skills. But however well he adapts, he will not survive unless he continues to provide those human qualities which people need — a caring approach and a commitment to the primacy of the person. Whatever else happens, he must continue to be the embodiment of *cum scientia caritas*.

Acknowledgements

I wish to acknowledge the assistance given to me by State and National planning groups in the Family Medicine Programme in the clarification of a number of the issues described in this chapter. My thanks go to Nadia Del Romano for her painstaking typing of this manuscript.

REFERENCES

Arthur Andersen & Co and American College of Hospital Administrators 1984 Health care in the 1990s: Trends and strategies. Arthur Anderson & Co and American College of Hospital Administrators, USA, p 36
Australian Bureau of Statistics 1983 Australian Demographic Quarterly Bulletin, December
Australian Bureau of Statistics 1980a Social indicators, Australia, Australian Bureau of Statistics, Canberra, 3, p 9–10
Australian Bureau of Statistics 1980b Social indicators, Australia, Australian Bureau of Statistics, Canberra, 3, p 11
Australian Bureau of Statistics 1980c Australian Health Survey 1977–1978: Doctor Consultations. Catalogue No 4319.0, Australian Bureau of Statistics, Canberra, p 6
Australian Bureau of Statistics 1980d Social indicators, Australia, Australian Bureau of Statistics, Canberra, 3, p 55
Australian Bureau of Statistics 1980e Australian Health Survey 1977–1978: Doctor Consultations. Catalogue No 4319.O, Australian Bureau of Statistics, Canberra, p 9
Bridges-Webb C 1981 How many GPs is enough? Australian Family Physician 10: 678–689
Bridges-Webb C 1976 The Australian general practice morbidity and prescribing survey, 1969–1974. The Royal Australian College of General Practitioners. Medical Journal of Australia (Suppl) 2:9
Bridges-Webb C 1974 The Traralgon Health and Illness Survey. International Journal of Epidemiology 3:37, 3:323

Bridges-Webb C 1973 The Traralgon health and illness survey. International Journal of Epidemiology 2:67

Commonwealth Department of Health 1984 Health care expenditure: Are we getting value for money. Health Reporter 1: (August) 3

Commonwealth Department of Health 1979 Health 30: 24–27

Family Medicine Programe 1984 Quarterly statistics, June 1984. RACGP, Melbourne

Fry J, Brooks D, McColl I 1984 NHS data book MTP Press, Lancaster, p 132

Permail Pty Ltd 1984 Mailing list of medical practitioners in Australia. Permail, Sydney

Royal Australian College of General Practitioners & Arthur Andersen & Co 1984 Working party report on general practice: 'the standards and current practice'. RACGP & Arthur Andersen & Co, Melbourne

Royal Australian College of General Practitioners 1984 Review of the schedule of Medicare benefits: Submission to the Commonwealth of Australia. RACGP, Sydney

Royal Australian College of General Practitioners 1985 Interpractice comparison study. RACGP, Melbourne

Rowe I L, Carson N E 1984 Distribution of general practitioners in Victoria 1982. Monash University, Melbourne

New Zealand

INTRODUCTION

New Zealanders often refer to their country as 'God's own', counting themselves singularly blessed to enjoy not only a temperate, or in some parts an almost subtropical climate, but also an astonishing variety of scenic and natural wonders, low levels of atmospheric pollution and for its size, marked underpopulation.

Most able-bodied New Zealanders revel in the opportunities for outdoor pursuits and sporting activities receive high priority.

Improved means of travel and communication have greatly reduced the isolation from the outside world that once characterized the nation, and ties with the UK remain strong, so that many of the older generation still refer to Britain as 'home', even when they have never visited that country.

The threat of nuclear war has recently brought a greater awareness of international events, while other clouds on the horizon relate to the rapidly increasing international debt that the country is incurring and, for the first time since the depression of the 1930s, a significant unemployment problem.

By most standards, productivity per capita is low in this country with a population of only about 3.5 millions and a total area slightly greater than the British Isles. Inflation is high and, as a result, the country is finding it ever more difficult to remain competitive in overseas markets. During the last 5 years, a small but significant fall in the standard of living has occurred and the disparity between the well-to-do and the lower socioeconomic groups appears to have widened, although it is not as marked as in North America and many other parts of the world.

A notable feature in the New Zealand scene is the high percentage of Maoris and non-Maori Polynesians in the community. Not only do these ethnic groups have their own individual cultures but they also have a different pattern of disease susceptibility and morbidity. This appears to be due to innate differences in response to diseases and the fact that most are in the lower socioeconomic brackets. Traditionally their families tend to be large and less emphasis is placed on the European values of scholarship and competitiveness.

OUTLINE OF CURRENT HEALTH SYSTEM

New Zealand has an international reputation for its innovative welfare policies. Notable among these has been the introduction of universal superannuation for the aged and a subsidized health care service at the primary care level together with a completely free service at secondary level.

General practice is still the usual entry point to health care services and, as such, still provides most first-contact care.

Currently, a patient seeking medical care may visit any general practitioner he or she wishes. The doctor will charge a fee that seems appropriate for the service, but the state contribution is fixed and at present represents only about one-tenth of the usual total fee charged for a working adult and about one-third of the usual total fee for a child or a person on any sort of pension, including the unemployment benefit. Accidents represent a special category and all medical services provided in respect to injuries are totally state subsidized.

The patient requiring secondary care is also expected to see first a general practitioner, who can then provide a referral to either a private or a public-hospital based specialist. In the case of the former, the patient or insurer will pay most of the fee, whereas all services provided through the public hospital system are free.

Thus, the New Zealand health system which once successfully combined private enterprise with a universally available state-run health insurance has been allowed to shrivel to an almost completely patient-paid system at the primary care level.

As in other developed countries, with increasing sophistication in medicine, there is a greater tendency to refer patients to secondary care so that patients are not denied advantages in modern diagnostic and therapeutic techniques. This trend is balanced by a greater need for a 'pilot' to guide patients through tortuous and often potentially dangerous medical seaways. There is a need for a trusted counsellor who can provide support and understanding and who can make known to the patient the available options and their likely consequences, so that he or she can make an informed decision in a supportive environment.

Private enterprise

The general practitioner remains a bastion of private enterprise in a nation of predominantly salaried health workers. He fights a rearguard action defending his chosen territory from hoards of voluntary and statutory workers whose activities impinge upon his, and who usually work for a salary and, as a result, are able to provide their services without charge to the patient.

Many such workers have provided care only between 9 and 5 p.m. and the general practitioner has used his greater availability as a weapon to counter such services. Unfortunately, many general practitioners now use deputizing services to provide out-of-hours cover and this previously telling argument has lost much of its force.

Most allied health professionals are salaried by the government directly or indirectly, and most have a significant role to play in the community. It is the demarcation disputes which tend to lead to friction, especially when they are able to compete with the general practitioner service in cost to the patient.

Although general practitioners are independent, they have to accept some control from government departments. Thus, the Health Department places some constraints on general practitioner prescribing and, although many prescriptions are completely free to the patient, there is a part-charge imposed by the Health Department on some varieties of drugs where cheaper generic preparations are considered to be equally effective. This need not necessarily have any effect on a practitioner's prescribing but, if patients regularly complain about the expense of pharmaceuticals, most doctors would feel obliged, when they believed a cheaper alternative was equally or almost equally effective, to select that in order to maintain the goodwill of the patient.

Increasing competition

General practitioners continue to have the right to practise where they like, but fewer are entering the more popular residential areas, because of pressures of competition. This should lead to better service in areas previously underdoctored. Whether there will be a surplus of general practitioners remains to be seen. As yet, no real attempt has been made to determine what actually constitutes a surplus, and debate centres around what is understood by excessive servicing of patients.

The future role of female graduates also remains an unpredictable factor.

There is a wide variation in the time individual doctors spend with their patients. There is also a variation in demand from patients for in-depth consultations. As in Britain, some doctors who spend very little time in history-taking, examination and explanation have a large practice. Presumably they serve those patients whose expectations are limited and whose confidence in their doctor is absolute. Apparently such patients are prepared to accept a short waiting time and a brief encounter as adequate exchange for a basic consultation, with very little educational or health-promoting content. Some such doctors run what is little more than a glorified pharmacy. Unfortunately, the system of payment tends to reward such doctors better than those who are liberal with their time and give much of themselves.

MONITORING THE QUALITY AND COST OF HEALTH CARE

Currently there is little check on the quality of care and even more difficulties in measuring outcomes. Questions of peer review and/or medical audit are under discussion and debate.

Prescription monitoring

The Health Department has an efficient system of monitoring the prescribing of general practitioners and, from time to time, presents doctors with data on their prescribing costs, comparing these anonymously with the costs of other doctors practising in the same area. Should a practitioner's prescribing costs be notably in excess of his or her fellows, special attention is drawn and the doctor will be required to explain.

Because he is an independent operator there are few checks.and balances to ensure continuing high-quality care. The doctor who works in a group practice is theoretically likely to have more opportunity for peer review, as his work will from time to time be observed by his partners. Thus, when he is on holiday, or when he is off duty, they will assume his role and have access to his records. However, it is not uncommon to find a sort of folie-a-deux or folie-a-trois situation developing where each of the doctors in the group follows the other down the slippery path of mediocrity or worse.

The RNZCGP

The Royal New Zealand College of General Practitioners was established as an offshoot of the Royal College of General Practitioners (UK) and has as its aim the development of better quality primary health care for the people of New Zealand.

It sees better educated general practitioners as the principle means of achieving this.

The College provides a two-part examination which is designed to establish an acceptable level of competence for those who are entering general practice. It remains voluntary, but a substantial proportion of those who plan to go into general practice do sit and pass it. There is currently no attempt to develop any form of periodic review, such as re-examination.

Undergraduate and professional training

A willingness to accept family medicine trainees, or even medical students, into their practice for a significant time is, for some doctors, both an opportunity and a stimulus to review their own work. Many have freely confessed that they find the experience salutary and an incentive to keep abreast of recent developments.

Many general practitioners regularly attend courses for professional refreshment. The support for these courses, attended by practitioners largely at their own expense, suggests that they are meeting a need.

Effect of economic recession

Development of energy-related projects by the government has crippled the economy and it may be many years before good returns for initial outlays are seen. Money is not available for imaginative new developments in health or health-related fields. Furthermore, subsidies developed for primary health care, which initially were designed to represent 75% of the fee, now cover less than 10%.

The hospital component of the health-care system remains completely free to the patient, although, for those who seek them, private facilities are available either through insurance or at their own expense. Lack of adequate subsidies has placed great strains on general practice during the current major recession and many in the lower socioeconomic groups have been unable, or unwilling, to seek care. General practice incomes have fallen compared with other professional groups and so also has morale.

Private insurance

One consequence of Government's failure to increase the subsidies and provide adequately for primary health care has been a phenomenal growth in private health insurance.

Several companies are in the field and have secured membership of over 900,000 in a country with a population of only 3 million and with a supposed welfare state. For the majority, only private surgery and not primary care is covered.

Changes in subsidy

The socialist government, which has now regained power, claims that it intends to raise the quantum of the subsidy, but has declared that this will not be done unilaterally and that any increase will be accompanied by a fixing of maximum fees for primary care services. Such a move would probably effectively trap the general practitioners and presumably eliminate the principle of a fee commensurate with the service. As it is, most general practitioners have undermined this principle by charging a fixed fee for almost all services and, in so doing, have demolished one of the few arguments which could have prevented such a development.

General practitioners, mindful of the 31 years which passed before there was even a trivial increase in the subsidy for primary health care, are naturally fearful of any government which seeks to introduce such restrictions, but which would probably be prepared to compromise on the level of subsidy and the level of the extra the doctor is allowed to charge the patient, if both were subject to regular reviews based on the cost of living index.

One obvious danger of a fixed fee is that, if it is set too low, doctors would almost inevitably attempt to increase their patient turnover. This can lead to patients receiving insufficient time and sometimes unnecessary services are performed. It can also lead to doctors performing tasks which are more properly the province of allied health professionals.

PRIMARY CARE TEAM

The concept of team work is not one that receives much attention in medical schools, particularly in the general practice context. On the whole, the enthusiasm of practising doctors for extensive team-work waxes and wanes depending on how busy they are. In New Zealand, any general practitioner who also provides a receptionist is entitled to a practice nurse with salary paid by the Health Department. Most have taken advantage of this offer, which has become for many doctors a very important subsidy. From time to time successive Ministers of Health, when displeased with what they consider to be lack of co-operation from the profession, have threatened to remove this support. Some practitioners have been able to build themselves, their practice nurses and their reception-ists, together with the district nurses (who are paid by the hospital boards and who work in the community) into an acceptable team. Occasionally social workers or other allied health professionals are incorporated. Such teams can work well where each sees him or herself as complementary to the others and each respects the contribution of the others. Too often it is the doctor who cannot cope with the concept of sharing tasks, believing that if you want a thing done well, it is always best to do it yourself.

Many practice nurses (but by no means all) feel frustrated that so little use is made of their skills. Some would give up the job were it not for the fact that the hours of work are more convenient than in the hospital service.

Latterly, a number of courses designed for doctors and their practice nurses have been held and these hold the promise of a more co-operative approach than in the past. In the future it may be that the early training of nurses and doctors could be to some extent amalgamated with the hope that this would encourage a greater appreciation of their respective roles.

Involvement of the public in primary health care

Of recent years there has been a worldwide dissatisfaction with primary health care, which has been disease orientated and totally dependent on pharmacological remedies.

This has led to a proliferation of lay healers and quacks and a renewed interest in herbal remedies and alternative lifestyles. Amongst the Maoris and Polynesians, the traditional healers have always been a first port of call for some. In response to all this, some general practitioners have explored the unorthodox and have sought to apply what they perceive to be the best of it to their own practices. Thus many now offer acupuncture and some have embraced the theories of homeopathy. Referral to chiropractors is also permitted, but is still uncommon as most doctors still regard the theories of chiropractic as bogus, although few would deny the value of back manipulation for certain back disorders.

One clinical school provides a brief course in acupuncture techniques which have now achieved a wide level of acceptance.

The thin line that separates the pragmatic approach to medicine from the scientific has been breached at times and there is always the danger, when this occurs, that some will get carried away with their enthusiasm and not realize that their results are really the products of powerful suggestion rather than the specific techniques used. Few still believe that this applies to acupuncture.

Consumer input

New Zealand has not seen the spontaneous development of patient participation groups in relation to general practice but a few doctors have tried to stimulate dialogue by inviting groups of patients to meet to discuss mutual interests.

It is the policy of the Health Department to foster the concept of area health boards (see below); these would be responsible for all health services at a peripheral level. A global sum would be provided by the Health Department for division between the various elements of the health services, according to need as perceived by the local area health board. It is felt that, by decentralizing responsibility for health care, the system will be rendered more efficient.

In a recent trial of the area health board concept, there was considerable public support for the development of an effective feedback mechanism whereby the performance of the primary health care services could be monitored and hopefully improved. The next decades should see considerable progress in this direction.

Scope for prevention

Preventive health care is receiving a new emphasis, although, apart from inoculations which are subsidized, the Health Department does not reckon to pay doctors for such services unless they are associated with a curative function. Thus, a doctor who encouraged his patient to consult him purely for health education purposes would, strictly speaking, not be entitled to claim subsidy from the Health Department for this. Most doctors attempt to incorporate some health education into their discussions with patients but this usually takes the form of secondary rather than primary prevention. Improved recall facilities, via computers and reduced workload due to a better doctor/patient ratio, are likely to lead to better surveillance of at-risk patients.

A recognition of the limitations and cost of many screening procedures has meant that few practitioners offer their patients the very extensive check-ups provided by American health maintenance organizations and screening clinics. On the other hand, most of the recommended case-finding and screening procedures are widely practiced by doctors as part of their day-to-day work.

In the main centres, occasional attempts have been made to introduce screening clinics for executives and others, but these have been vigorously opposed by most of the profession and, as far as the writer is aware, none has been established.

Where there is a competent, well-organized primary health care service available, there seems little evidence to support the development of such clinics, and the people who benefit most appear to be those who run them.

Of recent years, medical practitioners have become less reluctant to speak to groups of the public, or communicate through the media helping to assuage the unquenchable thirst for medical knowledge that seems to exist in the community.

How to make the best use of finite resources in primary health care

The claims of primary health care, vis-à-vis secondary health care for a share of Vote Health will remain a hot issue. Those who believe good primary health care leads to a diminished need for secondary health care strongly advocate a greater injection of financial support for the former. On the other hand, secondary care is so sophisticated, so costly and so compelling that it is hard for the public to ignore its demands.

Doctors' incomes represent only a relatively small component of the total cost; pharmaceuticals and investigations cost much more in primary health care and both could be used with more discrimination. Over-investigation and over-treatment are two faults that the New Zealand general practitioner tends to share with counterparts in other developed countries. If costs continue to rise, there seems little doubt that more restraint in these areas will have to be exercised and, if the profession does not monitor itself, it is in danger of having restrictions imposed.

The value of such ancient skills as good history-taking, careful examination and the exercise of clinical acumen may well need to be re-emphasised by teachers, thus reducing the dependence of doctors on high technology. Similarly, a more rational and conservative approach to prescribing could well lead to considerable savings.

Some aspects of preventive care also have the potential to save the nation much expense. As one example, the recognition and successful discouragement of early alcoholic tendencies could make a tremendous impact on the health budget and save much suffering.

More effective use of allied health professionals could also lead to the doctor having more time for those matters that demand personal attention.

THE YEAR 2000

Crystal ball gazing is seldom easy and it is hard to predict the changes that the next one and a half decades may bring. One would like to think that more studies would be made by the academic community into the needs of the population, so that medical training may be directed to meeting real, rather than perceived needs. Doctors who are responsible for teaching tend to plan their training on the supposition that their own health and medical needs correspond to those of the community at large, and often forget the huge gulf between their knowledge and background and that of most patients. Even among teachers there seem to be few doctors who truly see themselves in the role of servant to the public, and yet in this country not only are general practitioners paid most of their fee directly by the patient, but the cost of the doctor's training is paid almost entirely out of the public purse.

Throughout most of the Western world there appears to have been a considerable disenchantment with doctors, who have often come to be seen by the public as a group who are self-seeking and greedy. Doctors are also perceived as the lackeys of the pharmaceutical companies, having been educated to suppose that the answer to most medical problems is either a surgical or a pharmaceutical one, or perhaps a combination of both.

New Zealand has followed this trend, and the considerable

success of practitioners of alternative medical philosophies is testimony to this.

Counselling skills

A new emphasis on interpersonal skills and some training in counselling techniques has resulted from the introduction of behavioural sciences into the hallowed and very traditional halls of academic medicine. Coupled with pressure from enlightened general practitioners both within and without the medical schools, this has brought some changes, but not enough.

The clinical years still see many teachers deriding this sort of instruction and, by their example, undoing much of what has been achieved earlier. In an effort to minimize this and enhance the relevance of what is taught, the teaching of behavioural sciences will in future straddle both the preclinical and clinical years.

One would like to think that, in the future, much more undergraduate education will be provided away from the base hospital and in the community. Logistically this is difficult, too difficult for most traditionalists even to contemplate, but not impossible. As the hospital becomes more technologically orientated, it becomes more irrelevant to the undifferentiated doctor. It is possible, too, that we will see an increasing emphasis on one-to-one apprentice-type learning, which really will reflect a full turn of the circle back to what occurred in earlier times.

Post-graduate training

It seems likely that, as in Britain, New Zealand will shortly make postgraduate training programmes specifically directed toward general practice obligatory for all who wish to make this discipline their career. General practice is not easy and only those who have not experienced it, or whose insight and experience is very limited, would argue with the wisdom of such a development.

Self-confidence in their own medical ability is something which a surprising number of general practitioners lack. In the past this has sometimes been well founded and one has been led to wonder how, given the raw materials — usually a well-motivated person and an above-average intellect — universities could produce such an inferior product after 6 or more years of tertiary education.

In the future, with better training programmes, it is to be hoped that general practitioners will have a new confidence in their own abilities and in their role in the community and that this will be well justified.

Regionalization

Regionalization of medical services is likely to occur. Some experimental work in this direction has already taken place and it is Health Department policy to encourage further development. The aim is to establish in all major regions, local area health boards. These will be constituted much as local hospital boards are at present, namely elected representatives of the public, providing general direction and supervision of trained professionals who would, together, be responsible for the health needs of the whole community. They would provide surveillance at all levels of health care, including preventive medicine public health, primary, secondary and tertiary health care. The chairman of the health board would combine the functions currently undertaken by the medical officers of health and the superintendents-in-chief of the hospital boards. Each area board would be allocated a share of Vote Health budget from central government on a population basis and would be responsible for the way in which monies were spent in their area. What consequences such a development might have for primary health care remains to be seen. Among other things it could lead to a variety of experiments into the way in which general practitioners were paid; it could also lead to a greater rationalization of services and a change in the allocation of resources.

However, with hospital care being so very expensive and so politically sensitive; with taxation levels among the highest in the world and, as a result, little prospect of more money being available to Vote Health, it seems unlikely that there will be much room to manoeuvre. Primary health care seems likely to remain the poor relation, receiving the fallen crumbs.

Freedom

Perhaps of greater concern to the practising doctor, would be questions of professional freedom. Will he continue to be free to practise where he wishes, as at present, or will he be told that certain areas are closed to him? Will patients be free to attend the doctor of their choice and, if they wished, several in one day, as at present, or will they be allocated to or registered with one doctor? Will the medications that are available to the doctor be limited and will he be hedged about by a protocol for management which, in the interests of economy, must be followed assiduously, leaving little room for individuality, innovation and experimentation? And if he does step out of the routine required by him will he be confronted by litigation problems as is not uncommon in some countries, where it seems that doctors practise law and lawyers practise medicine.

SUMMARY

Present problems

1. An emphasis on the treatment of established disease rather than the prevention of illness.
2. A degree of fragmentation of medical services.
3. An underfunded primary care service.
4. A system which tends to reward brief, multiple services rather than comprehensive but less frequent encounters.
5. Medical education based on educators' personal perceptions of the community's needs.
6. Limited research into health care needs.
7. An underfunded postgraduate education programme for general practitioners.
8. Inadequate training in human relationships at undergraduate level

The needs for 2000

1. A greater orientation towards health rather than disease.
2. A better integrated health service.
3. A review of priorities in budgetary distribution of Vote Health.
4. A system of payment which rewards good and penalises poor practice.
5. A more appropriate medical course with doctors trained to meet the real needs of the community.
6. A greater emphasis on determining what are the needs of the community as distinct from the needs and wants of the medical profession.
7. A properly established and funded postgraduate training programme for general practitioners.
8. Doctors who are skilled counsellors, well-versed in the human dimensions of medicine, yet competent clinically.

FURTHER READING

Davis P 1981 Health and health care in New Zealand. Longman Paul
Geyman J, Fry J 1983 Family practice, an international perspective in developed
    countries. Appleton Century Crofts
Richards J 1979 The general practitioner in New Zealand. Longman Paul
Richards J 1981 Primary health care and the community. Longman Paul
Trends in Health and Health Services (1983) National Health Statistics Centre,
    Department of Health publication

13

J. C. van Es

Netherlands

HISTORY

In the Netherlands during the first two decades after World War II, the position of general practice was a very difficult one. This situation originated from two factors. The first one is that in 1942 the government decided to introduce a new *sickfund system*, which was already initiated before the war. The consequence of this system was that about 70% of the population — wage earners with a limited income — became members of a compulsory insurance system and each one of them came on the list of a general practitioner. Before only a voluntary system existed. This new medical care became available for all, without financial barriers and, after a short time, overall medical consumption rose to the levels of upper classes before the war. The result was that general practitioners were confronted with a very heavy increase in doctor–patient contacts. The second factor which influenced the position of general practice was the rapid *development of specialist medicine*. As elsewhere, this was the result of scientific and technical progress, but in the Netherlands the health insurance systems stimulated hospital medicine in an indirect way: the costs of specialist care were not limited: the remuneration of specialists was on a fee-for-service system, while general practitioners were paid by capitation fees.

The tension created by the increase of doctor–patient contacts was relieved by general practitioners referring patients to specialists, who accepted them with pleasure, because they were paid fees for their service. Universities were not limited in the acceptance of numbers of medical students; many of the young doctors wanted to become specialists, and there almost no limitations on the education of future specialists.

Around 1956 the first signs of a rebirth of general practice became noticeable. In that year the Dutch College of General Practitioners (NHG) was started. 10 years later a National Institute for General Practice (NHI) celebrated its second anniversary and the first chair in general practice in Utrecht was created. In the same year, the remuneration of general practitioners, after a deep conflict with the government, was increased by 50%. In the same crucial year, the government published a White Paper on the organization of health care, in which general practice was given an important role. Nevertheless further development of general practice was very slow.

FIGURES AND TRENDS

The population of the Netherlands increased from 10 million in 1950 to 14.3 million in 1983. About 5% of the population came from abroad: Surinam, Turkey, Morocco and other Mediterranean countries. The population density in 1983 was 423 inhabitants/km^2. Table 13.1 shows the slow increase of general practitioners; it also shows that the numbers of practising specialists doubled in 18 years.

Table 13.1   Practising doctors

	No.	1965 per 100 000	No.	1975 per 100 000	No.	1983 per 100 000
General practitioners	4249	31	4809	35	5634	39
Specialists	4518	33	6635	49	9937	69

The disproportion in the increases of general practitior.ers and specialists is partly due to the progress in the specialization in medicine, which resulted in an increase of subspecialization and, as a result, in a request for specialist examination and treatment by the population.

Historically, general practice was a private enterprise; nearly all general practitioners were singlehanded. Recently there has been an increasing interest in partnership, group practice and health centres. In 1983, 12% of all general practitioners worked in a partnership of more than 2 general practitioners, 26% in a partnership of 2 and 62% in singlehanded practice.

Nearly all practising specialists have a hospital appointment. General practitioners have no regular hospital appointments, but there are privileges for obstetrics and to use the services of the departments of pathology, radiology and electrocardiography. On

Table 13.2 Health care expenses

	1978 millions DFl.	1978 millions £	1983 millions Dfl.	1983 millions £	% increase
Hospitals and other intramural institutions	13 785	3243	19 537	4597	41
Specialists	1567	368	1989	468	26
General practitioners	1172	275	1442	339	23
Extramural costs	2572	605	3830	901	49
Drugs, bandages, hearing- and other aids	2299	541	3186	750	38
Prevention	598	141	768	181	30
Other services and administration	1375	323	2128	501	54
Total expenses	23 368	5496	32 880	7737	40

the other hand, specialists can only work in hospitals and in their outpatient departments, they are not allowed to make home visits. The result is that first line care and specialist medicine have strongly divided territories.

The average gross income (excluding practice expenses) of general practitioners is 144 000 guilders a year (£34 000). To draw a parallel: the average gross income of specialists is 225 000 guilders (£53 000), with a range from £40 000 for lower paid specialists like rheumatologists and pediatricians to more than £60 000 for the higher paid specialists like radiologists. The gap between the income of general practitioners and specialists is slowly narrowing. The total expenses for health care have shown a rapid increase. From 1975 till 1983 the costs increased by 93%. Table 13.2 provides a comparison between the expenses in 1978 and 1983. This table shows that the costs of first-line care, including general practitioners, are 16% of the total expenses, and intramural sector costs 65%.

MEDICAL EDUCATION AND VOCATIONAL TRAINING

In 1966 the first chair in general practice was established in the State University in Utrecht, the second following that in Edinburgh. This chair was created by a lucky combination of factors: the activity of the Dutch College of General Practitioners, the intention of medical faculties to change the undergraduate curriculum and the existence of a 3-year-old National Institute of General Practice in Utrecht which could serve as a matrix for a department of general practice. The most important factor was the reorganization of the medical curriculum. The original curriculum, of 7 years, was compressed to 6 years. A seventh year was available for new, additional programmes. This situation created the opportunity to introduce a compulsory vocational training of 1 year. It was evident that this period was too short, but the chance to introduce, from the beginning, a *compulsory* vocational training was considered important.

The consequence of this situation was that each of the other six universities had to establish a chair in general practice, and subsequently a department of general practice. These departments became responsible for the vocational training. Each contracted about 120 teaching practices. The existence of all these departments made it possible for medical faculties also to use them for undergraduate education and training. The result is that, in each medical faculty, general practice is responsible for approximately 5% of the curriculum time.

Meanwhile, the government decided in 1970 to found a new medical faculty in Maastricht, the basic philosophy of which implied an orientation towards primary health care. A professor of General Practice was in the first group of six appointed professors.

Continuing education

In the past, hospitals and professional bodies provided continuing education for general practitioners. In 1975, the Minister for Education intended to lay the foundation for a continuing education for all medical and other professions. By law, the tasks of the universities were expanded: together with professional bodies, they will have to provide a continuing education. For all disciplines preparatory commities were set up. In the medical field the continuing education of general practitioners was given priority. The preparatory work has been completed and a definite committee will function very soon.

A handicap for the realization of this excellent design is that the cost of continuing education has to be paid for 100% by the users.

RESEARCH IN GENERAL PRACTICE

The College of General Practitioners has promoted research in general practice from its start. The College organized several large research programmes. In 1964, the Dutch Institute of General Practice was founded to give support to these programmes and to develop new ones. But the foundation of eight university departments in general practice drained the most competent general practitioners from the College. Research moved to the departments. On the other hand, these departments were limited in their capacity, because they were deeply involved in the development of undergraduate and vocational training programmes. Most of the research developed in Nijmegen and Utrecht. The influence of social scientists in general practice research is large. Many research projects are on morbidity studies, studies in prevention, doctor–patient relationship, patient's behaviour, and diagnostic and therapeutic procedures in general practice. There has been a slow start in more fundamental research.

GOVERNMENT POLICY

In 1966, the government showed for the first time its awareness that a health care system without financial feedback mechanisms was unmanageable. A rapid increase of the total costs of health care was an ominous signal. In 1974 the Minister for Health delivered a White Paper (Nota eerstelijnsgezondheidszorg 1973) in which proposals were made for a restructuring of the health care system. In this paper the intention to give the general practitioners a central place in the health care system was the main theme. Since 1974 this intention has been many times avowed, but without being given concrete forms. The reasons are many, but two predominate. In the first place, the way back to general practice in the referral habit seems to have been difficult. The remuneration system and a lack of coupling in the work of GPs and specialists have prevented a more important role for first-line care in health care. In the second place, the creation of primary teams has been slowed down. The fact that GPs are free enterprisers, the public health nurses in the service of voluntary organizations and the social workers employed by county councils has discouraged progress.

Two years ago, however, it became absolutely clear that dramatic reductions in government expenditure were inevitable. In a new White Paper (Volksgezondheidsbeleid bij beperkte middelen, Verhaudelingen, 1983–84) on first-line care, the government expressed its intention to limit the finances of specialist medicine and to promote first-line care. In this second White Paper the promotion of self-reliance by patients was the basic aim. Thus, primary health care is an important target in the governmental policy. In this policy, general practice fits very well, and, in its footsteps, first-line care. However, there is no doubt that these intentions of the government are inspired by the expectation that first-line care is cheaper than hospital care, and, as hospital care covers two-thirds of all health care costs, financial cuts in this field should be most effective. The Ministry of Health took four measures:

1. A temporary moratorium on new building of hospitals, followed by a very strong restriction.

2. The closure of 8000 hospital beds to the limit of 3.7 per 1000 inhabitants. This has to be realized within 5 years.

3. Limitation of the income of specialists by introduction of a regressive remuneration scale.

4. Introduction of a controlled budget finance system for all hospitals.

These four measures in specialist and hospital care are of utmost importance for the division of work between general practitioners and hospitals. In the first place, a decrease of hospital beds, in combination with a budget system for hospitals, will make it less attractive than before to hospitalize patients: in the past it was a financial advantage for hospitals and specialists both to treat patients in hospitals. In the second place the regressive development of the incomes of specialists make an unnecessary prolongation of treatment and control less attractive.

At the other side of the balance, the government intends to promote self-care, primary health care and care by general practitioners. These efforts are very limited by the lack of a solid basic and integrated structure for first-line care. Home helps and home nurses are available only on a limited scale and not enough to compensate the lack of self-care by family members. The unrealistic policy of the government is to try to restore 19th century family life. But these difficulties could create new opportunities for a further development of general practice. Negotiations between the government and the Dutch Medical Association seem to be moving in the direction of a reduction of the mean size of the patient list of general practitioners from 2500 to 2200 or even 2000. As a compensation, general practitioners will accept a compulsory job description designed by the professional body itself, strongly influenced by the Dutch College of General Practitioners. In this job description the clinical competence of general practitioners is a more central issue than it has been in the last 10 years.

The role of the Ministry of Education

In the appliance of the axe in government expenditure, the role of the Minister for Education is an important one. He planned to cut down the costs of universities, based upon an evaluation of their scientific productivity. This resulted in a reshuffling of faculties and, in some cases, the closing of faculties (such as semitic languages and dentistry). All medical faculties were saved, but had to cut 100 million guilders (£235 million) yearly. Only general practice is considered an important developing discipline. It has been decided that two medical faculties have to improve a first-line orientation: the Free University of Amsterdam and the University of Maastricht. These medical faculties have to increase teaching in general practice and develop research in this field. The government allocated yearly 11 million guilders (£2.6million) for the promotion of these activities. From this new innovation fund 1 million guilders a year will be allocated for the development of training programmes for well-selected young general practitioner-research workers. A very limited part of the fund will be used for innovating or continuing research projects of the other medical faculties in the field of first-line care. The innovation fund offers the opportunity to intensify the relationship with research and teaching practices.

ON THE WAY TO THE YEAR 2000

The emphasis laid upon external influences in the above information is in accord with the results of a sociological study on the professionalization of general practice in the Netherlands (van Hove-Baeck 1978). One of the conclusions is that the present state of general practice in the Netherlands is the result of societal processes and decisions which cannot be influenced or challenged by the profession. The continuing process of job definition, according to this study, is more an adaptation process than a self-defined process. This agrees with Freidson's opinion that the influence of social environment limits the targets of people and groups: '. . . what survives and thrives is that which happens to be adapted to the environment' (Freidson 1970). However, challenges and responses are both crucial elements in our expectations over the next 15 years.

Involvement of patients in health care has created many formal patient organizations. Some of these have been powerful politically, e.g. the Heart Patients' Organization and, to a lesser extent, the Diabetes Patients' Organization. In primary health care, groups of patients have endeavoured to influence processes and decisions, e.g. the euthanasia movements. Smaller groups try to promote self-care, such as those for patients with hypertension or hyperventilation. Some health centres have formed patient organizations, in several cases doctors themselves promoting the foundation of such groups. Until now, the influence of these groups has been marginal, but a national 'platform' of patient organizations is slowly increasing their political influence.

Based upon demographic predictions, we can expect that, up to the year 2000, our population will increase by 10%. The percentage of elderly people will increase from 11.7% to 13.3%, and the percentage of people older than 75 years will increase to 5.9%. Assuming that the age-related need for primary care will be the same as today, the total of doctor–patient contacts will increase by 15% (10% by population growth, 5% by aging). Based upon the assumption that the mean patient list of general practitioners in the year 2000 will be 2000 patients, an increase of general practitioners from 5643 (in 1983) to 7200 (in the year 2000) can be expected.

One can expect that the economic situation will improve by the implementation of high technology and by the recovery of the international market. However, more than 1 million Dutch inhabitants will remain unemployed for many years. It depends on the political colour of future governments if the widening of the financial gap between employed and unemployed people will or will not continue. We can expect changes in the social security systems and, as a consequence, in the health insurance systems.

With reference to the role and the position of the general practitioners, two opposing developments are conceivable:

1. The pressure of the development of high technology in medicine, with a further *concentration of medical care in hospitals*, will be so strong that the governmental policy, as described, will be shipwrecked. In that case general practice increasingly will be the distributor of medical care amongst specialists of many types, and the general practitioner will come in a position in which he will allowed to provide medical care for minor ailments, common diseases, psychosocial problems and a selection of chronic diseases.

2. Government policy will follow a *strong support for first line care*, including the development of research in general practice, the realization of a longer vocational training (promising to be 2–3

years soon) and a well organized continuing education, and the financial limitation of hospital medicine. The increase of group practices, health centres and interdisciplinary co-operation for single-handed general practitioners will increase opportunities to delegate time-consuming care for patients with psychological and social problems. This will provide the general practitioner with more time for medical work. Besides this, one can expect that self-care and self-reliance will increase, perhaps as a byproduct of unemployment. There is an increasing interest in a closer co-operation between general practitioners and specialists in which the specialist has a more consulting function for the general practitioner and in which he takes fewer responsibilities for the patient. This co-operation between general practitioners and specialists has to be based upon a mutual regard and an awareness of each others expertise. To improve this relationship, general practice needs a scientific development of its specific knowledge and experience. This specificity can only be discovered when general practitioners are confident of their own value and identity. Only this awareness can make general practice an influential factor in the social process which defines the content of health care. However, multidisciplinary primary teams will only develop when general practitioners, primary health nurses and medical social workers have a common organizational base. To achieve this, drastic structural changes are needed.

When the latter happens one can expect that the Dutch general practitioner in the year 2000 will be one who works in a close co-operation with, on one the hand, a multidisciplinary team to provide primary health care and, on the other, with specialists from the local hospital. Both forms of co-operation will form a network with the general practitioner in a central position. Related to the hospital and to primary care, hospitals for chronic ill people will function as today. But the selection of their patients will be better than today. This is of utmost importance, because the population will include many very elderly people and many chronic ill patients. There will be a tendency to keep patients out of hospital as long as possible. This will be possible because new ways of living together in the community will develop: communals in which self-care and caring for each other will develop as in large families in the past. Under these conditions the role of the general practitioner will continue and the general practitioner will help to provide health care with a human face.

REFERENCES

Friedson F 1970 Professional dominance; the social structure of medical care. Aldine, New York

Hove-Baeck A van 1978 Het professionaliseringsproces van de Nederlandse huisarts. Politica 28: 319–70

Nota eerstelijnsgezondheidszorg 1973 Ministerie van Welzijn, Volksgezondheid en Cultuur, Staatsuitgeverij, Den Haag

Voksgezondheidsbeleid bij beperkte middelen, Verhaudelingen 1983–84, 181808, nr nr 1, en 2, Staatsuitgeverij, Den Haag

Norway and Nordic countries

HEALTH IN THE NORDIC COUNTRIES

When health care systems are discussed, a 'Nordic' or 'Scandinavian' model is sometimes referred to. People from other countries might have the impression that Denmark, Finland, Iceland, Norway and Sweden have identical health services. This is not so. There are many similar traits, and a similar social and cultural basis for the services, but a closer look will reveal important differences in the way health services are organized. One country cannot be considered a copy of another.

The Nordic region has a population of 22.5 million people. In terms of land the area is larger than the rest of Western Europe put together. The countries are democratic societies, where the population can move freely within the region and do not need a work permit to live and work in another Nordic country. If one moves from one country to another within the region one receives the same social benefits as that nation's own citizens.

By international standards, all the countries must be considered rich, and the citizens enjoy a high standard of living. The national policies are committed to the welfare society, where public authorities play an important role, e.g. in education and delivery of health services.

Their languages, with the exception of Finnish and possibly Icelandic, can be understood in the other countries.

As pertaining to health, the countries have compulsory national insurance that covers most of the expenses for health care.

The countries have developed planning systems for health services during the last 10 years that aim at nationally equal distribution of resources on the one hand, and local involvement in organizing the services on the other. There is a general commitment to decentralize political power as well as the distribution of services.

Comprehensive primary health services have become regulated

by law in Finland (1972), Iceland (1973), Sweden (1983) and Norway (1984). General medical practice is considered more and more a part of local health services with general responsibilities towards prevention, medical treatment, nursing care, health education, research and development, and planning and management.

Chairs for general practice, family medicine or community medicine are being established at the universities in all countries. Programmes for vocational training are instituted, although these are not identical, and not of the same statute. In Iceland, Finland and Sweden, there are recognized specialities in family medicine or general practice. In Norway there is a semivalid recognition by the Medical Association that has to be renewed every five years, whereas no speciality has been recognised in Denmark. Norway has established a speciality in community medicine in 1984.

In the 1980s, the disadvantages of a doctor surplus are being felt, whereas in all countries there was a doctor shortage in the beginning of the 1970s.

Infant mortality is below 9 per 1000, and life expectancy is more than 70 years for men and 77 years for women. The challenge for primary health care now lies in prevention of cardiovascular disease, cancer and accidents, and care for the increasing elderly population.

The differences in the health services may be exemplified with the contrasts between large Swedish multispeciality health centres, often linked to hospitals, on the one side, and small private, often single practices in Denmark on the other. Sweden has no system of referral to specialized health care. In Finland and Denmark this is an integral part of the system. In Iceland and Norway it is a virtue of geographical necessity. In Finland there are well-equipped health centres, and so few house calls that they can count the grand total (30 000 in 1980, relating to 7.5 million consultations). In Norway it is estimated that there is a house call for every 10 consultations. In Finland and Denmark, consultations are free of charge to the patients, whereas in Sweden, Norway and Iceland there is a personal fee to pay.

In Denmark, general practitioners are largely paid on a capitation basis, whereas in Finland and Sweden they are mostly salaried, and in Norway and Iceland there is a combination of both salaries and fee for services rendered.

There is a tendency in all countries to link general practice closer to a defined population. In Denmark each doctor has a list of patients, whereas in Iceland, Norway and Finland the population is mostly geographically defined by the communes, the communes or the municipalities being the smallest administrative units of the countries. In Sweden, general practice is linked to the counties, the practice population is large and thus only to a small extent the defined responsibility of any general practitioner.

Against this background, the reader should bear in mind that, although the Nordic countries are close to each other — not only geographically but also culturally and politically, the details of their health systems do not apply everywhere. In the following attempt to describe primary health care in Norway, this country might be considered as a valid example of health care in the Nordic countries. However, few of the Norwegian institutions are identical to those in any of the other countries.

NORWAY — NATIONAL FEATURES

Norway is a country that extends from far beyond the arctic circle to a southern latitude that corresponds to Moscow or Anchorage. The geography is characterized by mountains and fjords. The country is sparsely populated, with 4 million inhabitants and an average density of 12 people per km^2. It would have been even less populated if it was not heated by the Gulf Stream, creating a temperate oceanic climate with relatively mild winters. The waterways, fjords and rivers have been important for the development of small, local societies based on farming and fishing. Modesty and solidarity were basic cultural virtues. Towards the end of last century the population was relatively poor, and 25% of a generation left for America to seek a brighter future.

Today the Norwegians have the technology to exploit their surroundings. Fish is frozen and exported, Norwegian fisheries being the fifth largest in the world. The forests provide raw material to a highly diversified industry. Cheap hydropower has been exploited to the extent of 20 000 kW.h per inhabitant per year, and more than half of this goes to profitable metallurgical and electro-chemical production. An important merchant fleet has helped to balance foreign trade. In the last decade, there has been a boom in the North Sea oil industry, and Norway has become an important exporter of oil and natural gas.

The present constitution of the country dates from May 17th 1814. The country is ruled by a constitutional monarchy, with a government by parliamentary majority. The government is a three-tier system, with the national government at top, and the 19 county councils and the 452 municipal councils being the other two tiers.

The Norwegians are passionate believers in decentralization. The median size of the municipalities have less than 5000 inhabitants. They govern themselves on all matters that are not better organized on a larger scale, and they do not readily accept regulations from above.

On a national level, 12 political parties are struggling for influence. Until recently, the Labour party, which collected 40–45% of the votes, has ruled with various allies. The result has been:

1. A social democracy which involves people in government
2. A mixed economy, some of it capitalist and some planned public efforts
3. A welfare society based on heavy taxation.

The Norwegian society has a high degree of solidarity and social responsibility. It is a well-organized society with very little corruption, a high standard of living and considerable individual freedom. The problems are the ever-growing public involvement, public expenses and public services. This has brought in a conservative, or mildly conservative, government in recent years, which has a less expansive health and social policy on their programme.

HEALTH SYSTEM — EVOLUTION AND FORMAT

The Norwegian health system was founded 350 years ago, when the Danish King, ruling over Norway then, appointed a physician to Norway. It was a fully socialistic arrangement — the physician was salaried and expected to give care to the indigents, and was responsible to the King on public health matters. However, one physician left his job for a better paid position as a judge in Trondheim.

An important step in the development was taken when the Health Act was passed in 1860. The Act still regulates matters of hygiene and public health today. On the basis of this legislation, local boards of health were to be established in every municipality. The boards of health were less dependent on the municipal council than other municipal bodies or boards. The activities of the board was to be led by a state-appointed district medical officer, who also presided over the board meetings. He received a salary for his public health work, but was expected to practice as a general practitioner on a fee-for-service basis in the district as far as his time would allow.

The boards of health are appointed by the municipal council and it was ruled from the beginning that at least one member should be a woman. The combination of a medical expert as appointed chairman, and elected representatives of the local community, ensured both a scientific foundation, as far as medical knowledge would go at the time, and local acceptance; at times even committment to the resolutions of the board.

The decisions were not always popular. They might mean condemnation of old housing or temporary closing during epidemics of infectious diseases of schools and other places where people would be assembled. The board could stop production or distribution of food if it was considered to be unsafe for hygienic reasons.

Another important step in evolution of health care was taken in 1911, when a compulsory sickness insurance was introduced for employees in the lower wage groups. After a gradual extension, the sickness insurance scheme was made compulsory for the whole nation in 1957.

The underlying principle that has been generally accepted in Norway since the end of the 1930s, is that financial aid should be rendered independent of private charity and poor-relief, by giving the individual citizens legal rights to benefits during illness, other unforseen loss of income and old age.

At the the turn of the century, with the advancement of medical knowledge and skills, the need to finance and build hospitals on a larger scale became apparent. The post-World War I period was a very expansive period, where the state, larger cities, some voluntary organizations and some county councils were building and operating hospitals. From 1970, all hospitals under the sickness insurance coverage would have to be included in a county health plan, exceptions made only for a few teaching hospitals run by the state. The financing of hospitals were at first on a daily charge reimbursement basis. Since 1980 the county councils are granted a block grant according to the size of the population.

In the mid-1980s, there are approximately 20 000 general hospital beds costing NOK 6000 per citizen per year, which corresponds to roughly half the average monthly Norwegian wage.

Primary health care

It is significant for the status of primary health care that the term, until very recently, was 'health services outside institutions': the left-overs.

The distribution of general practitioners was of national concern, but the practice of the district medical officers more or less guaranteed access to health services all over the country. In the cities, there were private practitioners. Both district medical officers and private practitioners served on a fee-for-service basis, the fees being partially reimbursed by the national insurance. The same would apply to physiotherapists.

Over the last decades, the concept of primary health care has broadened and, slowly, the services have been made subject to legislation. Thus, school health, mother and child health clinics, home nursing and, to some extent, occupational health were regulated by law.

In the 1970s, in a period of rapid extension of hospital services, the general practitioner saw his field of responsibility shrinking, and felt he (or she) might end up with only the common 'flu, tears and night calls as the professional basis. In 1977, representatives for the private general practitioners and the district medical officers came together and issued a statement of purpose. The general practitioner, fee-for-service or salary based, should be part of comprehensive, continuous and personal services. This facilitated the further development of primary health care in Norway. The municipality had already, at that time, started to organize primary health care in a more integrated fashion in local health centres. They even had employed salaried physicians, the long-time dread of the Medical Association.

From 1984 primary health became 'commune health services' in Norway. The Commune Health Act of 1982 obliges the Municipalities to give primary health services to everyone who lives, or is residing temporarily, within the community. The municipality shall, through its health services, further public health, personal health and welfare. It shall seek to prevent and treat illness, injury or defects. Efforts for this purpose shall be organized as preventive services (health board services, maternal and child health clinics, school health services and health education and information), diagnosing and treatment of illnesses, medical rehabilitation, care and nursing. This means that the communities will provide:

1. General practitioner services, including emergency ambulatory care
2. Physiotherapy
3. Nursing services, including public health nurse and health visitor services.

The municipality may also, at its own discretion, organize services for the disabled, midwifery services and industrial and occupational health services. They may organize these services by employing its own personnel, or contracting services with private practitioners.

At the time of introduction of the new legislation, private practitioners and physiotherapists who were practicing full time, or had private practice as their main occupation, had a right to a contract with the municipality. Through the contract, he or she is paid an estimated 40% of average earnings as a monthly sum. The rest of the income will be fees-for-service, partly reimbursed by the national insurance. In practice, the doctor or physiotherapist will collect the deductable amount from the patient, and bill the insurance for the rest.

The private practitioner is obliged to work the hours and weeks he or she has agreed to in the contract. But they work on their own premises, and are free to decide how to work, as long as they can be said to be an extension of the municipal health services. They must be willing to see new patients, participate in emergency services and co-operate with other health personnel.

The fee paid by the patient corresponds to 1 or 2 hours average earnings. The total cost of primary health care is roughly one-tenth of hospital services, but is growing at a much higher rate. More than 2000 of the total 10 000 Norwegian doctors work in, or are connected to, the health services of the municipalities. For physiotherapists, the share is greater, and for nurses, the proportion who work in primary health is little more than 10 per cent of the 27 000 economically active nurses.

THE CHALLENGE FOR YEAR 2000

In Norway, primary health care has a well defined and broad basis in the Municipal Health Act. Resources, both manpower and money, are on hand. Supporting systems, like referrals to hospitals, transport for patients, drug control and distribution, and national insurance are well organized. The challenge now is to fill the framework of primary health care with relevant, well co-ordinated activities of high quality. This might be difficult for a number of reasons:

1. Health personnel, doctors more than others, are trained to diagnose and treat diseases that only cause a fraction of disability and death in Norway. The important health problems today are difficult to treat successfully. They are accidents, cardiovascular diseases, cancer, chronic musculoskeletal pains and nervous disorders. They are influenced by human behaviour and are potentially

preventable. We have to find the best preventive strategies to influence them, however.

2. Care is becoming increasingly more important than cure. The increasing proportion of elderly people, calls for more nursing at home and education towards self-care.

3. Knowledge and skills are not enough if the goals for the Municipal Health Act shall be realized. There needs to be a new emphasis on attitudes that support preventive strategies and this must be team-work. This again means that professional self-sufficiency and independence have to be played down, beginning at the medical schools and nursing colleges.

4. The health services must give priority to the most important health problems. New information systems and computer technology will give a clearer picture of distribution of diseases and variations among the communities.

5. The basis for medical decisions is medical knowledge. It will become increasingly clear that many decisions on health, choices for health, are not purely medical decisions, but also must be based on personal or local preferences. Health in Norway towards the year 2000 will depend on our ability to take this into account appropriately.

Finland

INTRODUCTION

Finland is one of the Nordic countries. It has common land boundaries with Sweden and Norway in the west and with the Soviet Union in the east. It has been independent since 1917. From the 13th century until 1809 Finland belonged to the Swedish kingdom, since 1809 until 1917 it was a part of the Russian czardom. Both these historical periods have influenced the later development of the Finnish society. The Swedish language still is the second official language in Finland, although only about 6% of the population are Swedish speaking. Since the Finnish language is not spoken nor understood in countries outside Finland, Swedish formed a kind of link between Finland and other Scandinavian countries. The population of Finland is about 4.8 million and the area about 337 000 square kilometres. The average population density is about 16 persons per km^2, which density, however, varies greatly in different parts of the country. In the northernmost part, Lapland, this ratio can be as low as 0.8 persons per km^2. The distance from south to the northernmost point is about 1100 km. About 60% of the population live in cities and towns and at present about 13% are at least 65 years old. The country has a market economy, a president, 8 political parties and a non-socialist parliamentary majority.

THE HEALTH CARE SYSTEM

At present there are 456 local authority areas, communes, in the country. These local authorities have their own taxation powers and a relative autonomy, which means that they have initiating and executive powers but the central authorities have the obligation of controlling and directing, largely through legislative and purposeful subsidy procedures.

The principle of local self-government was established in 1865. Under this principle, the local authorities have been obliged to provide primary medical services in their areas (in addition to services such as education and social welfare). Until 1972 this was accomplished by establishing positions for local medical officers of health who were responsible for both curative and preventive care. The first post was established in 1882. These doctors received a small salary as well as free housing and, in addition, they received fees from patients on a fee-for-service basis. In addition to doctors, the local authorities hired other health personnel, such as public health nurses and midwives. Since 1956 the specialized hospitals have been owned by the local authorities, who, for this purpose, form federations of communes which run the hospitals and are accountable to the local authorities whom they represent. The average number of hospital beds (all hospital types) is about 15.5 per 1000 population. The proportion of private hospital beds is about 5%. In 1964 the universal sickness insurance scheme was adopted in Finland. It operates on a reimbursement basis and covers the whole population (Kekki 1976a).

The apex of the health services administration is the Ministry of Social Affairs and Health under the Cabinet and the Parliament. Under the Ministry there are two central agencies: The National Board of Social Welfare and the National Board of Health. Under the National Board of Health there are the health divisions of the 12 provincial governments with departments of social affairs and health. The local authorities are responsible for the local health services under the control and supervision of the provincial governments and the National Board of Health.

PRIMARY HEALTH CARE

During the 1950s and 1960s, the focus in the development of the Finnish health services was in hospitals. Primary care was left undeveloped. By 1971 the number of the local medical officers of health was around 700. Usually they worked single-handed with a very heavy workload. Towards the end of the 1960s the communal medical officer establishment was probably at the end of the road. Although relatively well liked by the population, these doctors were not very much appreciated by their colleagues working in the teaching hospitals, whose attitudes were reflected in the minds of the students who graduated from the medical schools. The situation was worsened by the fact that there were no career opportunities whatsoever for local medical officers, and their possibilities for continuing education were poor. Under these circumstances it was reasonably clear that research interests were almost non-existent.

The development of current primary health care

Since the beginning of 1960s planning was carried out in order to implement improvements in primary health services, especially in the rural areas. This planning, which was initiated by the National Board of Health, and the increasing demands for the improvement of primary health services, finally led to an entirely new legislation in 1972 and the reorganization of the primary care system. The general aims of the 1972 legislation were:

1. To increase the use of primary care services.

2. To increase the availability and accessibility of health services and make the various parts of the country more equal in this respect.

3. To promote the health of the population by putting more emphasis on prevention.

4. To control the costs of health services, especially hospital services.

The goals were to be achieved by using the national health planning as a tool to allocate and direct the available resources.

Two basic principles of the 1972 Community Health Care Act were;

1. The health centre concept for provision of primary health care services to the whole population of a defined administrative area.

2. Systematic planning controlled at the national level. Each year a national 5-year plan is enforced and extended by 1 year, so that a 5-year plan is always in force. This plan is approved by the Cabinet. Each health centre district must have a plan and this plan must fit in the framework of the national plan.

Further, a change was made in the central government subsidy system so that subsidies now ranged from 39–70% (10 grades), of the approved costs according to the wealth of the local authority.

The hospital sector was also covered in the planning system, which made it possible to control the resource allocation to the hospitals from the national and provincial levels.

In 1979 the service fees were abolished in the health centres and services are free and doctors are paid by monthly salary.

The health centre

As mentioned above, the health centre concept was created by the

1972 legislation. This concept meant a tool through which the local authorities were to act in order to meet their health care responsibilities at the local level. Thus, the health centre was not a building but a functional organization, whose activities include:

1. Health education, maternity and well baby clinics, family planning
2. Medical care and rehabilitation, transportation of the sick
3. School and student health care
4. Dental health care
5. Occupational health care.

These services the health centre offers to the population of the local authority districts, or districts, who maintain the centre. The health centres also employ a number of personnel other than doctors, and offer good diagnostic facilities. The majority of health centres have a small hospital unit attached to them. At present there are 213 health centres, which cover the whole country. Of these centres, about 75% have a population basis of 20 000 or less. The largest centre is formed by the City of Helsinki, with about 480 000 inhabitants. This centre is divided into 25 basic districts, each with its own health station.

The total number of personnel working in primary health care in the health centres in 1983 was about 41 000, compared with about 58 000 working in the hospitals. The number of personnel in primary health care has more than tripled since 1973. The personnel structure of a typical health centre is shown in Table 15.1.

Table 15.1 The personnel structure of a 'typical' health centre (population 20 000 or less)

Personnel	No.
Doctors (general practitioners)	5–10
Registered nurses	8–15 (if hospital unit)
Public health nurses	10–15
Physiotherapists	1–2
Psychologists	1–2
Dentists	5–6
Speech therapist	possibly 1
Social worker	possibly 1
Auxiliary nurses	depending on the hospital unit
Health centre aids	4–6
Laboratory technicians	2–3
X-ray technicians	1–2
Office and administrative personnel	
Catering and maintenance personnel	additional
Total number of personnel	160

The doctors

Currently, Finland has about 11 000 doctors (1 to 440 persons). In 1970 this number was 5000. In 1983, about 42% of these doctors were working in hospitals, 22% in health centres, 6% were full-time private practitioners, and about 3% were working in private occupational health services.

From a primary health care point of view, the most important group consists of doctors who work in health centres as salaried medical officers employed by the local authorities. Since the reorganization of 1972, the number of health centre doctors increased from about 900 in 1973 to about 2500 in 1982. During this period the number of hospital doctors increased from 3600 to 4100. The official long-term goal is a health centre doctor to population ratio of 1:1500 (it is now 1:1900). The majority of health centre doctors can be regarded as basic doctors, since in Finland it is still possible for a newly graduated doctor to get a permanent position in the health centre, in contrast to some other countries, where specialization in general practice is required. This fact still reflects the attitudes towards work in primary care as compared with work in hospitals.

Besides the health centres, the population can use private medical services. Private sector utilization is high, especially in big cities where the health centres are still relatively undeveloped (Kekki 1982). However, in an average Finnish health centre district it is the health centre doctor who renders most of the medical services to the population. Table 15.2 is based on the results of our study from a typical health centre district, where we collected all visiting information during one year (Kekki 1983). The result showed that

Table 15.2 The population's use of health services during 1 year in a Finnish health centre

Population at risk	1000
Consulted a health centre doctor	548
Treated exclusively in ambulatory care by the health centre doctor	474
In addition, consulted a private doctor without a referral	82
Non-urgent referral to the central hospital outpatient clinic	33
Admitted immediately to the health centre hospital	28
Urgent referral to the central hospital	26
Non-urgent referral to a private doctor	16
Urgent referral to the mental hospital	2
Consulted exclusively a private doctor	58

the general practitioners alone took care of about 90% of persons visiting during that year. Only about 10% of persons visiting were referred either immediately or as non-urgent cases to other sources of care. These figures include only visits to doctor's offices, they exclude preventive visits to clinics, schools and occupational health.

With regard to the expected effects of improving public primary care services, a study was conducted by the author in the late 1970s (Kekki 1979), which covered the whole population of the country and focused on the relationships between availability of resources and use of health services. The special points of interest were the associations between the development of primary care resources and use of various types of health services. Table 15.3 gives the main results of the study, in which the unit of analysis was the population of the health centre district and the method the multiple linear least squares regression. The general practitioner seemed to be the most important single factor in these associations, when all the other variables were controlled. The findings of this, and the subsequent study (1982), strongly supported the ideas behind the development of primary health care services. As the study covered the whole population and all the health centres the results can be considered highly reliable.

Present problems

The problems can be categorized as educational and organizational. General practice, as a medical specialty, was first recognized in

Table 15.3   Effect of an increase in an independent variable by one unit (in absolute numbers) when in each case all the other variables are unchanged

1. An addition of one health centre physician is associated with:	2. An addition of one Public health nurse is associated with:
a total increase of 2846 health centre doctor visits	a total reduction of 92 health centre doctor visits
an increase of 2238 illness-related health centre doctor visits	a reduction of 48 illness-related health centre doctor visits
a reduction of 1332 private doctor contacts	a reduction of 39 private doctor contacts
a reduction of 1201 outpatient visits to general hospitals	a reduction of 67 outpatient visits to general hospitals
a reduction of 106 admissions to general hospitals	a reduction of 7 admissions to general hospitals
a reduction of 467 days in general hospitals	a reduction of 70 days in general hospitals
an increase of 7.5 days in health centre hospitals	a reduction of 122 days in health centre hospitals

1970. At present it is the third largest specialty with a membership of about 750. The annual increase is about 60, which means that in a few years time it will become the most important medical specialty for the size of its membership. However, contrary to the situation in some other countries, general practice specialty has lacked the support of a strong specialty association, and especially the support of academic departments. Until 1981, teaching of general practice was given by the departments of Public Health Science in the Finnish universities, which meant that general practice was not clearly identified by the students, nor the other academic disciplines. When this identification was weak, the postgraduate or vocational training system also remained weak in contrast to other clinical specialties. There was no clearly definiable vocational training programme and there were no general practitioner trainers. It was only in 1981 that the first Chair in general practice was established in Finland in the University of Helsinki and, in 1982, the first independent university department of general practice. Although not yet adequately manned, this department has now the position of national leadership in the development of general practice education in Finland.

Due to the confusion caused by the departments of public health science during the 1970s, the understanding of the ideology and philosophy of primary health care-oriented general practice in the medical faculties and among the students — even general practitioners — is weak. The traditional attitudes and ignorance are the main problems to be solved when developing both the undergraduate and vocational education in primary health care. This may be easier, however, with vocational training, which becomes the responsibility of the university in 1986.

As for other educational problems concerning primary health care, it seems relatively clear that there are educational shortcomings also in the education of other health personnel, especially the nurses. The current common problems focus on aspects such as the ability to collaborate and work in teams, communication between various personnel groups and understanding each other's roles in primary health care. There seems at the moment to exist a kind of competition between the doctors and nurses, focusing on the question of who is the leader. Basically this whole problem can be traced back to educational shortcomings of both the doctors and the nurses.

In the Finnish system, consumer participation and intersectoral collaboration are relatively good. However, questions such as the motivation of personnel, quality of care, continuity of care, arise and are among the organizational problem areas. When we studied the provider continuity, we found that the continuity index (K) was about 42%, or the COC index about 0.35. The co-ordination between different levels of care was relatively poor, with a referral letter return rate of 56% from general hospitals to the health centre, 18% from private practitioner specialists. Also, the follow-up visit compliance was lower than expected (Kekki 1983). The research results have also shown that quality of care in primary care settings in Finland may sometimes be problematic.

Due to the low self-respect and weak role identification of the primary care workers, doctors included, the motivation and the feeling of achievement are not as good as they could be. The lack of understanding of the chief goals and objectives of primary health care activities, and how these goals and objectives can be achieved, seem to be the major obstacles in the development. A very important element in this respect is the education of doctors and other health personnel. The basic medical and nursing education are still strongly hospital oriented.

PRIMARY HEALTH CARE BY 2000

Summary of planned development

The Finnish primary health care system is well structured; through specific legislation the basis for the development is strong and, more important still, there is a strong support for primary health care concept at the highest national decision-making level. All these facts will guarantee the necessary developments. In the draft of the Finnish Strategy of Health for All by 2000 by the Ministry of Health and Social Affairs and the National Board of Health (1985), the detailed strategy programme is based on three spheres of action, all complementing one another. These are: promotion of healthy life habits, reduction of preventable health risks and development of health services. It is stated that health care policy can only be carried into effect with the support of other sectors. When the health care part is considered, the following developments are some of those mentioned: the GNP share of health costs was, in 1982, 6.8%, which is the same level as in 1977. According to a projection based on an economic growth of 3% per year, the number of posts in health care would be increased by 20% from the current level. The increase in primary health care would be 28% and in specialized health care 13%. The total health care expenditure, as the percentage of the GNP would be 7.5% in the year 2000. If the present financial structure is to be maintained, the health care costs to the central government and the communes will grow, at constant costs, by 77% from 1984 to 2000. The growth and development will be highest in primary health care, so that allocated funds will double by the year 2000. During the same period, the scope of medical education will have to be developed. It is clearly stated that, according to the health political priorities, more attention will have to be paid to primary health care within the basic education of physicians. Considering all the facts, people working in primary health care can look forward optimistically to the developments by the year 2000 A.D. in Finland.

REFERENCES

Finland: Ministry of Health and Social Affairs, The National Board of Health 1985 The Finnish Strategy for 'HFA-2000'. A draft
Kekki P 1976a Same goals — different philosophy. British Medical Journal i: 205–206
Kekki P 1976b General practice in Finland. Journal of the Royal College of General Practitioners 26: 853–859
Kekki P 1979 Analysis of relationships between availability of resources and use of health services in Finland. A cross-sectional study. Doctor of Science dissertation, The Johns Hopkins University, School of Hygiene and Public Health, Baltimore, Maryland; and The Research Institute for Social Security, Social Insurance Institute of Finland, Series M, No 34, Helsinki
Kekki P 1982 Use of illness-related ambulatory physician services in Finland. Medical Care 20(8): 797–808
Kekki P 1983 Use, content and provider-specific continuity of health centre physician services. Conference proceedings, 10th WONCA World Conference on Family Medicine. WONCA, Singapore; p 250–254

United Kingdom

THE COUNTRY

The United Kingdom (UK) is a democratic monarchy of four countries; England, Wales, Scotland and Northern Ireland, each having strong ancient historical roots that have been submerged, but not forgotten, to form a single nation.

The United Kingdom is an old nation with new roles. The great British Empire of the 19th century has dispersed and become a loose British Commonwealth of nations, each free and independent. Since 1975, UK is an off-shore island of the European Economic Community (EEC). During the past 25 years there has been a mass immigration from Commonwealth countries, West Indies, Asia and Africa. Such immigrants number almost 3 million (5% of the population). In some districts, recent immigrants make up around one-half of the population.

Once the world's wealthiest nation, the UK now is relatively 'poor'. Apart from its natural resources of North Sea oil and coal, UK's income comes from trading, manufacturing, science, technology, education, commerce, banking and insurance.

The 'mother of parliaments', the UK always has had a strong social conscience for fairness and equality. Nevertheless, still there tend to be 'two societies' — upper and lower classes; the north and the south; and white collar and blue collar workers. Social inequalities exist.

The UK is a small country (233 100 km^2/90 000 square miles), densely populated with almost 56.5 million people. England 47 million, Wales 3 million, Scotland 5 million, N. Ireland 1.5. The population has been static for the past 5 years and is not expected to change.

HEALTH SYSTEM

Recognized organized health care goes back almost 1000 years and can be followed through a series of steps to the present.

Originally it was the Church that provided shelter, succour, care and hospitality in monasteries and other places. Personal care was provided by untrained persons who acquired skills and reputations as lay-healers.

The feudal-agricultural system of the middle-ages produced landlords who provided paternalistic responsibilities for their workers.

At about this period universities began to teach 'physic' (medicine) but it was quite unsuitable for general care of the people.

In the 15–16th centuries colleges and guilds were established, each interested in and concerned with the status and opportunities of their fellows. Physicians were university graduates and surgeons were craftsmen. Neither were involved in primary care of ordinary people. It was the apothecaries (pharmacists) and lay-healers who provided such care.

The second half of the 19th century, with the industrial revolution and mass migration to grimy cities, saw the beginnings of organised primary care. By now the colleges and universities were producing increasing numbers of general doctors who were working alone in the communities for fees. The poor could not afford fees so employers supported 'sick clubs', the forerunners of prepaid health insurance.

In 1911 National Health Insurance was created. This entitled working men and women (below a certain level of income) to receive prepaid care from general practitioners. It established patient registration with a doctor who undertook to provide necessary care for all those on his 'panel'. Payment was by annual capitation fees.

During World War II the Welfare State was conceived (1942). This included a National Health Service.

In 1948 the National Health Service (NHS) provided 'free' medical care. General practice was one of its three parts; the other two were hospitals and public health.

THE NATIONAL HEALTH SERVICE (NHS)

Almost all the population (98%) is registered with a general practitioner. The NHS costs £300 ($350) per person per year, which is just over 6% of GNP. General practice accounts for almost 10% of

NHS costs and prescribed drugs for another 12%. The revenue sources for the NHS are chiefly from indirect taxation.

Parliament is responsible for the NHS. The Department of Health and Social Security (DHSS) includes services such as pensions, unemployment and supplementary benefits for the poor.

The NHS is administered through regional and district health authorities for hospital and public health services. General practice has independent administrative family practitioner committees (FPC). Each general practitioner is in contract with a local FPC to provide services for those patients registered with him/her.

Patients have free choice of doctor and doctors free choice of patient.

The general practitioner is free to arrange and organize his work as he/she wishes in premises of his choosing, which have to be approved by FPC. For his services he/she receives:

1. Annual capitation fees.

2. Item-of-service payments for maternity care, immunizations, cervical cytology, contraceptive services and night visits.

3. Extra fees for elderly persons

4. Reimbursement (70%) of salaries of his employed staff and for rent of his premises.

5. Various other fees.

At present (1985) the average net annual income is £25 000 ($30 000) and his NHS prescribing costs £50 000 ($60 000). This average income is in the upper national quartile. In addition to his regular income he will receive a pension on retirement related to his total lifetime NHS earnings.

General practitioner in NHS

The average general practitioner has some 2000 patients. He works in a group (partnership) of 3–4 doctors. Most practices work from their own premises and one-quarter work from public health centres. General practitioners provide:

1. Directly available and accessible care; each is responsible for 24-hour cover by rotas or deputizing services.

2. Portals of entry into the NHS; referral to hospital specialist is only by referral from general practitioner.

3. Long-term and continuing personal and family care.

Their work tends to be 'as it comes' from patients who decide when to consult. The annual consultation rate is 3–4 which means 6000–8000 consultations or 25–30 per working day.

Most of the work is with minor and chronic disease. Most general practitioners carry out some formal preventive work — antenatal care, immunization, cervical cytology and family planning, as well as much informal advice and anticipatory care.

Practitioners are able to *organize* their own practices as they wish:

1. Arranging their work schedules and rotas.

2. Employing their own staff (for which they are reimbursed 70%).

3. Providing their own equipment — but having free access to local hospital radiology and pathology services.

4. The great majority of practitioners do not have hospital privileges for treating their own in-patients.

Education and training

All university medical schools include *undergraduate teaching* on general practice. There are departments of general practice at almost all medical schools.

Vocational training is compulsory for all general practitioners seeking NHS appointments. This is over 3 years (1–1½ years in general practice and 1½–2 years in approved hospital work). The training programme is supervised and administered by the Joint Committee for Postgraduate Training in General Practice (JCPGTGP). Stress is laid on clinical, behavioural, social, epidemiological and organizational skills.

On completion of their training, young doctors can enter general practice by private selection and appointment to group partnerships, or by public competition through FPC to solo practices.

Postgraduate education is widely available at local post-graduate medical centres, one or more in each district. It is quite voluntary. In addition, there are many free medical journals and an increasing choice of audiovisual educational resources.

Present state

The NHS is an inviolable part of British society. Within the NHS the general practice is an essential part. It is impossible to foresee British general practice changing very much by 2000 A.D.

The present patterns of general practice have evolved gradually but definitely over the past century. The general practitioner of the latter part of the 20th century is the doctor-of-first-contact in the community. He has no inpatient hospital privileges. He works independently, without major incentives or any real controls or directives, as he/she thinks fit.

Conditions and facilities for good care are there, but the ranges of services and their quality are variable between doctors and between practices. There are real inequalities of general practice care and standards, with few ways of achieving quick improvements.

Practice team

The practitioner working alone is a rarity, only 12%. General practitioners work in groups. They work with their own staff and with NHS nurses and other health workers attached to the practice. Thus, a practice may have attached nurses, health visitors, midwives, social workers, clinical psychologists, counsellors and others. Sharing and delegation of work tends to be traditional with each working independently and with poor communications. There are, however, practices where these highly skilled workers are being used to their full potentials (see also Chapters 8 and 9).

Prevention

In the future much more emphasis will be put on prevention, health maintenance and promotion. At present, prevention does not figure large in most practices. However, there are examples and leads that will be followed in using age-sex registers and computers for ensuring complete community immunization and cervical cytology, and for hypertension, diabetes, thyroid disease and asthma screening and supervision.

Quality assessment and promotion

Reliable data on professional performance in general practice are scant. Regular recording of general practice work, its processes and outcomes are not generally available. It is impossible to find out whether resources are being efficiently, effectively and economically used.

Records and computers

It is a startling fact that the form of records used are those introduced more than 75 years ago in 1911 and after. They are too small and quite inappropriate for modern medical record keeping.

Attempts are being made to pass from the old to the new in one large jump. Computers are being provided for general practice, but it is unlikely that machines such as these will ever completely replace the need for good, traditionally recorded medical information. Experiments and trials with computers are demonstrating the special opportunities for using the potential of PHC.

Patients

General practitioners generally pride themselves as approachable, kindly, sympathetic personal and family doctors, yet are resistant to involvement of patients in their practices. In a NHS, presumably for the benefit more of the public rather than doctors, there are only the beginnings of patient groups and others in influencing the nature and quality of care. 'Consumerism' is a major factor in British society and has to be taken seriously by those in PHC. (See also Chapter 7).

Alternative medicine

For whatever reasons, and there are many suggested, the public is moving more to alternative forms of health and medical care. Homeopathy, naturopathy, osteopathy, chiropractice, acupuncture and many other types of care are becoming increasingly popular. 'Holistic medicine' is a new arrival that seeks to provide care for the whole person, perhaps because the public feel they are not receiving it from general practitioners.

Women doctors

Although now only 1 in 8 of general practitioners are women, by 2000 A.D. it may reach as many as 1 in 2. About one-half of medical students now are women and more women doctors than men are likely to opt for general practice.

Professional organizations

There are two major general practice professional bodies: the Royal College of General Practitioners (RCGP), largely an academic body interested in standards; the General Medical Services Committee (GMSC) of the British Medical Association, medicopolitically concerned with conditions of service.

Deficiencies exist in applying known clinical and operational facts to PHC practice. Through weaknesses in management and organization, there has been a failure to seize opportunities to promote better health and prevent disease in a known registered population.

FUTURE NEEDS

The future of general practice in the NHS is likely to be eventful and changing. For a long time general practice has had much freedom with few responsibilities.

The recent state of the British economy is such that controls of expenditure will increase and that these will involve general practice. Attempts are being made to reduce expenditure on prescribing and other items of service. General practice has had very much an open-ended budget that NHS controllers have found impossible to check. It is evident that general practice will have to act to anticipate government actions and to introduce reasonable methods to improve efficiency, effectiveness and economies.

In the *clinical field* it is necessary to continue to develop voluntary systems of self-checks and audit to measure quality and volume of work, to define weaknesses and introduce improvements. Such checks need to be on-going and repeated.

There is much that general practice can contribute to *research* to add to the understanding of the common conditions that are seen chiefly in general practice. Such research must include clinical trials to decide on best ways of management.

It is necessary urgently to examine *manpower (womanpower) needs and to rethink the roles of various members of the team.* We do not know how many doctors or other PHC workers we need, nor do we know who can do what work best. The answers will only come from intensive and extensive studies and trials.

Prevention of disease is the ultimate goal but has to be tempered with realities. It is necessary that we know what is preventable, how best to do it and who should do it, if finite resources are to be deployed usefully.

Patients' roles and responsibilities need to be examined and assessed. It is good to think of more patient involvement in the work of general practice but it is even more important to re-emphasize the individual's own responsibilities for self-help and self-care.

Possibly the most urgent need is to improve the *medical recording system* and to use it as the basis for analytical examination of what we are doing, how we do it and to what effect.

Plans and protocols — all the major diseases demand good collaborative care between general practice and the hospitals. To provide the best care and make best use of available resources, hospital doctors and general practitioners should come together to prepare guidelines for step-by-step care for early diagnosis and subsequent care of conditions such as hypertension, arthritis, asthma, cancers, peptic ulcers, strokes, heart attacks, pregnancy and others.

United States of America

THE COUNTRY

The United States is a young country, of little more than 200 years in age. Its development as a world power and industrial giant has been rapid and vigorous, especially in the last 75 years. This growth has been made possible by an abundance of land and natural resources which, until recent years, have seemed to many to be without limits.

The land mass of the United States, including Alaska and Hawaii, embraces well over $7\frac{3}{4}$ million km² (3 million square miles). Most of this land is productive, with only about 10% of the total area classified as 'wasteland' (compared to a world average of 45% 'waste'). This land includes all types of terrain and climate, including desert, mountains, plains and coastal regions (Estall 1972).

The population of over 226 million people is likewise heterogeneous, representing many ethnic and racial backgrounds. On average, there are only about 24 people per km² (60 per square miles), a lower population density that all but 3 of the world's 20 most highly populated countries. Again, this population density is highly variable, ranging from extremely sparse populations in remote areas to as many as 4000 people in a single block in some parts of New York City (Schnell & Monmonier 1983).

Americans are of very mixed origin; almost 20% of the white population in 1960, for example, were either foreign-born or children of foreign-born parents. About 10% of the US population is black, and another 2% include other races, especially American Indians, Japanese, Chinese and Filipinos. As is the case with many of the world's developed countries, the proportion of elderly people over 65 years of age is steadily increasing and presently is over 10% of the population.

The per capita gross national product in the United States is higher than in any other country in the world, and high levels of both production and consumption have been sustained for many years. More than 25% of all employment is in manufacturing. The total labour force is now about 102 million people. The last 20 years have seen a steady increase in the number of working women, and women now represent about 42% of the labor force. As the country has become more industrialized, marked increases in employment have taken place in managerial, professional, technical, sales, and clerical positions, whereas the growth of employment was less for semiskilled jobs and minimal for unskilled jobs.

Although the early years in America stressed agrarian life in a frontier society, a major shift has taken place since 1900 from rural to urban areas. The population living on farms typifies this shift, decreasing from 31 million people in 1940 to about 10 million people today. Whereas the farm industry provided about 33% of all employment in 1910, farming now provides less than 5% of US employment. Thus American society has now become one of the most urbanized in the world; as the big cities became densely populated and became afflicted with all of the environmental and socioeconomic problems of these communities, a large shift of many people has occurred from metropolitan areas to rapidly growing suburban communities on their fringes.

THE HEALTH CARE SYSTEM

Evolution

The evolution of both the medical profession and the changing health care system in the United States over the last 200 years closely paralleled the larger trends in this young, rapidly growing society. The rugged individualism of the early frontier was reflected in the predominance, for many years, of solo practice. Medical practice in the US has tended to be entrepreneurial by nature, though recent years have seen increasing efforts toward a more collective or 'system' approach to health care problems.

Medicine in early America drew its traditions and content largely from Europe, particularly England. Some of the earliest advances in American medicine, not surprisingly, took place in rural and frontier settings. Thus, the first laparotomy (oophorectomy) was carried out in a frontier state, as was the earliest use of ether for general anesthesia. The latter part of the 19th century saw the development of major medical teaching centres in some of the cities, of which Boston, Philadelphia and New York were the best known. By the start of the 20th century, US medicine was on solid ground and had contributed major advances to medicine, particularly in surgery, anesthesia, obstetrics, public health, and the control of infectious diseases.

The American Medical Association (AMA) was organized in 1847 as an association of physicians with the overall goal to improve medical care throughout the country. After 1900 it became actively involved in promoting improved educational and training standards. Medical education in the United States at the start of this century was highly variable in quality and content, with an emphasis on experiential training through preceptorships. The AMA's Council on Medical Education led a drive to close inferior or unnecessary schools, and almost 100 medical schools were closed between 1904 and 1929 (Shryock 1936). The Flexner Report of 1910 was a major catalyst to this reformative process. This report led to the introduction of premedical education, an increased emphasis in the medical schools on the biomedical sciences as a foundation for medical practice, and the requirement of postgraduate training in the form of an internship. The inevitable result of these changes was the subsequent development of biomedical research, specialty boards, and formal residency training programmes in the various specialties.

The growth of specialization has been the dominant feature of American medicine in the last 50 years. The first specialty to be established was ophthalmology in 1917. During the 1930s specialty boards were established in obstetrics-gynaecology, paediatrics, internal medicine, surgery and psychiatry, together with several other medical and surgical subspecialties. In 1979 the most recent specialty board was established in emergency medicine, bringing the number of primary specialties to 23. The result of this emphasis on specialization was the dramatic reversal in the proportion of general practitioners to specialists from 80:20% in 1931 to about 15:85% today.

Specialization in medicine has had a profound influence, both good and bad, on hospitals throughout the country. Improved standards of education have undoubtedly led to improved standards of care in hospitals of all sizes. On the other hand, particularly as a result of an increasing surplus in many specialties, there is now in many communities substantial redundancy and excessive competition among hospitals, associated with an incremental increase in marginal or unnecessary health care services.

The allocation of health care services has undergone major changes in the United States, particularly during the last 20 years. Based on the private practice model and the patient's ability to pay, most medical services were traditionally provided on a fee-for-service basis. This often resulted in a system of two standards of care, one involving private physicians and hospitals, the other involving municipal or charity hospitals. In the last 20 years, major national efforts and substantial progress have been made in improving the availability and quality of health care services for the entire population. The Medicare and Medicaid legislation of 1967 provided supplemental governmental funding for the health care needs of the elderly over 65 years of age and the economically disadvantaged younger population, respectively. Recent years have seen a growing public recognition that health care, at least at a basic level of services, can and should be the personal right of all citizens.

Other significant trends over the past 20 to 30 years, which have considerable impact on today's health care system, include expansion of the country's biomedical research effort through the National Institutes of Health, various research institutes and medical schools; the steady expansion in the number and types of allied health fields; the continued growth of group practice; and the increased emphasis on alternatives to fee-for-service private practice, particularly involving various new forms of prepaid practice.

Present system

The health care industry today in one of the largest, most diverse, and fastest growing industries in the United States. Over 4 million people were employed by this industry in 1973 in over 100 discrete occupations, including about three-quarters of this number in allied health fields. National health expenditures have almost doubled in the last 20 years, and now comprise more than 10% of the GNP. Hospital care represents the largest single part of national health expenditures (about 40% of the health care dollar). The average length of stay has decreased in recent years, but the numbers of hospital admissions and hospital days per 1000 people per year have generally increased. Physician services represent about 20% of the health care dollar, and this figure has remained stable for many years. The US saw an 8-fold increase in per capita expenditures for health care between 1950 and 1976, from about $78 to about $638.

The government now pays for approximately 40% of health care costs, principally through the Medicare and Medicaid programmes.

Over 75% of the population has some private health insurance, but this coverage is usually incomplete and spotty. Most health care in the country is provided through a free choice of physician on a fee-for-service basis. During the last few years, however, there is an increasing trend toward the development of various alternative approaches to the delivery of health care, including health maintenance organizations, large prepaid group practices, and independent practice associations. Various forms of national health insurance have been hotly debated periodically over the last 25 years. Although there may be substantial public support for some kind of national health insurance, especially coverage for catastrophic illness, the large and uncertain price tag for a major national programme has so far delayed the enactment of such legislation.

20 years ago, there was general agreement that physicians were in short supply. As a result, there was a concerted effort by government and medical schools to increase the number of physicians being trained. Today there are about 450 000 physicians in the United States, which represents more than a 68% increase since 1960 and a 30% increase since 1970. It is now widely acknowledged that a surplus exists in the aggregate number of physicians, that this surplus will become much greater in coming years, and that maldistribution of physicians (both by specialty and by geographic location) is the major problem. Various recent national studies have called for the reduction in number of many specialties, particularly in the surgical and other non-primary care fields.

There is also a surplus of hospital beds and excess utilization of hospital services in the United States. Many health planners believe that the current national average of about 4.4 non-Federal short-term general hospital beds per 1000 population should be reduced to not more than 3 beds per 1000. As is true of other parts of this pleuralistic health care system, there are many different types of hospitals available to different population groups, including various federal hospitals (e.g. Public Health Service, Veterans Administration), state hospitals (e.g. mental hospitals), academic medical centres, county hospitals, non-profit community hospitals, and proprietary hospitals.

The trend toward overproduction of physicians in non-primary care fields, together with overbedding in the hospital sector and incentives in various third-party reimbursement systems favouring utilization of high-technology, procedure-oriented use of hospitals and emergency rooms, has led to a crisis of spiralling costs of health care. Because of an increasing surplus in many of the limited specialties, many non-primary care specialists provide some incomplete primary care services which are outside of their training or principal interest. Since the health care system lacks any systematic structure for primary care (i.e. the patient can see any type of physician for any kind of problem), discontinuity and fragmentation of health care are the result for many patients.

Despite the developing surplus of physicians in many fields, the abundance of hospital facilities and related resources in most parts of the country, and major advances in technology of medical care, numerous inequities exist. Although 4 out of 5 Americans have some kind of health insurance for general hospital care, many do not have coverage for drugs, diagnostic studies, preventive care, counselling, or nursing home care. Least likely to have adequate health insurance are the poor, minorities, young adults, the elderly, and residents of rural areas. The Medicaid and Medicare programmes, initiated almost 20 years ago, have greatly improved access and utilization of health care services for the poor and elderly, but these groups have higher prevalence of serious health problems with only partial coverage of needed health care.

FAMILY PRACTICE AND PRIMARY CARE

Although there was some initial groundwork in the 1950s for the development of family practice as a specialty, it was not until the 1960s that real progress was made in this direction. This specialty was finally established in 1969 with the formation of the American Board of Family Practice and many factors were responsible for its creation. Unlike most other specialties in medicine, the specialty of family practice was created, not because of the development of new knowledge or techniques, but in direct response to well-recognized deficits in primary care. The American Academy of General Practice, founded in 1947 to improve the standards of US general practice, played an important leadership role in creation of the specialty. Family practice was a logical, even inevitable, response to a basic problem in US medicine — the loss of its generalist base. It is interesting that four major, broadly representative, Commissions issued reports independently and simultaneously in 1966, each calling for basic changes in medical education to train an increased number of family physicians.

The development of family practice in the US since 1969 has been remarkable in many respects. In just 15 years, teaching programmes in family practice have been instituted in over three-quarters of the nation's medical schools, together with more than 380 family practice residency programmes. The federal government and many states have strongly supported this effort. A high level of student interest in family practice has been developed and sustained.

The American Board of Family Practice, as the certifying body of the specialty, is the first American specialty board to require (every 6 years) recertification by examination. To be eligible for examination, a candidate must have completed an approved 3-year family practice residency programme. In addition, during the first few years of the Board's activity (until 1978) a candidate could be board-eligible on the basis of a minimum of 6 years of practice as a family physician, together with at least 300 hours of continuing study acceptable to the board. There are now over 30 000 Board-certified family physicians in the US. Since 1978, all newly certified family physicians have been required to be graduates of family practice residency programmes.

It is perhaps not surprising that many specialties have claimed a stake in primary care as federal priorities have shifted to fund primary care programmes and as the surplus in many specialties has led to intense competition among physicians and hospitals. The definition of primary care has been hotly debated, and the claims to 'primary care' roles by non-primary care specialties have been based on limited definitions of primary care (e.g. first-contact care without long-term continuity of comprehensiveness of care).

The following definition suggested by Alpert draws from the contributions of many and represents a general consensus within medicine (Alpert 1976).

> Primary care can be defined as being within the personal rather than the public health system, and is therefore focused on the health needs of individuals and families — it is family-oriented. Primary care is 'first-contact' care, and thus should be separated from secondary care and tertiary care, which are based on referral rather than initial contact.
>
> Primary care assumes longitudinal responsibility for the patient regardless of the presence or absence of disease. The primary care physician holds the contract for providing personal health services over a period of time. Specifically, primary care is neither limited to the course of a single episode of illness nor confined to the ambulatory setting. It serves as the 'integrationist' for the patient. When other health resources are involved, the primary care physician retains the co-ordinating role. He or she cares for as many of the patient's problems as possible, and, where referral is indicated, fulfills his longitudinal responsibility as the integrationist.

Table 17.1   Distribution of ambulatory visits to office-based US physicians, by patient age and physician specialty (%)

Physician specialty	Patient age				
	<17	17–44	45–64	> 65	all age
General and family practice	32.6	38.0	39.1	40.0	37.4
General internal medicine	1.5	8.6	17.9	22.1	11.6
Paediatrics	44.5	0.7	0.1	0.0	9.6
Obstetrics and cynaecology	1.0	18.8	4.4	1.3	8.7
General surgery	2.8	6.0	7.9	7.7	6.1
Psychiatry	0.6	4.6	2.6	0.6	2.6
Other specialties	17.3	23.3	28.0	28.3	24.0
Totals	100.0	100.0	100.0	100.0	100.0

Source: Rosenblatt R A, Cherkin D C, Schneeweiss R et al 1983 The content of ambulatory medical care in the United States: An interspecialty comparison. New England Journal of Medicine 309:892.

The federal government has defined only three fields as primary care disciplines: family practice, general internal medicine, and general paediatrics. The American Medical Association has also classified obstetrics-gynaecology as a primary care field, but many view this as a surgical specialty and not primary care. Although the 'contract' for primary care is not entirely settled, the US is likely to retain a pleuralistic approach involving family physicians, general internists and general pediatricians.

There are now about 55 000 general/family physicians in the United States. Their activities in ambulatory care have been extensively studied as part of a National Ambulatory Medical Care Survey. The most accurate portrait yet available of the distribution of ambulatory care by specialty in the US is provided by a study of almost 100 000 diagnoses recorded by more than 3000 physicians responding to the National Ambulatory Medical Care Survey in 1977 and 1978 (Rosenblatt et al 1983). Table 17.1 displays the distribution of ambulatory visits by patient age and physician specialty. It can be seen that general/family physicians account for three-eights of all visits, representing more than three times the ambulatory volume of internal medicine, and even exceeding the combined ambulatory volume of general internal medicine, paediatrics, and obstetrics-gynaecology. Interestingly, general/family physicians account for almost twice the number of ambulatory visits for the geriatric population than provided by general internists.

15 diagnosis clusters were found to comprise 50% of all ambulatory care visits. Only a few specialties handle the majority of all ambulatory visits. General/family physicians, general internists, and general pediatricans together account for well over one-half of all

Fig. 17.1 Most frequent ambulatory diagnoses in American medical practice by rank order and physician specialty (NAMCS 1977, 1978). (From Rosenblatt R A, Cherkin D C, Schneeweis R et al 1983 and *The New England Journal of Medicine*.)

Contribution of Each Specialty (in percent) to Total Care Rendered for Specific Diagnosis Cluster

Rank Order	Percent of All Ambulatory Encounters	Cluster Title	Contribution of each specialty (percent)
1	8.9	General Medical Exam	GP/FP (34) · IM (7) · Peds (31) · Ob-Gyn (16) · Other (12)
2	7.3	Acute Upper Respiratory Infection	GP/FP (59) · IM (8) · Peds (24) · Other (9)
3	4.4	Pre- and Postnatal Care	GP/FP (25) · Ob-Gyn (73) · Other (2)
4	4.4	Hypertension	GP/FP (57) · IM (32) · Other (11)
5	3.1	Depression/Anxiety	GP/FP (29) · IM (12) · Psychiatry (46) · Other (13)
6	2.7	Soft Tissue Injury	GP/FP (52) · IM (5) · Peds (8) · GS (14) · Orth (7) · Opth (5) · Other (9)
7	2.7	Medical and Surgical Aftercare	GP/FP (21) · IM (4) · Ob-Gyn (13) · GS (23) · OPth Ur (4) · ENT (4) · Other (27)
8	2.6	Ischemic Heart Disease	GP/FP (41) · IM (38) · Card (14) · Other (7)
9	2.4	Acute Sprains and Strains	GP/FP (53) · IM (8) · GS (7) · Orth (24) · Other (8)
10	2.2	Acute Lower Respiratory Infection	GP/FP (56) · IM (14) · Peds (22) · Other (8)
11	2.2	Otitis Media	GP/FP (27) · Peds (49) · ENT (21) · Other (3)
12	2.0	Dermatitis/Eczema	GP/FP (37) · IM (7) · Peds (16) · Derm (28) · Other (12)
13	1.8	Fractures and Dislocations	GP/FP (26) · GS (6) · Orth (56) · Other (12)
14	1.8	Chronic Rhinitis	GP/FP (23) · IM (6) · Peds (8) · ENT (15) · Allergy (43) · Other (5)
15	1.7	Diabetes Mellitus	GP/FP (52) · IM (31) · GS (4) · Other (13)

Source: Rosenblatt R A, Cherkin D C, Schneeweiss R, et al: The content of ambulatory medical care in the United States: An interspecialty comparison. **N Engl J Med 309:892, 1983**

patient visits for the 15 most common medical problems combined. The three primary care specialties together account for 58.6% of all office visits to physicians and 65.9% of all visits for the 15 most common diagnosis clusters. General/family physicians alone account for more than one-quarter of the visits in 12 of the 15 most common diagnosis clusters. Figure 17.1 displays the comparative contributions of the various specialties to the ambulatory care of patients presenting with problems included in the 15 most common diagnosis clusters. Of special interest are the findings that general/family physicians account for more than one-half of all office visits for 6 of the most common diagnosis clusters, including hypertension, diabetes mellitus, acute upper and lower respiratory infections, soft tissue injury, and acute sprains and strains. Most studies have shown that the average referral rate is in the range of 2–3% of all visits for general/family physicians in the US.

Hospital work is also an important and integral part of the practice of the great majority of general/family physicians in the United States. Most spend about one-quarter of their time caring for patients in the hospital, involving the care of paediatric, general medical and geriatric patients. Many family physicians are involved with some surgical procedures, surgical assisting and obstetric care, but there is considerable regional variation in this respect.

A recent trend is the development of growing numbers of clinical departments of family practice in community hospitals. Guidelines have been prepared by the American Academy of Family Physicians (before 1971 the American Academy of General Practice) for the organization and operation of such departments. Two major functions of these departments involve the monitoring of quality of care provided by family physicians and the delineation of their hospital privileges conjointly with other clinical departments.

About one-quarter of all general/family physicians in the US today are in group practice (defined by the AMA as including at least three physicians). Some of these are multispecialty groups and many are family practice groups. Solo practice has become the exception, and the proportion of family physicians in one or another form of group practice is steadily increasing.

Today's family physician works with a larger and more diverse team of allied health professionals and office staff than was the case in earlier years. The offices of most family physicians employ individuals in the following areas: nurse and/or licensed practical nurse, secretary-receptionist, book-keeper, and laboratory technician. Some offices have X-ray facilities and employ an X-ray technician (often a laboratory technician with additional training). The average number of support staff working in these areas is more than 2.5 per physician in family practice groups. Some family physicians also work with physician extenders (i.e. physician assistants, nurse practitioners). Under variable degrees of physician supervision, these physician assistants and nurse practitioners diagnose and manage uncomplicated illnesses; provide screening, preventive services and patient education; and assist with or carry out various office procedures (e.g. laceration repair). A more recent development, but still quite uncommon, is the inclusion of other disciplines in the group practices of some family physicians, usually on a part-time basis, including medical social workers, clinical psychologists, and/or clinical pharmacists.

The typical US family physician accounts for an average of 125–175 patient visits each week. Most of these are in the office, about one-quarter are in the hospital and/or emergency room, and a few involve home visits. The duration of the average office visit is about 13 minutes, which is comparable to office visits in paediatrics and obstetrics-gynaecology.

Practice satisfaction among US general/family physicians is generally quite high. A recent study found that 96% of over 3000 recent graduates of family practice residency programmes are satisfied with their hospital privileges, and the great majority of graduates surveyed were generally satisfied with their practices (Geyman 1980).

Academic family medicine

Starting without an established place in medical education in 1969, it is impressive how much progress has been made in the development of academic family medicine in its first 15 years. Educational programmes have been designed and developed at all levels; faculty have been recruited to serve as teachers, administrators and role models; a clinical and teaching base has been started in many schools, and a beginning has been made in family practice research.

Perhaps the most important advance has been the development of departments of family practice in about three-quarters of the nation's medical schools. These departments comprise the natural base for patient care, teaching and research in family practice, including linkages to other disciplines and to affiliated teaching programmes and practising family physicians in the community. It was just this medical school base that was missing in the 1950s when an unsuccessful effort was made to develop and sustain good general practice residency programmes in community hospitals. These programmes were isolated in unaffiliated hospitals, were relatively unattractive to graduating medical students and most had floundered by the end of the 1960s. Experience during the 1970s has shown that medical schools, with organized departments of family practice and required clinical clerkships in family medicine, attract the highest number of their graduates into family practice residencies.

Although there is considerable variation in undergraduate teaching in family medicine in US medical schools, most departments of family practice offer a co-ordinated curriculum over a 4-year period, with provision for progressive levels of responsibility for patient care. Many such departments are involved in the 'introduction to clinical medicine' courses in the preclinical years involving the teaching of patient interviewing, history-taking and physical diagnosis. Preceptorships are invariably offered in various community-based family practice settings, as well as family medicine clerkships during the third and fourth year of medical school in affiliated residency programmes and/or group practices of family physicians. Many departments also offer electives in such areas as geriatrics, sports medicine, preventive medicine, community health, and related areas.

At the graduate level, 3-year family practice residency programmes provide a balanced experience in both ambulatory and hospital care, with the first year replacing the traditional internship. These programmes are based upon the *Essentials for Graduate Training in Family Practice*, a document jointly prepared by the American Academy of Family Physicians, the American Board of Family Practice, the AMA Section of General/Family Practice, and the AMA Council on Medical Education. There are now over 7400 family practice residents in training in 386 approved family practice residencies. Over one-half of these programmes are located in community hospitals in affiliation with medical schools.

The family practice centre is the clinical and teaching base of the family practice residency programme. It replicates as much as possible a community-based group practice of family physicians. Here each resident cares for an increasing number of families over a 3-year period, including continuity of care into the hospital when hospitalization is required. Hospital teaching rotations are required on all of the major clinical services, including internal medicine, paediatrics, obstetrics-gynaecology and general surgery. Additional teaching experiences (some hospital-based, others ambulatory) are also required in emergency medicine, the medical subspecialties, the surgical subspecialties, and community medicine. Behavioural science (often including a rotation on psychiatry) is presented as a longitudinal experience over at least a 2-year period.

Continuing medical education was established in 1947 as a high priority by the newly formed American Academy of General Practice, which has since required of its members 150 hours of accredited study every 3 years. The emphasis during earlier years was upon attendance at formal conferences as the principal method of continuing education. Recently, the limitations of relying on a single approach to continued learning have been more widely appreciated. The emphasis today is to recognize that continuing education is a highly individual matter, that it should be tied as closely as possible to patient care needs, and that physicians may have quite different learning styles and needs. As a result, a number of approaches to continuing education are used today, including self-assessment, medical audit, learning through teaching, and even collaborative research. There is now an increasing effort to centre continuing education as an ongoing process in each group practice and in each hospital's department of family practice. The American Board of Family Practice has encouraged the practice of office-based audit by utilizing, as part of the recertification examination, audit of a total of 20 patient records representing 5 selected categories of illness.

Although the quality and amount of research in US family practice is still at a comparatively rudimentary level compared to most of the established specialties, considerable progress was made during the 1970s in the development of methods and concepts for family practice research. Examples of progress include the increasing interest and more positive attitudes toward research among many family physicians; the development of various research methods, including classification systems, data retrieval systems, and indices for health status; the organization of the North American Primary Care Research Group as a forum for sharing research techniques and results; and the successful completion of collaborative research projects involving medical school departments of family practice and community-based family physicians.

CURRENT STATUS OF FAMILY PRACTICE

Although the development of family practice in the United States during its first 15 years has been remarkably successful, the development of any specialty is inevitably a long-term evolutionary process. Accordingly, it is useful to briefly list some of the strengths and weaknesses of US family practice today as a means of clarifying its present status and problems.

Strengths

1. Breadth of patient care services
2. Hospital practice
3. Continuity and comprehensiveness of care
4. Group practice
5. Regional variations of practice patterns based on needs
6. Public and governmental support
7. Board certification and required recertification
8. Organizational development with complementary roles (e.g. American Board of Family Practice, American Academy of Family Physicians, and Society of Teachers of Family Medicine)
9. High level of student interest
10. High calibre of residents
11. Congruence of graduate training to practice needs
12. Quality control of teaching programmes
13. Emphasis on continuing medical education
14. Clinical departments of family practice in hospitals
15. Practice satisfaction of family physicians

Weaknesses

1. Lack of systematic and accepted national plan for health care system
2. Redundancy and waste within the system
3. Overlapping and competitive roles among specialties
4. Lack of clear-cut responsibilities for primary care within the system
5. Reimbursement policies favouring high technology and procedure-oriented care, with disincentives for breadth of primary care
6. Inadequate number of family practice residency positions

7. Unstable funding base for family practice teaching programs
8. Shortage of qualified family practice faculty
9. Medical education system still more oriented to tertiary care than to primary care
10. Weak family practice base in many medical schools
11. Inadequate research base
12. Persistent view among many family physicians of family practice as a 'derivative' specialty, not as an academic and a clinical discipline in its own right

FUTURE NEEDS FOR THE YEAR 2000

In order for family practice ultimately to develop to its full potential in this country, as an effective response to the needs of the public for primary health care, the health care system itself will require considerable remodelling to strengthen the role of primary care at the foundation of the system. This will require formulation of a co-ordinated national plan for the health care system, restructuring of medical education at both undergraduate and graduate levels, and fundamental changes in the reimbursement system and incentives affecting practice patterns. A new working partnership will inevitably be required between government, organized medicine, and the medical education system. A system must be found to redistribute the 'mix' of residents in training and practicing physicians by specialty consistent with the public interest. Ideally, this process would involve clarification of the 'contract' for primary care, which logically might include family physicians, general internists and general pediatricians as 'gatekeepers' to the system. The extent to which these issues are actually addressed will, to a large extent, shape the future role and character of family practice in the year 2000 and into the next century.

There is considerable evidence that a new 'contract' for primary care is beginning to take shape. The last few years have seen rapid growth of various forms of prepaid health care, increasingly based upon the 'gatekeeper' role of the primary care physician. Within such programmes, the role of primary care physician is strengthened, all consultative services require authorization, and direct self-referral by patients to consultants is discouraged or eliminated. Many observers now believe that one or another form of prepaid practice will replace fee-for-service practice as the dominant form of reimbursement in the US by the year 2000. This will inevitably produce increased conflict between and among physicians, hospitals, third-party payers, and others involved in the health care system. New patterns of referral and consultation will emerge, and the present emphasis on hospital care will shift toward ambulatory care and integrated systems of care involving various types of facilities and settings. Utilization of hospital services is already decreasing, partly as a result of prepaid capitation insurance programmes and partly as a result of a recent change in the method of reimbursement of hospitals from retrospective cost-based reimbursement to prospective reimbursement based on fixed payments for specific diagnostic-related groups (DRGs). The DRG system presently applies only to Medicare patients, but is being seriously considered by other third-party payers, and shifts the incentive from providing more to providing less hospital and ancillary services.

The rapid and continued escalation of health care costs in recent years has led to a variety of cost-containment measures. Increasing use of copayment by patients for selected services can be anticipated, and various forms of direct and indirect 'rationing' of services are certain to evolve. Fee-for-service reimbursement systems, as well as some of the prepaid systems now in operation, tend to preferentially reimburse secondary and tertiary care services, and many important primary care services are either not reimbursed or only partially reimbursed (e.g. preventive and counselling services). Future reimbursement patterns are needed which assure an appropriate share of the health care dollar for primary care services while limiting the application of high technological services to those with demonstrated positive outcomes of care within limits of what the entire health care system can afford.

While hardly a panacea for all of the problems of the health care system, the performance of family practice already provides considerable evidence that the further development of this field will go a long way toward alleviating many of the deficits and inequities of the present system. The growth of family practice has led to improved geographical distribution of physicians, particularly in underserved rural areas. Numerous studies of family practices have demonstrated high levels of physician and patient satisfaction. Studies of cost-effectiveness and quality of care have so far been more limited, but available evidence shows that family physicians are performing well in both of these areas as well. Since a sizeable proportion of internists and pediatricians continue to subspecialize, it is clear that the single best investment to strengthen primary care is to further develop family practice, the only specialty with an undivided commitment and interest in primary care and the one specialty trained in breadth to provide comprehensive care with continuity to a population, regardless of age, sex, or presenting complaint.

Within family practice, several future directions seem clearly needed, including:

1. Taking an active leadership role in development of cost-effective high-quality primary care within varied organizational structures, including various kinds of prepaid practice.

2. Maintaining an integrative and patient advocacy role based on a continuing physician–patient relationship as the foundation of a changing health care system.

3. Developing more specific and clinically useful standards for measuring quality of primary care.

4. Developing improved information management systems in primary care, including clinical, administrative, educational and research applications of microcomputers.

5. Strengthening the medical school base for family practice, including a solid clinical base, an established role in the required undergraduate curriculum, adequate number of faculty, and ongoing research programmes.

6. Increasing the number of family practice residency positions from their present level of 13% to at least 25% of US residency positions.

7. Increasing the emphasis on various kinds of faculty development programmes focused on both teaching and research skills.

8. Expanding the role and priority for family practice research in both medical school and community settings.

9. Developing a more active and direct teaching role for family physicians at undergraduate, graduate, and postgraduate levels.

10. Maintaining and improving interactive links between medical school departments, affiliated residency programmes, and practicing family physicians in the community.

11. Developing new alliances with other specialties based on complementary rather than competitive roles.

REFERENCES

Alpert J L 1976 New directions in medical education: Primary care
    In: Purcell E F (ed) Recent trends in medical education. Josiah Macy Jr.
    Foundation, New York, p 166
Estall R 1972 A modern geography of the United States. Penguin Books,
    Baltimore

Geyman J P (ed) 1980 Profile of the residency trained family physician in the
United States 1970–1979. J Fam Pract 11:715
Rosenblatt R A, Cherkin D C, Schneeweiss R, Hart L G 1983 The content of
ambulatory medical care in the United States: An interspecialty comparison. N
Engl J Med 309:892
Schnell G A, Monmonier M S 1983 The study of population: Elements, patterns,
process. Charles E. Merrill Publishing Company, Columbus
Shryock R H 1936 The development of modern medicine. University of
Pennsylvania Press, Philadelphia

Canada

THE COUNTRY

By the year 2000 Canada will be 133 years old as a nation. Her $3\frac{1}{2}$ million square miles will be inhabited by just under 30 million people (Gordon 1984). Of the population, three-quarters will live in urban communities with less than 0.5% scattered over 40% cent of the land mass in the northwest and Yukon Territories (Canada Year Book 1975). English and French continue to be the largest cultural groups (the country is officially bilingual) but the indigenous groups of Inuit and Indian and substantial immigrant populations of many other cultures will maintain the country as distinctly cosmopolitan.

Currently, rich natural resources sustain industrial and agricultural developments in mining, forestry, farming, and fishing. Unemployment ranges about 11% (Kirsh 1983). 40% of the workforce are women of whom 40% are single, widowed or divorced. (Byers 1984a). Day care centres for preschool children are increasing. There is 1 divorce for every 2.8 marriages (Byers 1984b).

A tax-sharing system permits the federal government to influence what are primarily provincial jurisdictions of health and education. As it interfaces with the individual citizen, the health care system reflects the problems of bureaucracy and political interactions at many government levels. Nonetheless, by generally accepted standards of health care, and in comparing the cost of health care with other similarly developed nations, Canada's health care system is one of the most cost effective in the world. This is somewhat remarkable given the wide disparity of demands which result from varied societal expectations and geographic hardships (Bennet & Krasny 1977).

THE HEALTH CARE SYSTEM

Historical background

The medical care system in Canada began in the 1600s with surgeons and apothecaries, who were initially army surgeons, ship surgeons and a few physicians who came to the continent as early settlers (Heagerty 1928).

Early *medical education* depended primarily on apprenticeship without regulation until standards were laid down in the Province of Ontario in 1815 when a licensing examination was first established. Medical schools, founded first in Toronto and Montreal by the 1840s, essentially graduated general practitioners (Biehn & McWhinney 1983). Following the time of William Osler, one of the first 'consultants' (Cushing 1925), and with the impact of the Flexner Report (Carnegie Foundation 1910) (which closed many of the apprentice-type schools in North America between 1910 and 1920) the medical schools began more specialized training, and the certification of specialist-consultants came about with the formation of the Royal College of Physicians and Surgeons in 1929 (Woods 1979a).

The *Canadian Medical Association*, which was itself established in the year of Canadian Confederation, 1867, supported the establishment of the College of General Practice in 1954 (Woods 1979b) (subsequently The College of Family Physicians of Canada).

Changing needs

Presenting symptoms and common diagnoses in primary care by Canadian family physicians reflect patterns studied in other developed countries (Curry & MacIntyre 1982). The emphasis on prevention by the family doctors of Canada is well represented in the recent publication of the College of Family Physicians' Blue Book on Health maintenance (CFPC 1983) Recent studies in the Maritime Provinces show that 15% of services provided by family physicians are primarily preventive in nature and that, for patient visits for cardiovascular problems, preventive advice is given in 2 out of 3 cases (Stewart 1982).

The Lalonde Report by the Federal Government in 1974 recommended the pursuit of two broad objectives:

1. To reduce mental and physical health hazards for those parts of the Canadian population whose risks are high.

2. To improve the accessibility of good mental and physical

health care for those whose present access is unsatisfactory (Lalonde 1975).

In 1979 a special task force on the periodic health Examination identified those preventive strategies, which might occur in doctors' offices to identify high-risk situations for treatable conditions (CMA 1979).

In the last decade, the improving standards of fitness in Canada, have reflected a general societal appreciation for the importance of health maintenance (Canada Fitness Survey 1983).

Counteracting this, however, have been the pressures of unemployment and the gloom of the future in the face of nuclear war threat, which have combined to demoralize youth. Recent surveys of mental illness show there is a substantial pool of unidentified but treatable mental illness (about 40%) in the community (Leighton 1982). Of all ambulatory psychotherapy and counselling services, the percentage provided by family doctors in Canada increased from 35% in 1972–73 to 45% in 1978–79 (Mental Health Services in Canada 1982). If the currently unidentified and treatable pool of mental illness becomes identified, this would require twice as many family practice counselling services simply to meet current needs. The identification of such problems and their management will fall for the most part on the family physicians of the medical team.

Health-related task forces and commissions of the early 1980s, agree that the year 2000 will see a significant increase in the proportion of elderly citizens. The projected increase between 1981 and 2001 of persons between 65 and 74 years of age is 39% and of persons over 75 is 95% compared with a total population increase of 19.7% (Woods 1984). Again, the greatest proportion of this increased workload will fall on family physicians.

Education for family physicians

Specific training for family practice came about when the College of Family Physicians of Canada established pilot family practice training programmes at the Universities of Calgary and Western Ontario in 1966 and subsequently developed an educationally sound certification examination in 1969 (Woods 1979c). Currently, all 16 medical schools have departments of family medicine and training programmes at the postgraduate level.

In 1984 there were approximately 44 000 physicians in Canada licensed for the practice of general medicine, of whom half are specialists. Nearly 8000 are members of the College of Family Physicians and 5000 have successfully passed their Family Medicine certification exam. In 1983, the specialist Royal College (not of Family Physicians) granted just over 1000 members their specialty by examination, whereas the College of Family Physicians granted just under 500 family doctors their certification by examination in family medicine (RCPSC 1984, Canadian Family Physician 1984).

FUTURE PATTERNS OF PRIMARY CARE

The pattern of primary medical practice in Canada has been traditionally one of the family physician as the doctor of first contact and the specialist acting as a consultant. In urban medical school centres, there has been an increasing practice of Royal College trained specialists taking on greater amounts of primary health care responsibilities. Parallel with this trend has been reduced involvement of family physicians in hospitals that are dominated by those specialists. This is shown by reduced privileges and reduced opportunities for the family doctor to admit patients directly to hospital and care for them independently. This trend is supported by tightening up of the availability of hospital beds, especially in large urban communities, increasing proliferation of those communities by specialists who demand beds, and economic payment systems which reward family physicians to work out of their community-based offices but not to offer hospital-based care. This reduced participation in hospital care is paralleled by a reduced participation in obstetrical care by family physicians (Klein et al 1984).

Primary health care by other health professionals, is substantial, though poorly organized. Typically, urban centres have hundreds of community agencies supported on marginal budgets (funded by charitable donations and insecure government grants). Nurses, social workers, psychologists, physiotherapists, respiratory therapists and others work out of such agencies providing various primary care services. Even nationally credible organizations such as the Victoria Order of Nurses have somewhat insecure financial support and depend to a large extent on fee for service payments by patients. Osteopaths and chiropractors make up a relatively small proportion of primary care practitioners. Pharmacists conduct considerable amounts of primary care from their retail outlets, occupational health nurses and physicians provide primary care in the workplace. Hospital emergency rooms, staffed by full-time emergency room physicians, are the rule in major urban centres,

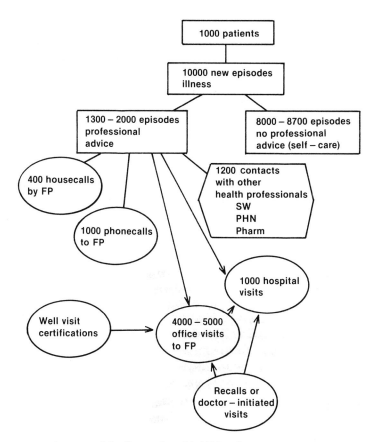

Fig. 18.1 One year of family practice with 1000 patients

with family doctors from the community having variable involvement and responsibility in those departments.

Figure 12.1 outlines a diagrammatic representation of primary health care in developed countries such as Canada, England and Australia (Hennen 1982).

Educational programmes for nurse practitioners do not exist in Canada now with the exception of a small programme for remote nurses out of Dalhousie University. From the point of view of training programmes, the nurse practitioner movement in Canada in 1984 is dead, but there is much political pressure by the nursing profession to revive it (Spitzer 1984).

The task force on the allocation of health care resources (supported as an independent review by the Canadian Medical Association) (Watson et al 1984), suggested ways of controlling costs while providing the care necessary for the year 2000. These included reducing institutionalization of the elderly and of the mentally ill, reducing the average length of stay in acute care hospitals for non-elderly patients and reintroducing nurse practitioners. All of these solutions place the greatest demand for increased resources on primary care medicine and suggest a greatly increased need for family physicians. As the Report reads,

> Medical schools have a new challenge before them, to maintain the kind of new thought and leadership that is needed to produce a sufficient number of well-rounded doctors who are, in the best sense of the word, 'generalists'.

Standardization of services by family physicians

Primary medical care services by family physicians are provided in most provinces by independent practitioners in an entrepreneurial fashion. The family physicians organize themselves in groups (with or without specialists) or as solo practitioners. Except for having to provide services in a manner that will be accepted by the payment system, there is little standardization required. Members of the College of Family Physicians have some collective guidelines which are voluntary. The College offers a record system to its members, which is purchased by less than 10% of them. A Health Maintenance Guide was recently distributed to all members, but its use is completely voluntary and it will likely only become a major part of practice organization for some. The Committee on Practice Assessment of the College has completed a feasibility study (Committee on Practice Assessment 1983) to develop methods for assessing ambulatory medical care services. Such methods may ultimately be used to establish acceptable standards of care given by family physicians. The College of Family Physicians requires its members to complete 50 hours of continuing medical education each year. College members, who have acquired their certification by examination, are required to complete a practice log and self-assessment examination at 5-yearly intervals.

Individual provinces, through their own licensing bodies, can apply checks and controls of quality. The Ontario licensing body has developed an audit programme which includes a record review, a visit by an auditing team to individual practices, and interviews with those practitioners whose quality of care, as demonstrated by the record and visitations, seems questionable. One of the statistically significant predictors of satisfactory performance on the assessment of 800 practitioners (family physician and consultant) randomly selected from the Ontario doctor pool, is certification by examination of either the Royal College of Physicians and Surgeons or the Canadian College of Family Physicians (Klotz 1982).

The Canadian Medical Protective Association has recently increased its fees substantially because of increased numbers of cases to be investigated and dealt with. Doctors believe they are being forced to adopt a more costly style of practice of defensive medicine, through the increased use of diagnostic tests, because of substantial increases in the number of litigation cases.

PAYMENT OF MEDICAL SERVICE

Remuneration for medical care in Canada has, since 1970, been based primarily on a comprehensive government insurance scheme or medicare plan. The federal share of taxes related to health care is assigned to provinces on the understanding that the individual citizen is assured access to necessary medical and hospital care with universality of service, regardless of which province the individual happens to be in.

The provincial share of taxes related to health care is incorporated in some provinces as a tax-based service (in Nova Scotia and Newfoundland no extra premiums are collected) while other provinces continue to charge individuals premiums setting aside variable amounts from general taxation into the support of the health system in different ways, such as research and development, or home care services. Drugs are provided for the elderly, but dental care is variably provided depending on the province.

Recent federal legislation requires that physicians accept the fees negotiated between their professional medical organizations and their provincial governments without maintaining the right to bill patients anything privately (Government of Canada 1984). This has created a major medical-political conflict, and provinces which allow their doctors to charge beyond that negotiated amount will be financially penalized through a reduction of federal payments into the provincial system. This remains untested in most provinces, although at least one province (Nova Scotia) immediately imposed legislation on the physicians making it illegal for them to bill the patient directly any amounts (Government of Nova Scotia 1984)

Payment to physicians is based on a fee-for-service, with each fee negotiated individually between the profession and the province. Other patterns of payment are experimental. For example, in Ontario about 3% of family physicians participate in a Health Services Organization (HSO) based completely on a global budget, which is calculated according to a capitation formula (Seidelman et al 1982). This system encourages health promotion activities (which are poorly paid for in the fee-for-service system) and allows for the effective use of other health professionals within a family practice setting. Such health professionals are not eligible under the basic fee-for-service system for payment of services they provide un-supervised directly by physicians.

FUTURE EDUCATION FOR FAMILY PRACTICE

The educational standards for primary medical care education have recently been highlighted by a special task force of the Canadian Medical Association, which has recommended improvements in training with the responsibility resting with the College of Family Physicians (Wilson et al 1984). More consultation is suggested for the College of Family Physicians with other branches of medicine. Ambulatory training in family practice is considered an essential part of the education of all family physicians. Also emphasized is the need for family doctors to continue to provide primary medical obstetrical services and hospital-based personal medical services to their patients.

If the recommendations of this task force are to be fully imple-mented, two major trends must be reversed. These are the reduced participation by family doctors in hospital care of their patients and the reduced participation by family doctors in obstetrical care, especially intrapartum hospital-based care. The degree of success in reversing these trends will determine by 2000 whether or not Canadian medicine will be one of primary care by family doctors and consulting care by specialists or will be one of fractionated primary care, according to speciality, with general care only being provided by remotely placed family physicians in communities which could not support the complex of specialists required to provide care for all body systems.

PATIENT INPUT INTO DECISIONS

Public involvement in health care matters is increasing. Health coalition groups and patient advocate groups are becoming increasingly organized and increasingly vocal. Hospitals are developing more patient advocate and patient information services. Over 30 Canadian hospitals employ ombudspersons (Watson et al 1984). The role of the family physician as a patient advocate is the one particular role that is not controversial, even in the tertiary care hospitals (Premi et al 1980). A Bill of Rights for patients has been widely publicized, which includes the right to be informed, the right to be respected, the right to participate in both individual patient-care decisions and in health organization decisions, and the right to equal access to health care (Watson et al 1984).

PROBLEMS OF THE NEXT 20 YEARS

For the medical profession, particularly as it relates to primary care, the priority problems include:

1. Education that is appropriate for primary care physicians.
2. Concomitant preparation for appropriate primary care roles for other health professionals.
3. Development of accurate predictors of manpower needs of the future.
4. Cooperation of provincial licensing bodies with the development of the educational systems of medical schools, the Royal College of Physicians and Surgeons and the College of Family Physicians.
5. Very special problems in the appropriate training for family doctors in obstetrics and geriatrics.
6. A continued and active participation by family physicians in their patients' hospital care.

Future needs for 2000 then require greatly improved co-operation amongst the health care disciplines and, within the medical profession, between the specialists and generalists. Appropriate educational programmes must be developed through which professionals can undertake co-operativley the application of their best skills in meeting the health care needs of the population. Improved attitudes, better information, and more rational provision of services by government and the professions are essential to establish better home care services. The appropriate distribution of hospital services must be balanced with community home-based programmes. The continued development of improved lifestyle strategies will depend on professional leadership, but be implemented primarily by lay or public participation.

REFERENCES

Bennett J E, Krasny J 1977 Health care in Canada. The Financial Post (Mar) 26

Biehn J F, McWhinney I R 1983 Family practice in Canada. In: Geyman J P, Fry J (eds) Family practice: an international perspective in developed countries. Appleton-Century-Crofts, Norwalk, Connecticut, ch 3, p 30

Byers A R (ed) 1984a You and the law, 2nd edn. Canadian Automobile Association in conjunction with the Reader's Digest Association (Canada) Ltd, Montreal, ch 12, p 522

Byers A R (ed) 1984b You and the law, 2nd edn. Canadian Automobile Association in conjunction with the Reader's Digest Association (Canada) Ltd, Montreal, ch 10, p 449

Canada Fitness Survey 1983 Fitness and lifestyle in Canada. Government of Canada, Department of Fitness and Amateur Sport

Canada Year Book 1975. Information division, Statistics Canada, ch 1–5

Canadian Family Physician 1984 Executive director's page. Canadian Family Physician 30

Canadian Medical Association 1979 Canadian task force on the periodic health examination. Canadian Medical Association Journal 121: 1193–1254

Carnegie Foundation for the Advancement of Teaching 1910 Medical education in the United States and Canada. Updike D B, the Merrymount Press, Boston

College of Family Physicians of Canada 1983 Health maintenance guide. Committee on patterns of practice and health care delivery. The College of Family Physicians of Canada

Committee on Practice Assessment Assessing the quality of care in the practices of family physicians. College of Family Physicians of Canada

Curry L, MacIntyre K A 1982 The content of family medicine. Do we need more studies? Canadian Family Physician 28: 124–126

Cushing H 1925 The life of Sir William Osler, Oxford University Press, Oxford

Government of Canada 1984 Canada Health Act, (Bill C-3, April 9)

Government of Nova Scotia 1984 Health Services and Insurance Act, ch 50, (Bill 106)

Heagerty J J 1928 Four centuries of medical history in Canada. MacMillan, Toronto

Hennen B K 1982 General practice in the Newcastle undergraduate curriculum. Faculty of Medicine, The University of Newcastle, New South Wales

Kirsh S 1983 Unemployment, its impact on body and soul. Canadian Mental Health Association, p ix

Klein M, Reynold J L, Boucher F, Malus M, Rosenberg E 1984 Obstetrical practice and training in Canadian family medicine: conserving an endangered species. Canadian Family Physician 30: 2093–2099

Klotz P G 1982 Peer assessment program educational, not punitive. Ontario Medical Review (Jan): 21–22

Lalonde M a 1975 A new perspective on the health of Canadians. Information Canada, 66

Leighton A 1982 Caring for mentally ill people. Cambridge University Press, Cambridge

Mental Health Services in Canada 1982 edn. Health and Walfare Canada, table 11

Premi J N, Johnston M A, Shea P E, Tweedie T 1980 The role of the family physician in hospital. IV. FP's attitudes towards their hospital role. Canadian Family Physician 26: 521–524

Royal College of Physicians and Surgeons of Canada 1984. Submission to task force on allocation of health care resources

Seidelman W E, Moore C A, McLean D W 1982 Paying for primary care: innovation in Ontario. Canadian Family Physician 28: 893–894

Spitzer W 1984 The nurse practitioner revisited: slow death of a good idea. New England Journal of Medicine (April)

Stewart M 1982 Factors affecting patients' compliance with doctor's advice. Canadian Family Physician 28: 1519–1526

Watson J, McGibbon P, O'Brien-Bell J, Richard L, Romanow R 1984 Health, a need for redirection. A task force on the allocation of health care resources. Canadian Medical Association Journal

Wilson D L et al 1984 Family practice training: an evolutionary plan. Report of the Canadian Medical Association task force on education for the provision of primary care services to Canadian Medical Association General Council

Woods D 1979a Strength in study. The College of Family Physicians of Canada, Toronto, p 3

Woods D 1979b Strength in study. The College of Family Physicians of Canada, Toronto, p 7

Woods D 1979c Strength in study. The College of Family Physicians of Canada, Toronto, p 170

Woods Gordon 1984 Investigation of the impact of demographic change on the health care system of Canada. A commission of the Canadian Medical Association task force on the allocation of health care resources, table 12

USSR

THE COUNTRY

Although often described as 'Russia', the Soviet Union is an enormous multinational state in which ethnic Russians account for only just over half of the total population. It has a federal constitutional structure consisting of 15 Union republics whose boundaries coincide, to varying extents, with major historical homelands.

A glance at a map confirms that one republic clearly predominates over all others: extending from Baltic Sea to Pacific Ocean, the Russian Soviet Federated Socialist Republic occupies 17 million out of the country's total area of 22 million km^2. Its population at the beginning of 1983 was 141 million as against 271 million for the whole Union. Next down the scale comes the Ukrainian republic with a territory of 604 000 km^2 and a population of just over 50 million persons. Excluding Uzbekistan and Kazakhstan, the other republics contain fewer than 10 million inhabitants.

Its federal structure notwithstanding, the Soviet polity is characterized by a high degree of centralization. While that key feature represents an element of continuity with the Russian imperial past, it should be explained primarily in terms of the unifying control exercised by the Communist Party of the Soviet Union (CPSU). To quote from Article 6 of the 1977 Constitution, the Party is 'the leading and guiding force of Soviet society, and the nucleus of its political system and of all state and public organizations'. The concept of 'democratic centralism', which underlies the Party's mode of operation, serves to legitimate concentration of decision-taking at the highest levels of authority in Moscow.

Over the decades, the CPSU leadership has attempted to foster the emergence of a 'new Soviet man', and state institutions, especially educational ones, are expected to influence sociocultural values to this end. According to Marxist-Leninist ideology, attitudinal change constitutes one prerequisite for the emergence of full communism, society being currently at the stage of 'developed socialism'.

If the Soviet Union's political structure conduces to uniformity, its geography must be classed as a factor working in the opposite direction. Occupying almost a sixth of the world's inhabited surface, this vast land mass contains a fascinating diversity of topography, vegetation and climatic conditions. In many regions, for example the far north, the physical environment can hardly fail to influence the inhabitants' outlook and life-styles. The existence of thousands of remote villages (called 'bears' corners' by the Russians) poses difficult organizational problems for the delivery of public services.

Responsibility for those services rests unequivocally with the State, in keeping with the ideological imperative of public owner-ship of the means of production and distribution. Thus they are planned as integral elements in the total socioeconomic infrastruc-ture: the pace, extent and character of their development is deter-mined by decisions of the CPSU and government.

THE HEALTH CARE SYSTEM

Turning now to the system of health care (*zdravookhranenie*), the first point to be made is a methodological one. While official accounts of social institutions in any country may call for discrimi-nating interpretation, that caution applies with uncommon force to the Soviet Union. A one-party state with the geopolitical role of a superpower, it has compelling reasons to convey an idealized picture of its health service to both its own population and the outside world. As I have demonstrated elsewhere, the standard Soviet descriptions are substantially misleading unless accompanied by detailed explication and qualification (Ryan 1978).

Since the early days of industrialization and urbanization in the 1920s and 1930s, a vast quantitative increase has occurred in health care facilities. While that achievement must not be under-rated, it is essential to recognize the heavily instrumental justification for the expenditure entailed: provision of medical care was and still is perceived as a factor contributing to the productivity of the current labour force and to potential productivity in the younger generation.

Very large increases in basic 'inputs' have continued to be recorded since the end of the Second World War. As Table 19.1 shows, during the period 1950–1982 the number of doctors and

Table 19.1 Basic indicators of health service development 1950–1982

| | In thousands, end of year: | | | | |
	1950	1960	1970	1980	1982
Doctors	236.9	385.4	577.3		
Dentists with:				997.1	1071.2
higher education	10.4	16.2	39.6		
intermediate education	17.7	30.1	51.5		
Middle-grade medical personnel*	719	1388	2123	2814	2963
Hospitals	18.3	26.7	26.2	23.1	23.1
Hospital beds	1011	1739	2663	3324	3443
Units providing ambulatory-policlinic care	36.2	39.3	37.4	36.1	37.0

* This category consists mainly of feldshers, feldsher-midwives, midwives, environmental health officers, nurses, medical laboratory staff, radiotherapists and dental technicians.
Sources: Tsentralnoe Statisticheskoe Upravlenie SSSR 1971 and 1983

dentists rose sharply from 265 000 to 1 071 200, i.e., by 304%. Paramedics, or middle-grade medical personnel, to use the Russian terminology, increased by 312% and the total complement of hospital beds rose by 241%. Whatever the quality of care provided, access to it has greatly improved, at least for the majority of people.

In the same time-frame, the ratio of hospital beds to population rose from 55.7 to 127.1 per 10 000 and the ratio for paramedics from 39.6 to 109.4 per 10 000. Doctors and dentists taken together increased from 14.6 to 39.5 per 10 000. (Only an aggregate figure is published for recent years but it can be estimated that the two grades of dentists now account for about 14% of the total.)

These data, which represent averages for the Union, conceal marked spatial variations, both as between individual republics and as between urban and rural areas. Republican governments and their health ministries receive planning targets for these inputs from the USSR Ministry of Health but have the right to exceed them.

It should also be noted that the data relate not to a single civilian health service but to several. This plurality exists because certain ministries and departments run schemes for their own employees throughout the USSR. In general these absorb relatively few staff and capital resources although it is interesting that the service for railway workers, started in the 1920s, operates on a fairly extensive scale.

Even the main health service, subordinate to the USSR Ministry of Health, is multiform at local level. Thus facilities for both ambulatory and inpatient care are found at industrial plants, mines and other workplaces, in addition to the units serving specific territorial areas, such as the district of a town. A third subsystem exists for the country's elite, in particular for high-ranking officials of the Party and government.

Primary health care

Some indication of the balance between primary health care and other elements in the service emerges from Table 19.2. Admittedly what it reproduces are planning norms published in 1974 and intended for implementation by about 1990. However, the current position is unlikely to diverge from that picture to any great extent. From the table it can be calculated that ambulatory-policlinic care was assigned just over half (52.2%) of the total medical manpower.

In *urban areas* primary care is delivered, not exclusively but to a large extent, from *policlinics*. It should be emphasized that though they are generally quite sizeable units, many of them do not treat all categories of disease or admit the full age-range of the population. In addition to separate policlinics for children, there is also a range of dispensaries for specific disease categories including cardiology, tuberculosis, dermatovenereology, oncology and psychoneurology. The existence of other specialized facilities fragments the first line of health care still further.

In the *countryside*, district-centres also contain *policlinics* but many smaller settlements are served by what are termed *ambulatories*: these function with much lower levels of staff and equipment. Patients in the most sparsely populated and outlying areas receive initial diagnosis and a certain amount of treatment at *feldsher or*

Table 19.2   Norms for staffing levels in the main divisions of the health service

	Doctors per 1000 persons
Hospital care for urban and rural population total	11.35
Ambulatory-policlinic care: total	20.78
within which for: urban population	23.57
: rural population	14.29
First aid and emergency medical care	1.29
Sanatoria — health resort institutions	1.06
Sanitary — prophylactic institutions	2.04
Other health service instituttions	0.58
Educational establishments, scientific research institutes, organs of health service administration	2.7
Average for USSR as a whole	39.8

Source: Malov & Churakov 1981

feldsher-midwife posts. Shortage of doctors in rural areas represents a long-standing problem which would be more acute but for the 'drafting' there of newly qualified staff for a period of three years.

The salience of policlinics and ambulatories can be assessed by reference to two key statistics. In 1980, according to one textbook, these units represented over 75% of all non-hospital institutions and accounted for about 85% of non-hospital consultations conducted by doctors (Serenko & Ermakova 1984). That second figure almost certainly includes home visits.

The same source points to the very high degree of integration which exists in the physical structure of health care plant: as many as 93% of hospital and non-hospital institutions are described as 'unified'. In practical terms this means that policlinics are frequently sited within the curtilage of hospitals, with one head doctor having overall responsibility for both. During recent years, it should be added, a number of 'self-standing' policlinics have been constructed in order to facilitate access for patients.

Quality controls

The treatment of ambulatory patients, like other forms of medical practice in the USSR, is subject to a number of checks and investigative procedures which range from 'in-house' supervision by a hierarchical superior to a full legal trial. Whether or not a complaint has been received, each health service unit is required to investigate any fatal outcome of care provided in its catchment area and, if gross errors are discovered, the matter must be considered by the relevant machinery. What are termed treatment control commissions, composed entirely of doctors, can be set up at various levels to establish whether a breach of duty has occurred. Overlapping them to some extent are medicolegal commissions, also ad hoc bodies, which are linked to a branch of the legal system known as the Procuracy. Moreover, clinicians may find themselves subject to disciplinary measures following a third type of investigation — one undertaken by the Peoples' Control Commission, which has a watchdog role for all public services. However, to point out the existence of these forms of control is not to demonstrate that they raise the general standards of medical practice.

Payment of doctors

Given that all health service staff have the status of employees, their remuneration, predictably enough, is by means of salary. Wide differentials exist between senior medicobureaucrats and top academics on the one hand and the ordinary policlinic doctors on the other. Additions to the basic salary can be achieved in various ways, for example by working in the far north or by passing into a higher qualificatory category in the scheme of accreditation known as attestation.

The fact that the salary of many doctors is less than the national average wage directly reflects the low priority-tag attached by the Party leaders to this 'non-productive' sector of the economy. It would be most curious if that did not also affect the social standing of doctors or go some way towards explaining the very high proportion of women physicians and dentists. (In 1982 the figure stood at 68%.)

However, a doctor's 'command over resources' can far exceed his or her salary, thanks to favours and gifts in cash or kind from health service patients. Private practice is not prohibited but cannot be undertaken openly in purpose-designed and suitably equipped buildings.

Arguably, the prevalence of overt private medicine is an issue of less significance than the blurring of distinctions between health service and private consultations, which results from unofficial 'payments' for the former. Perusal of the Soviet press leaves little room for doubt that many health service staff expect to be rewarded in this way; there is a high probability that the well-publicized cases of extortion which come to court form only the tip of a large iceberg.

Vestigial generalists

Although Russians employ the phrases 'family doctor' and 'home doctor', important differences separate the relevant category of physician from the community general practitioner familiar in the United Kingdom. In the first place, no Soviet doctor trains as a generalist: in place of a single curriculum for all students, medical institutes have one or more basic specialist tracks — in 'curative medicine', paediatrics, environmental health, stomatology and, for small numbers, non-clinical medical science.

It is true that many of the *terapevti* (general physicians) at a policlinic are intended to act as doctor of first contact for specific microdistricts in the catchment area. The effectiveness of this strategy, however, must be substantially impaired when children normally make their initial visits to microdistrict paediatricians, and many employed adults consult a different *terapevt* at their place of work. In addition, patients have direct access to more specialized staff at the policlinic or elsewhere; thus many women will proceed straight to an obstretrician-gynaecologist. In the case of an accident or emergency, a patient will often be treated by personnel of the units created for such work.

References to a high turnover rate among microdistrict doctors can be found in Soviet sources. According to one article, only 3–10% of all such staff had worked in the same place for over 10 years. It also afforded revealing insights into the frustrations which they experience, as in the following passage:

> Many instructions which regulate the doctor's activities have long since become outdated . . . Why should the duration of a visit always be determined by an instruction and not by the doctor, having regard to the nature of the illness, the patient's condition, and so on? Hasn't the instruction prescribing an obligatory repeat visit on the third day become obsolete? What if a patient has a hypertensive disease or an aggravated ulcer? With such illnesses, it is not only unnecessary but harmful to interrupt the regime of bed-rest and go to the policlinic.
>
> (Paikin & Silina 1978)

Standards of education

Regarding the standards of medical education and quality of treatment, wide-ranging evidence to support generalizations is not easily obtained. Nevertheless, it should be mentioned that in 1983 a professor from Grodno lifted the veil a little when he spoke out about gross deficiencies in the work of medical institutes. His article contained this indictment:

> Whether we intend it or not, to all intents and purposes we have freed the student from responsibility for acquiring knowledge, and this is the origin of the professional incompetence, maladjustment and irresponsibility which are so often encountered.
>
> (Brzhesky 1983)

Perhaps following that lead, a subsequent article expressed strongly critical views about the competence of recently qualified staff. Among other things, the author stated:

> It transpires that a young doctor still requires years to be proficient in, for example, methods of resuscitation . . . Sometimes he gets confused over elementary questions in the diagnosis of acute cardiovascular diseases and acute diseases of the organs of the abdominal cavity.
>
> (Kaverin 1984)

Patterns of work

Data on common disease problems, as a rule, relate only to a specific town, rural district or the catchment area of one health service unit. Any attempt to summarize and synthesize such reports is precluded by considerations of space. However, reference should be made to the fact that a large proportion of all ambulatory and domicilary consultations (which came to an average of 10.9 per person in 1982) occur in connection with surveillance of chronic illness and routine health checks. Whether the heavy emphasis on screening and presymptomatic diagnosis should be endorsed is a matter for debate.

A range of factors influences the balance between ambulatory-polyclinic and inpatient care: most of them interact to work in favour of the latter. Perhaps the most crucial is the absence of a counterpoise to hospitalization in the form of holistic community-based practice. Moreover, the conventional wisdom has long regarded inpatient care as preferable on the 'external' economic grounds that it obviates the need for working women to stay at home caring for a sick relative, and that fewer work days are lost by the patient if he is treated in hospital. Poor housing conditions, which include overcrowding, also been an indication for hospitalization.

The generous provision of hospital beds is predicated upon and allows for high rates of admission. In 1982, taking the Union as a whole, 24% of the population became inpatients at some time or other. Mainly because ambulatory-policlinic care is less well developed in the countryside, the rural population has a somewhat higher hospitalization rate than town dwellers. For decades now, Soviet sources have repeated the statement that 80% of all episodes of diagnosed illness run their course in the community and 'only' 20% involve hospitalization.

The status of doctors

As for relations with the general public, the essential point (in this author's judgement) is that Soviet doctors do not form a cohesive, high-status, self-confident group who take collective initiatives locally or nationally on key policy issues. Their relative passivity, like that of other white-collar workers in the USSR, has been conditioned by the power and leadership role of the CPSU, and it is probably not an exaggeration to say that medicine in the Soviet Union has become deprofessionalized. Certainly, a sense of status deprivation emerges from a number of recent articles, including one which stated: 'It is necessary to consider how doctors can be protected against undeserved attacks, mockery and humiliation and to consider how their prestige can be increased and strengthened in every possible way.' (Yanushkevichus 1981) Lack of respect for a doctor, the writer considered, had a harmful effect on the task of protecting people's health and it greatly reduced the effectiveness of medical activity.

FUTURE NEEDS

Looking to the future, it can be seen that the quantitative planning targets for the 1990s are now within easy reach. So norms for staffing ratios, average number of ambulatory consultations and hospitalization rates should be achieved if not exceeded. Spatial variations between republics will probably become less marked, as is intended, and upgrading of the ambulatory-policlinic service for rural areas seems likely to be a high priority. Even greater attention will be devoted to prophylaxis, in line with the decision announced by Yuri Andropov in June 1983 that the entire population should have a health check every year.

It would be interesting to know what Soviet patients themselves perceive as the features of their health service which are most in need of improvement. In all likelihood, the majority would favour a two-fold change: a less fragmented and specialized system, and care that is far more sympathetic and personalized.

There can be little doubt that concern exists at a high level about doctors' lack of motivation and other factors which give rise to complaints of brusqueness, inattention and 'formalism', not to mention grosser deviations such as extortion. But the actions envisaged to deal with these phenomena are conceptualized in terms of a conflictual model which requires Party and government to 'wage an implacable fight' against them. It may well be that ideological considerations rule out the adoption of a more consensual model of relationships which would entail granting doctors greater opportunities for self-esteem and collective self-determination. Arguably, however, that represents the most effective method of raising the quality of primary medical care in the Soviet Union.

REFERENCES AND FURTHER READING

Brzheski V 1983 Pochemu ne strog ekzamenator. Meditsinskaya Gazeta 94:3
Kaverin N 1984 Bez skidok na molodost. Meditsinskaya Gazeta 24:1
Malov N I, Churakov VI 1981 Sovremennie osnovi i metodi planirovaniya
    razvitiya zdravookhraneniya. Ekonomika, Moskva, p 188
Paikin A, Silina G 1978 Uchastkovi vrach. Literaturnaya Gazeta 39:11
Ryan M 1978 The organization of Soviet medical care. Basil Blackwell and Martin
    Robertson, Oxford and London
Serenko A F, Ermakova VV 1984 Sotsialnaya gigiena: organizatsiya
    zdravookhraneniya, 2oe izdanie. Meditsina, Moskva, p 264–265
Tsentralnoe Statisticheskoe Upravlenie SSSR 1971 Narodnoe Khozyaistvo SSSR v
    1970g. Finansi i Statistika, Moskva, p 689
Tsentralnoe Statisticheskoe Upravlenie SSSR 1983 Narodnoe Khozyaistvo SSSR v
    1982g. Finansi i Statistika, Moskva, p 497
Yanushkevichus Z 1981 V osnove-doverie. Pravda 221:3

People's Republic of China

NATIONAL FEATURES

Recorded history in China extends back over 4000 years and a highly developed civilization, based on agriculture in China's great river valleys, has been in existence for well over two millenia. Social organization for much of this period was feudal, based on dynasties. A powerful, highly educated and wealthy elite, through most of China's history, has governed a little educated, relatively poor, powerless peasantry.

Culturally and socially, the teachings of Confucius on family and social hierarchy and responsibility have for centuries played a major role in Chinese life. A common written language has helped to unify China, just as diverse speech dialects have tended to divide it. Both social organization and cultural social patterns were profoundly altered by the taking of state power by Mao Zedong and the Chinese Communist Party in 1949, but many of china's deep-rooted patterns of family life, respect for the elderly and love of children, and community organization persist and, indeed, have formed the base for some of the changes.

China's mainland territory, an area approximately the same size as Australia, Canada, or the United States, is the home of what is by far the world's largest population, over 1 billion people. Of its land area, however, only a relatively small part is arable; China must feed approximately 20% of the world's population with only 8% of the world's cultivated land.

China's population is, furthermore, most unevenly distributed. The vast majority of the people live in eastern China, with its three great river basins; western China, with its mountains and deserts, is exceedingly sparsely populated. The four least densely populated sections — Inner Mongolia, Sinkiang, Tsinghai and Tibet — comprise just over half of the area of the country, but contain less than 4% of the population. Overall, some 80% of the Chinese people live in rural areas and only 20% in cities and towns.

China, technologically, is a poorly-developed country with a gross national product estimated at $400 per capita. Great differences exist in material well-being between the cities and the countryside, and especially in the past few years between different rural areas and even within areas, but far less than the chiasm that existed prior to 1949, not only between city and country but also between the rich and poor of the cities and between the landlords and peasants of the countryside. In agriculture, labour-intensive rather than mechanized methods are largely used. Employment is guaranteed by the state but a significant amount of unemployment does exist, particularly in the urban areas. Most of the economy is a structured and planned socialist economy, but elements of 'free enterprise' have been introduced since the end of the Cultural Revolution in 1976, and their importance in the economy is increasing.

China's health services thus have had to deal with the needs of a vast country and an even greater population, predominantly rural, unevenly distributed, and extremely poor in material goods compared to the people of the technologically-developed countries. Western visitors, returning to China in the 1970s after two decades, reported a nation of healthy-looking, vigorous people. There was no evidence of the widespread malnutrition or the ubiquitous infectious disease and other ill health that accompanies poverty in most other countries of the world and was so prevalent in China 30 years ago. Infant mortality has been sharply reduced, from over 200 in the 1940s to approximately 40 deaths in the first year of life per 1000 live births today, and life expectancy at birth has increased from some 35 to 68 years today.

These changes in health status are not solely the results of changes in medical care, or even in what is usually defined as health care; improvements in nutrition, sanitation and living standards are at least as important. But changes in health care and in medical care have undoubtedly played an important role. Among those elements of the health-care and medical-care system in China that are of special interest are:

1. The society's fundamental redistribution of wealth and power, which made possible many of the changes that have occurred.

2. The system's emphasis on preventive medicine.

3. Its utilization of traditional Chinese medicine in combination with 'Western' medicine.

4. Its training of part-time health workers who remain integral members of the community and, at least until recently, provide most of the primary care.

5. Its attempts to mobilize the mass of people to protect their own health and the health of their neighbours.

HEALTH SYSTEM — EVOLUTION AND FORMAT

The first four millenia

There are two distinct streams of medicine in China — 'Chinese medicine' and 'Western medicine'. Until the 17th century, the history of medicine in China was synonymous with the history of traditional medicine; external influences and invasions of foreigners were simply absorbed and transmitted into the Chinese way of thinking.

Chinese traditional medicine is probably the world's oldest body of medical knowledge, having a history of several thousand years of accumulated empirical observations and abstruse and complex theory. By virtue of its rich and ancient theoretical base, Chinese traditional medicine, which incorporates both diagnosis and therapy, differs from many other systems of folk medicine, which are based purely on empirical observations. Diagnostic methods include observation and questioning of the patient, and detailed and prolonged palpation of the pulse; therapy makes use of medicinal herbs, moxibustion, breathing and gymnastic exercises, and acupuncture.

The theoretical concepts of health and disease are based, for the most part, on a philosophical view of nature, on a belief in the unity of man and the universe. The human body is seen as constantly influenced by the complementary forces of *yin* and *yang*; if all the forces are in balance, in harmony with the season and even the time of day, the human body is in good health. If there is imbalance or disharmony, disease may result. The object of medical care is therefore restoration of balance, rather than a 'cure' of disease.

Physicians were first appointed to the courts of the grandees during the 4th century B.C. The primary responsibility of government physicians attached to the courts was the examination of the numerous personnel of the palace and the early detection of disease; they were also responsible for food control and general hygiene. Thus, the current Chinese emphasis on prevention is not a purely contemporary phenomenon, for traditionally the physician who knew how to prevent disease was more highly respected than one who waited until the patient was sick.

The first Jesuit missionaries began arriving in China at the beginning of the 17th century and initiated the introduction of Western medicine to China. With the expansion of Western medicine through the missionary efforts of the 19th century, there arose great conflicts between the practitioners of the two schools. On the one hand, stories were spread about the 'evil practices' of Western doctors; on the other, traditional medicine was condemned as false and superstitious. The Chinese people were often torn between their faith in traditional medicine and the evidence of the efficacy of Western practices, particularly in surgery and obstetrics. In the cities, while the status and prestige of Western doctors increased relative to that of traditional doctors, there were far too few of them to meet the needs of people, particularly the poor. In the rural areas, except for major provincial towns, Western-type medicine was almost non-existent.

Schools of Western medicine were established in China during the late 19th century and the early decades of the 20th century. The first was established in Tientsin in 1881 by a Scottish physician, and during the next 30 years several other medical schools were founded under the auspices of foreign governments. As part of the Boxer Rebellion and the accompanying hostility toward foreigners, medical facilities were destroyed during the summer of 1900 and more than 100 Protestant missionaries were killed. It became apparent that missionary groups would have to pool their resources; thus, in 1906 under the leadership of the London Missionary Society, the Union Medical College was founded. 15 years later, with funding from the Rockefeller Foundation, it was to become the famed Peking Union Medical College. By 1913 there were, in all, approximately 500 Chinese students studying Western medicine in China under the auspices of foreign powers and only a relatively small number of Westerners practising in China.

Health Care in China in the 1930s and 1940s

The Peking Union Medical College (PUMC) was to become symbolic as a centre of excellence in a country racked by poverty, hunger, disease and eventually war. While the teaching and research were distinguished in many departments, in both the clinical and basic sciences, the work in public health is particularly noteworthy. John B. Grant, born in China of Canadian parents and educated in Canada and the United States, began to develop a programme in public health at PUMC at the time the college was opened. There were essentially no national or municipal public health services in China, and Grant attempted to develop a community-based public health programme, establishing an experimental health centre in Peking supported jointly by PUMC and the municipality. A programme in maternal and child health, which included the training of midwives, operated out of the health centre; there was a desperate need for such a programme, since, while there were an estimated 200 000 untrained midwives in China during the mid-1920s, there were only 500 trained midwives. A school health programme was also developed stressing immunization, sanitation and health education.

Perhaps the most impressive aspect of Grant's public health work at PUMC was effort to develop a rural health programme in Ting-Xian (county) 100 miles outside of Peking. Village health workers were trained to work with the peasants in the areas of immunization, first aid, the registration of births and deaths, health education and the treatment of minor ailments. A physician was available at a district health station for referrals and the training of the village health workers. While this programme was in some ways a forerunner of the present-day Chinese rural health network, it could have little impact because of the political structure of the time and the poverty under which people lived. Nevertheless, some of its elements were nearly 20 years and a revolution ahead of their time for China and untold decades ahead of other developing countries. With the Japanese occupation in 1941, the PUMC faculty was dispersed to a number of hospitals in the rest of the country. The college reopened in 1947 and was nationalized by the new government on January 20, 1951.

There is common agreement that prior to 1949, the date of the formal assumption of state power by Mao Zedong and the Chinese Communist party — an event the Chinese refer to as the 'Liberation' — the state of health of the vast majority of the Chinese people was extremely poor and the health services provided for them were grossly inadequate. The people of China in the 1930s and 1940s suffered the consequences of widespread poverty, poor sanitation, continuing war and rampant disease. The crude death rate was estimated at about 25 deaths per 1000, one of the world's highest, and its infant mortality and life expectancy, as we have noted, were among the poorest in the world.

Most deaths in China were due to infectious diseases, usually complicated by some form of malnutrition. Prevalent infectious diseases included bacterial illnesses such as cholera, diphtheria, gonorrhea, leprosy, meningococcal meningitis, plague, relapsing fever, syphilis, tetanus, tuberculosis, typhoid fever and typhus; viral illnesses such as Japanese B encephalitis, smallpox and trachoma; and parasitic illnesses such as ancylostomiasis (hook-worm disease), clonorchiasis, filariasis, kala azar, malaria, paragonimiasis, and schistosomiasis. Venereal disease was widespread. Nutritional illnesses included most known forms of total calorie, protein and specific vitamin deficiencies, including beriberi, pellagra and scurvy. 'Malnutrition' was often a euphemism for starvation.

Preventive medicine was almost non-existent in most of China, except for areas where special projects, such as John Grant's work at PUMC, were conducted, usually with foreign funding. Therapeutic medicine of the modern scientific type was almost completely unavailable in the rural areas — where 85% of China's people lived — and for most poor urban dwellers. Estimates of the number of physicians in China in 1949 who were trained in Western medicine vary from 10 000 to 40 000; the best estimate seems to be about 20 000, or approximately 1 doctor for every 25 000 of the roughly 500 million people in China at that time. Most of these were either doctors from Western countries, usually missionaries, or doctors trained in schools supported and directed from abroad; they were mainly concentrated in the cities of eastern China.

Nurses and other types of health workers were in even shorter supply, and the minimal efforts in the 1930s to train new types of health workers to meet the needs of China's rural population were largely controlled from abroad, usually poorly supported by the people they were supposed to serve and poorly integrated with their lives and needs.

The bulk of the medical care available to the Chinese people was provided by the roughly half-million practitioners of traditional medicine who ranged from poorly educated pill peddlers to well-trained and widely experienced practitioners of the medicine the Chinese had developed over two millennia. These practitioners, and those who practised Western medicine, remained deeply mistrustful of each other and blocked each other's efforts in many ways.

Probably most important of all, 75% of the Chinese people were said to be illiterate. Cycles of flood and drought kept most of the people starving or, at the least, undernourished. And the limited resources that did exist were maldistributed, so that a few lived in comfort and the vast majority lived a life of grinding poverty. Feelings of powerlessness and hopelessness were widespread; individual efforts were of little avail, and community efforts were almost impossible to organize.

Experiments in meeting these needs were started during the 1930s and 1940s by Mao Zedong and the People's Liberation Army, first in Kiangsi Province and then, after the Long March, in the area around Yenan in Shensi Province. These efforts involved mobilizing the people to educate themselves and encouraging them individually and collectively to provide their own health-care and medical-care services.

Health care from Liberation to the Cultural Revolution

Following Liberation in 1949, the efforts of the 1930s and 1940s to provide health services were expanded into a national policy that included the following elements:

1. Medicine should serve the needs of the workers, peasants and soldiers, that is, those who previously had the least services were now to be the specially favoured recipients of services.

2. Preventive medicine should be put first, that is, where resources were limited, preventive medicine was to take precedence over therapeutic medicine.

3. Chinese traditional medicine should be integrated with Western scientific medicine, that is, instead of competing, the practitioners of the two types of medical care should learn from each other.

4. Health work should be conducted with mass participation, that is, everyone in the society was to be encouraged to play an organized role in the protection of his own health and that of his neighbors.

Some of the efforts of the 1950s and early 1960s were based on models from other countries, particularly the Soviet Union, which provided a large amount of technical assistance to China during this period. A number of new medical schools were established, some of the older ones were moved from the cities of the east coast to areas of even greater need further west, and class size was vastly expanded.

These efforts produced a remarkably large number of 'higher' medical graduates, including stomatologists (dentists), pharmacologists and public-health specialists as well as physicians. The physicians were trained, following the Soviet model, either to treat adults or children. It has been estimated that more than 100 000 doctors were trained over 15 years, an increase of some 500%. But by 1965 China's population had increased to about 700 million, and the doctor/population ratio was still less than 1 per 500 people.

At the same time large numbers of 'middle' medical schools were established to train assistant doctors (modelled in some ways on the Soviet *feldshers*), nurses, midwives, pharmacists, technicians and sanitarians. These schools accepted students after 9 or 10 years of schooling and had a curriculum of 2–3 years. It has been estimated that some 170 000 assistant doctors, 185 000 nurses, 40 000 midwives and 200 000 pharmacists were trained.

In addition to these efforts to produce rapidly many more professional health workers, people in the community were mobilized to perform health-related tasks themselves. A large-scale attack was made on illiteracy and superstition. By means of mass campaigns, people were organized so as to accomplish together what they could not do individually. Using these techniques of mobilizing the general population to participate actively in the provision of medical care and the prevention of illness, such diseases as smallpox, cholera, typhus and plague were completely eliminated. Venereal disease and kala azar were markedly reduced, and diseases such as malaria and filariasis are being rapidly brought under control. Tuberculosis, trachoma, schistosomiasis and ancylostomiasis are still not under full control, although their prevalence is being markedly reduced. In short, the successes in the prevention of infectious disease over a time-span of only one generation were truly monumental.

Health care during the Cultural Revolution

In 1965, in a written directive that was one of the forerunners of what came to be known as the Great Proletarian Cultural Revolution, Mao severely criticized the Ministry of Health for what he called its overattention to urban problems. He urged a series of changes in medical education, medical research and medical practice. His statement, known throughout China as the June 26th Directive, conluded: 'In medical and health work, put the stress on the rural areas!' As a result of this directive, and of the Cultural Revolution of 1966–69, much in medicine was markedly reorganized. Higher medical schools began to admit students who had had less previous schooling (often as little as junior middle school, but with considerable work experience) and the curriculum was markedly shortened and altered to emphasize practice in the rural areas and the combination of Western and traditional Chinese medicine.

The Cultural Revolution also brought about great changes in medical practice. Peasant health workers who came to be known as 'barefoot doctors' were trained in large numbers and given responsibility for the provision of primary care, environmental sanitation, health education and preventive medicine. Although 'barefoot doctors' actually wear shoes most of the time, and especially while performing their medical tasks, the term is used to emphasize the fact that these personnel are peasants who perform their medical work while maintaining their agricultural tasks.

Barefoot doctors, trained for relatively brief periods of time, generally work in health centres provided at the brigade level of the commune structure. They provide treatment for 'minor and common illnesses', are skilled in first aid and are available for medical emergencies. Their emphasis has also been on preventive medicine — sanitation, health education and the provision of immunizations. Barefoot doctors had a clear referral path, again embedded in the commune structure; patients who needed more expert care were referred for primary and secondary care by physicians in the commune hospitals. If more specialized care were needed, the patient could be referred to a hospital at the county level, the third level of the 'three tier' system in the countryside.

The urban counterparts to the barefoot doctor were 'worker doctors' in the factories, Red Medical Workers in the urban neighbourhoods. They, like the barefoot doctor, were given responsibility for first level care, for preventive medicine, and for health education. They were, in addition, responsible for family planning at the local level. Primary care by physicians was provided at neighbourhood medical centres, which usually also had some beds for inpatient care; tertiary care was provided at district and municipal hospitals.

Health care since the Cultural Revolution

During the late 1970s, following the end of the Cultural Revolution, there began to be open criticism of the barefoot doctors. Their training was said to be uneven, their supervision sometimes inadequate, and their practice at times incompetent. Examples of mistakes made by barefoot doctors appeared in the Chinese press and a few critics suggested that some barefoot doctors went beyond the limits of their technical knowledge. In keeping with the Chinese drive to improve technical quality, local departments of public health began markedly to upgrade the training of barefoot doctors, require the demonstration of their knowledge through examinations, define their role more narrowly, reduce their numbers, increase their supervison by more extensively trained medical personnel, and, to some extent, centralize the structure in which they work. Overall, Chinese estimates of the number of barefoot doctors in China fell from 1.8 million in 1975 to approximately 1.5 million in 1980, and to approximately 1.2 million in 1982.

In addition, since the late 1970s fundamental changes have taken place within Chinese society and particularly in the rural areas. As part of an attempt by the Chinese government to increase production, the 'contracted production responsibility system' has been introduced into the rural areas all over China, giving individual households responsibility for production on communally-owned land. Peasants now receive direct financial rewards for individual or family output and, as a consequence, the economic structure of the communes has been significantly weakened. Almost 80% of the brigades have shifted from a collective to a household-based system of production. Since the barefoot doctors and the co-operative medical services were largely financed by commune funds, the implications of these changes for health care in the rural areas are critical. Some recent visitors have reported instances of private fee-for-service practice by some barefoot doctors; other observers note that less attention is being paid to public health matters such as sanitation and safe water supplies. Furthermore, it is not clear that the barefoot doctor system, as it is now structured, can survive the emphasis on professionalism and technology that is characteristic of China's modernization effort.

CURRENT PRIMARY HEALTH CARE

Despite the reduction in their numbers and in the structure of their practice, barefoot doctors continue to be the main source of primary care in the countryside. They provide both preventive care and first-level treatment, working from health stations at the 'production brigade' level. As we have noted, the services in the brigade health stations — as well as in the commune and country hospitals — had largely been financed by the co-operative medical care system. At its peak, some 80–90% of China's rural population was covered by this method; as a result of the economic changes in the countryside, it is reported that only 40–50% of the rural population is now covered. Not only are some barefoot doctors shifting to fee-for-service practice, but it is said that in many areas their continuing education is being affected by the change. In the past the cost of their training, at the commune or county hospitals, and their salaries during this training were paid by the co-operative medical care system; now they have far greater difficulty obtaining continuing education.

The second tier of care for the rural population remains the commune hospital, staffed largely by 'assistant doctors' with 3–4 years of training or upgraded from the barefoot doctor level following examination, and by a few 'higher-level' doctors with 5–6 years of training. Facilities at this level, like the brigade health stations are technologically poorly equipped. Care at the third tier, the county hospital, is more technologically-based, but usually at a considerably lower level than in the urban tertiary care hospitals, to which a small percentage of rural patients are referred.

In the cities, the local primary health care workers called Red Medical Workers during the Cultural Revolution are now called Red Cross Health Workers. They work in what are now known as Red Cross health stations in the urban areas providing first-contact basic primary care. Patients with more serious problems (but those that would still fall in most countries under the heading of primary care) are referred, or are increasingly likely to go directly, to the neighbourhood hospitals. These are largely ambulatory care centres, but usually include some inpatient beds. They are staffed by assistant doctors, doctors trained in Western-style medicine, and doctors of traditional Chinese medicine. The Western-type doctors in the larger neighbourhood hospitals practise in the 'polyclinic' style, with different doctors concerned with pediatrics and with adult medicine and with a number of specialty clinics available. Most secondary and all tertiary care patients are referred to the urban third tier, the district hospitals and, when necessary, to municipal and specialized hospitals. The technological level of the municipal and specialized hospitals — particularly those affiliated with medical schools — are far superior to those at lower levels in the cities and to those at all three tiers of the rural system, but are still considerably below the level of comparable institutions in the technologically-developed countries.

Patients who work in government enterprises are covered entirely for medical care costs, and one-half the costs of their dependents' care is covered. Others must bear the cost of their own care, although most preventive care and some treatment are subsidized by government funds.

In large factories a highly-organized medical service provide both primary care, including preventive service, and secondary care. The 'worker doctors' who provided first-contact care during the Cultural Revolution have largely been replaced by assistant doctors and fully-trained doctors.

Overall, the intense control during the Cultural Revolution of local health services by committees of local people has been dissolved. Control of technical quality at local levels is now exercised hierarchically through professional channels, extending upward through the municipal or provincial ministries of health and through them to the Ministry of Health of China, which sets national policies and standards for most areas of preventive medicine and medical care. Specialty societies, largely inactive from 1965 to 1976 are now back in full operation and have increasing power (Sidel & Sidel 1982, Henderson & Cohen 1984, Hsiao 1984).

PRESENT PROBLEMS

Enormous progress has been made over the past 35 years in improvement of the standard of living of the Chinese people and in their health services and medical care services, with concommitant improvement in health statistics. Infectious disease, although causing a considerably smaller percentage of population morbidity and mortality than in comparably-poor countries, is still at a higher level than in affluent countries. Conversely, death rates from cancer and cardiovascular diseases are rising rapidly. Large regions, particularly in China's western provinces, still lack access to adequate medical care and technology is still primitive in many areas. Perhaps most important, the new drive toward high technology, particularly in the cities, and the recent economic changes involving dismantling of the communes are threatening the extraordinary efforts that have been made in China to ensure equity of access to human services (Sidel 1982).

FUTURE NEEDS

China's most urgent need is to find ways to maintain its commitment to providing equity of services and upgrading the quality of life of all its people while pursuing 'modernization' of its economy and of its medical services. Methods are required to continue its support of innovative public health and primary care systems in the face of rapid social and technological change, rapid change in the nature and distribution of illness, and rapid change in medical and health care.

REFERENCES

Henderson G E, Cohen M S 1984 The Chinese hospital: a socialist work unit. Yale University Press, New Haven, CT, USA

Hsiao W C 1984 Transformation of health care in China. New England Journal of Medicine 310: 932–933

Sidel R, Sidel V W 1982 The health of China: current conflicts in medical and human services for one billion people. Zed Press, London

Sidel V W 1982 Medical care in China: equity vs modernization. American Journal of Public Health 72: 1224–1225

Sidel V W, Sidel R 1974 Serve the people: observations on medicine in the People's Republic of China. Beacon Press, Boston, MA, USA

Latin America

INTRODUCTION

The name Latin America is given to those parts of the Americas
that were explored and settled by the Spanish and Portuguese. It
consists of Mexico, Central America, and South America, and
includes the Caribbean countries of Cuba and the Dominican
Republic. Its inhabitants — apart from those Indians who still use
native languages — speak Spanish or, in the case of Brazil, Portuguese. Some important Caribbean islands, such as Jamaica and
Trinidad, were originally settled by Spaniards, but were under the
control of Britain in the 17th and 18th centuries and are now
English-speaking; similarly, other islands were controlled by
France and Holland.

History

Although the dates are rather vague, the general pattern of development is reasonably clear. Furthermore, the history of Latin
America has direct relevance to the current problems of primary
health care.

The most notable of Indian civilizations in America was that of
the Mayas, who first flourished in what is now Northern Guatemala
and British Honduras in the 3rd century A.D.. They subsequently
migrated northwards to southern Mexico, where they came under
the influence of the Toltecs.

As Toltec and Mayan civilizations declined, the Aztecs began to
dominate the region. They were at the peak of their power when
the Spaniards reached Mexico in 1519.

The other important Indian civilization was centred on Peru. The
precise origin of the Incas is obscure, but they are known to have
existed around 1200 A.D.. Although the Incas were inferior to the
Mayas in scientific achievements, they had a calendar, could do

mathematical calculations, and were skilled healers and surgeons. Operations to mend the fractured skulls of warriors were one of their specialities!

Millions of South American Indians, however, lived in areas where the Aztecs and Incas never penetrated: they include the Chibchas of Colombia and the numerous Indians of Brazil and the Caribbean islands. Their civilizations were far inferior, culturally, to those of Mexico and Peru and their political organization, too, was very primitive.

Most of the maritime nations of Western Europe obtained overseas possessions between the 15th and 19th centuries. By the middle of the 16th century, the great empires of the Incas and the Aztecs lay in ruins and Spain and Portugal had created for themselves American empires that were to remain intact for 300 years.

The independence of Spanish America was secured at the cost of 15 years bitter warfare between 1810 and 1825, which caused much loss of life and massive economic destruction, except in Brazil, where, independence from Portugal was secured in 1822 with comparative ease. Brazil continued to be ruled by the Portuguese royal family until 1889, when the country became a republic.

The struggle for independence left a legacy of serious social, economic and political problems for the new states, which were the product of political fragmentation.

In consequence, most states have elaborate constitutions which have often been ignored by the strong presidents or dictators who have seized power. The use of general elections to provide for peaceful political change is still not established in some countries, where the only way to remove a president who has seized power by force, is to use force against him.

Furthermore, although the Latin American states seized political independence from Spain and Portugal in the early 19th century, they did not become economically free. They became dependent upon Britain in the 19th century and today are dependent largely on the United States of America.

Geography

The implications for primary health care of the geography of Latin America are considerable. The limits of this area extend north of the Tropic of Cancer, across the Equator, down through the southern hemisphere to the edge of Antarctica itself.

The terrain varies from the plains of Patagonia to the mountains of the Andes, the jungles of Brazil, the tropical forests of Central America and the islands of the Caribbean.

The culture of the various countries has evolved from the historical traditions of their antecedents, and the introduction of Christianity 400 years ago has obvious implications for the provision of primary health care today.

It must also be remembered that, although all the American Indians have the same Asiatic origin, wide differences in language, culture and architecture developed in the thousands of years between the first migrations and the arrival of European settlers. Even today, in Guatemala where the language is officially Spanish, there are also 3 Indian languages each with 10 dialects, deriving from the ancient Mayan civilization with its long-established medical traditions, which included midwifery and family planning. At one time its population was controlled.

In countries where a large minority of the population still live in remote areas and in small communities, these differences are highly significant. In Mexico, for example, there are 9000 communities of less than 500 inhabitants. This makes the general provision of primary health care very difficult.

Economic and political changes

The economic dependence of most Latin American countries on Europe and North America has had major implications for the way in which the countries have developed. Furthermore, the frequent changes of government have not contributed to a rapid improvement in the economic stability of some of those countries. The development of health services has been delayed in consequence.

The natural resources of Latin America are still being discovered. Oil and minerals abound and the area has enormous potential for becoming self-sufficient in the long term. However, the development of most countries is still very dependent upon financial backing from developed countries. This poses considerable problems where governments are unstable. Economic investment is considered to be high risk in many areas and the international banking community has become nervous about committing itself to future projects in many areas. Furthermore, high interest rates on loans already outstanding have had a major impact on the economy of some of the more developed countries. In Mexico, the investment in oil mining was considerable, at a time when oil prices were high. The fall in oil prices and simultaneous rise in interest repayments, has had a crippling effect on the Mexican economy, from which it is only now beginning to recover.

Nevertheless, new technology, particularly in the field of communication, is having a major impact on the development of countries in Latin America. The interest in establishing higher standards of living and health care, is stimulated by radio and other communications systems. In some countries this has resulted in the movement of large numbers of people towards centres of employment. The ability of cities to respond to the demand for employment is limited, and concentration of population in substandard housing adds to the problems of providing a basic level of health care within those communities.

DEVELOPMENT OF FAMILY MEDICINE

An increasing number of doctors providing primary health care have recognized the importance of family-based medicine. Throughout Latin America, like-minded doctors have been promoting this system of family care, with remarkable success.

In 1971, Mexico was the first country to establish a family medicine or general practice programme. In 1974, Bolivia started their programme, Panama in 1978, and in 1982 these countries were joined by Argentina, Chile, Brazil, the Dominican Republic, Jamaica and Venezuela.

In 1981, the International Centre for Family Medicine (ICFM) was established. Its main objective is to promote family practice delivered by qualified family physicians. It seeks to ensure that family physicians are correctly certified and trained in good educational programmes. It expects family physicians to be committed to family medicine as a philosophy of medical care, in which the patient has an active role. A life-long commitment to continuing medical education is also expected. The Centre seeks to assure the public, the consumer and the providers of health care services, that the family physician is worthy of their trust. It promotes the following activities, which it believes are important in achieving its goals:

1. The creation and evolution of a strong, professional and scientific association at national level.

2. The creation, development and support of postgraduate programmes to train family physicians.

3. The development of undergraduate programmes to expose medical students to family practice.

4. The expansion of continuing medical education programmes for family physicians.

5. Faculty training for family medicine educational programmes.

6. The production and distribution of publications on family medicine and related matters in Spanish and Portuguese.

SYSTEMS OF HEALTH CARE

Most Latin American countries have evolved systems of health care which are broadly similar.

The main providers of health care services are the Institutes of Social Security. It is these Institutions which have been primarily responsible for creating residency programmes for training family physicians.

The Institutes of Social Security are controlled by trade unions and restrict their services to members of the unions and their immediate families. Their funding is dependent upon the membership of trade unions, to whom the health service providers are accountable. Health service facilities are organized by the Institute and four tiers usually exist: a diagnostic centre, area hospital, regional hospital and super-regional hospital. The administration of these centres and the employment of staff, including doctors, is undertaken by the Institute. Running parallel to this system of health care, the Ministries of Health organize an alternative service for those who wish to subscribe to it. Funding is less readily available for this service, with consequent reduction in the standards of health care provision. Naturally, this duplication of services impairs the process of development of family medicine with opposition or resistance to change coming from several sections of society.

Finally, there is a substantial provision of health care services remaining under the control of the private sector. The access to this type of provision is restricted to the very rich or, ironically, the very poor.

In metropolitan areas, about 60% are provided for through the social security and state systems. The remainder go privately. However, in the rural areas, medical attention is not always available. Traditional healing methods form an important part of the primary health care services in these areas, although these are in no way properly organized.

Chile

The Chilean experience is worth particular comment, since it has a long tradition in the utilization of general practitioners. In the 1950s it established a National Health Service modelled on the British experience. Initially, it appointed general practitioners in rural areas, and in recent years it began to use the system in urban areas. However, lately the Chilean government has shown some reluctance to improve the family practice model and apply it more extensively. A change of policy will be necessary for this development to occur.

Cuba

Since the revolution in 1969, a National Health Service has existed in Cuba. It has one of the most comprehensive systems of primary health care, which is available to all its population. The influence of family medicine is playing an increasing part in the delivery of health care.

CHECKS AND CONTROL OF QUALITY

At present, health resources are not shared equally by all the people; significant gaps still exist in many countries and health is the privilege of the few.

It is certainly true that, by most parameters, the quality of care at national level is improving, but the rate of progress varies from country to country. International comparisons are helpful to a limited extent in determining the progress a particular country, or a group of countries, is making towards health for all.

The World Health Organization has identified a number of priority indicators to monitor progress towards health for all, as well as to illustrate the difference in health situations within the countries. However, for each country within Latin America, an accurate assessment based on these indicators is not currently available.

ALLOCATION OF NATIONAL RESOURCES

The single most important indicator of political commitment to strategies for health is the allocation of adequate resources, which in some countries requires substantial reallocation of resources.

However, before indicators of financial resource allocation can be established, it is necessary for each country to solve, in terms appropriate to its own situation, two problems of definition: which components are included under 'health', and within that, what is included under 'primary health care'?

There are such great variations in the way that primary health care is organized that each national health authority will have to work out the most practical basis on which to construct a national indicator of expenditure in this field.

It is unfortunate that a considerable element of corruption exists within many Latin American countries and this has to be recognized as a serious threat to the achievement of maximum efficiency in the use of those resources that can be afforded.

COMMON PROBLEMS AND PREVENTION

The problems of achieving health for all in Latin America are those common to all developing countries, namely: population control, water and sanitation, nutrition and availability of food, health education, maternal and child health, immunization, prevention and control of endemic diseases, treatment of common disease and injuries, provision of essential drugs, and accessibility of health facilities.

The commitment of governments to achieving health for all by the year 2000 is variable and in some cases insufficient for such a goal to be considered realistic. In Mexico, the Institute of Social Services recently suggested that the problems of pollution and population control are unlikely to be resolved within the next 20 years.

The effect on the population of providing information and education on health matters depends on how effectively this provision is disseminated.

Newspapers, television and other mass media outlet are not available to significant minorities in most Latin American countries. The radio is more nearly universal in its distribution and is singularly the most important of the media in many regions. Individuals promoting health education supplement mass media communication. In Guatemala they have a system of *promotores*, health promoters, and in Nicaragua, individuals appointed to look after well-defined neighbourhoods. These men or women are members of the local *comite* and liaise closely with the other public services available in the area.

Water and sanitation facilities vary considerably in their availability. A large percentage of the population do not have a clean water supply, nor are the sanitation facilities adequate. In some cities, where urban growth has been particularly rapid, development has occurred without any proper infrastructure. 10% of the population of Mexico City lacks drinking water in their homes and 30% do not have drainage.

Birth and fertility rates are also a major problem for Latin America. The population has risen from 322 million in 1975 to 410 million in 1985. It is expected to rise to 566 million by the year 2000. Most of this rise will occur in Central America and tropical South America.

In many countries the philosophical approach to family planning differs markedly from that adopted by developed countries. Family planning is not considered a prerequisite to improving standards of health care; indeed, the reverse is considered true, that is, if the ecology and the expectation of life are improved a reduction in the birth rate will result.

A number of programmes have been established linking family planning and population control with other aspects of health care. The Japanese Organization for International Co-operation in Family Planning (JOICFP) has established an integrated programme for family planning and parasite control which is organized by the International Planned Parenthood Federation (IPPF) in London. This is particularly active in Brazil, Colombia and Mexico and depends to a large extent on involvement with the community.

Immunization programmes are still far from complete, although major efforts are being made to improve the uptake of immunization programmes when they are available.

Integrated programmes of health care are likely to have a significant impact on the provision of primary health care.

INTEGRATED HEALTH PROGRAMMES

In developing countries, where infant mortality is high and children are not only valuable income earners but also the most reliable form of security in old age for parents, the rationale behind family planning is sometimes difficult to understand. Under these circumstances people's needs are not met by a family planning only approach.

It has been necessary, therefore, to add to an existing family planning programme something beneficial and fundamental to the daily life of people in order to make their response more positive.

Health is one of the primary, commonly felt needs of people and has been increasingly integrated with family planning and, in particular, maternal and child health over the past several years. For example, where a service for common diseases is already operating, family planning advice has been co-ordinated with it. Similarly, this can be arranged in areas where little funding or advanced technology is required. The opportunity to set up other programmes is also taken where those offering family planning advice can cope easily with the subject to be integrated and where immediate and visible results are obtained after treatment.

With such conditions in mind the integrated family planning and parasite control programme was initiated on the basis of the Japanese experience with pilot projects in Taiwan, Indonesia, Korea and other Far East countries under the auspices of JOICFP.

Community participation is an essential factor in mobilizing available human resources to the maximum, to promote effectively and sustain the project and to generate a self-help spirit for institutionalization of the project. For these purposes, a local steering committee can be organized from the beginning, or in the process of project development. This may be composed of local government administrators, health centre personnel, formal and informal leaders, school teachers, other community workers and project personnel.

FUTURE NEEDS FOR 2000

National and international organizations will continue to be important in Latin America for promoting continuing medical education and the concept of family medicine itself. The ICFM has a major role to play in this respect and will be able to co-ordinate thoughts and collate information and experience.

The governments of Latin American countries will have to establish those resources they intend to make available if their objectives in providing primary health care for all by the year 2000 are to be met. This will inevitably mean the reallocation of resources in some countries.

The future of family practice will depend on greater consumerism. Family practice will need to embrace the whole of the primary health care team and nurses and other health promoters, who will all need to be trained to be part of this team, thus allowing family physicians to expand their role.

Self-care will become one of the central themes of primary care. Modern technology will make self-care easier through better communication. Communication needs to be improved between the patient and the primary health care team as well as between individual members of the team itself. The new technology will aid education of both patient and doctor and will have a particular impact on small communities without immediate access to medical facilities.

Separate programmes for specific aspects of health care, for example, population control, immunization and parasite control, although they lead to some fragmentation of the primary health care services, should be encouraged since it is difficult to see how, with resources being restricted, adequate provision for these aspects of health care can be made.

Finally, in order that the hopes and aspirations expressed at Alma-Ata can be tackled with renewed vigour, a reaffirmation by governments of their intention to fulfil the objectives of Alma-Ata should be encouraged.

South Africa

NATIONAL FEATURES

Historical

South Africa is situated at the tip of Africa. It is a mixture of a third world developing country, as well as a developed country. Advanced technology and free enterprise contrasts sharply with the tribal areas which exist on income partly derived from migrant labour and partly from a subsistence economy.

Its population, at the last 1980 census (Department of Health, Welfare and Pensions 1979), consisted of (in millions):

Blacks	16.0
Whites	4.5
Mixed races	2.5
Asians	0.75
Total	23.75

The Gluckman Commission in 1944 recommended a health centre and community-based comprehensive primary health care (PHC) service for all sections of the population (Gluckman 1944). Its recommendations were never implemented. It received little support from the medical and allied professions due to its threat to the entrenched status of the private practitioner.

However, even at that time, many mission hospitals in the rural areas were providing a comprehensive primary health care system (Spencer 1984).

Cultural–social

The social and cultural background of the peoples of South Africa varies tremendously. To understand the medical system, one has to grasp the diversity of these cultures, languages and health-related behaviours among the different groups. Broadly speaking, almost all people in the country make use of the Western scientific health care system. However, there are nine main tribal groupings with a distinctive language and subdialect. Each has some variation of a traditional African health care system (Fehrsen 1983). Traditional medicine in Africa is as old as Black culture. Because society is dynamic and changing, these traditional healers are responding to these changes and have adapted to become part of city life. The traditional healer still plays a significant role in the delivery of primary health care.

The Coloured and Asian populations, who occupy an intermediate position between the Whites and Blacks, usually seek their medical care, like the Whites, through the Westernized scientific health care system. They also however, make extensive use of traditional and faith healing systems.

In order to understand the role of the *traditional healer*, it is necessary to consider African concepts of disease and healing. Behaviour (whether one is sick or healthy), health and medical care delivery systems are not isolated entities but integrated into a complex network of beliefs and values that are part of the culture of that society. God is the creator and sustainer of the human race, spirits influence the destiny of human beings, and animals, plants, natural phenomena and objects constitute the physical environment in which people live, thereby providing our means of existence.

It is also widely accepted in African culture that there is a force, power or energy permeating the whole universe, of which God is the source and controller. The spirits have access to this force but only a few human beings, such as priests and medicine men, can manipulate this energy for the good or ill of society (Karlsson & Moloantoa 1984).

Geographical

About 50% of South Africa is desert or semidesert, with an average rainfall of below 500 mm per year. Only 12% of the land is arable (Official Yearbook of South Africa 1980/81). It is a country with large distances between large towns, interspaced with small towns in the rural areas, where many Blacks live in their own communities. It is a land of sunshine in all seasons, leading to much outdoor life in a contrasting countryside; from deserts to subtropical and temperate fertile areas; from large Westernized cities, with all the modern conveniences and necessities, to small country towns and Black community areas with almost no modern technological facilities available.

Economic

In the last decade there have been marked social changes in many parts of Africa, and in some places these have been little short of dramatic. Possibly, the major factor has been the massive influx of money, expertise and materials, supplied from overseas, to exploit the mineral, agricultural and other wealth potential features of the continent.

In South Africa, the economy is fast growing, with a growth rate of 5.5% in 1980, prior to the present economic slump. There is a general shortage of skilled manpower. Monetary, technological and political power has been effectively contained in White hands but the process towards sharing power is gaining momentum, and a new political dispensation in this regard commenced late in 1984 (Fehrsen 1983).

The Black people are moving increasingly into skilled professional and leadership situations. The emergence of the Black executive is a reality. Blacks earned 22% of the total personal income in 1970; the figure in 1980 was 29% (Department of Foreign Affairs and Information 1981). The process towards possession of land and capital will be slower, as large tracts of land are still under tribal control with a communal land tenure system.

Government finances and facilities have helped to upgrade the nutritional and social circumstances of many previously under-privileged people; not only in the matter of direct earnings but also through State spending on housing, health and educational amenities. Thus, many living near the large industrial, mining and seaport areas are better off than before and these benefits have resulted in a satisfactory fall in infant and child mortality (Campbell et al 1982). This is not, however, true of periurban squatter and many rural communities.

HEALTH SYSTEM — EVOLUTION AND FORMAT

The first Western health station was inaugurated in April 1652 at the Cape of Good Hope by the Dutch settlers, headed by Jan van Riebeeck. It supplied fresh food for the ships rounding the Cape from Europe to the East and catered mainly for the sick seamen. During the 18th century, many ships' surgeons settled in the Cape and served the local settlers on a 'fee-for-service' basis. They practised medicine, surgery and obstetrics.

By the turn of the century, the Dutch East India Company's era was ended by the British occupation. This brought a new surge of settlers from Britain, adding to the Dutch and French complement already at the Cape. The settler moved far into the interior, where major clashes developed between the Black populations moving south from Central Africa, and the Whites moving north. The first contacts Blacks had with Western health care were with doctors attached to these migrating Whites, and those attached to the armed forces.

Towards the end of the 19th century, the first mission hospitals were started by the churches to cover almost the entire area occupied by the Black populations. From the 1930s onwards, the State accepted more and more responsibility for subsidizing the mission hospitals. This gradually increased to total subsidization by the 1960's. In the 1970s the State took over most of these hospitals from the churches and handed them over to Black self-governing bodies.

The bulk of the western health manpower in the 19th century was from the White population. These practitioners had qualified mostly in Europe and Britain. Initially, there was no restriction on barbers and others setting themselves up in medical practice, but in 1807 legislative control for registration was established by the Supreme Medical Committe. This was the forerunner of the present South African Medical and Dental Council, which was created in 1928.

With the discovery of diamonds in 1867 and gold in 1885, there was an explosive development. The Northern South African Republic, for instance, had 30 medical practitioners in 1885. Within 5 years, Johnnesburg was rising from barren veld, and it alone had more than 30 practitioners.

The rich mineral wealth, still an integral part of South Africa today, resulted in reintegration of these settlers. The whole area was formed into the Union of South Africa in 1910, after the Anglo-Boer War (1898–1901). At this time, there was little thought for health matters. However, the influenza epidemic of 1918 brought about the Public Health Act of 1919, when a three-tier system of medical care was formulated and only modified for the first time in 1977. The basic principle was decentralization. Local authorities were subsidized by the Central Government to control infectious diseases and environmental sanitation. The four provincial administrations were responsible for the hospitals. The Department of Public Health controlled and co-ordinated psychiatric care.

Personal medical services for the population were rendered by private practice physicians with honorary appointments in the hospitals. Now there is a mixture of private practitioners and part-time and full-time salaried doctors. Many hospitals are privately owned.

The first South African Medical Association (SAMA) was founded in 1883, and was an affiliated branch of the British Medical Association (BMA). An independent Medical Association was formed in 1897. In 1925, the BMA in South Africa and the Medical Association fused to form the Medical Association of South Africa and became independent of the BMA. These Associations have done much to foster the organization of medical care in South Africa, and have been responsible for the establishment of the South African Medical Journal and other journals.

The first medical school was established in Cape Town in 1912. Today, there are seven.

The Royal Colleges of the United Kingdom had branches is South Africa. In 1955, the College of Physicians, Surgeons and Gynaecologists was formed which included all the specialist groups.

The first academic general practice organization was formulated in 1959 as an overseas faculty of the British College of General Practitioners. In 1969, an independent South African College of General Practice was established, which amalgamated with specialist groups to form the the College of Medicine in 1970. This body involves all doctors in a unified academic body for post-graduate examinations, which have reciprocity with overseas Colleges. The College offers the MFGP (Member of Faculty of General Practice) and, up to 1984, 300 family physicians have obtained this diploma.

Until 1979, the College and the University of Pretoria, with a full academic department of general practice, had formed the spearhead of modern academic family practice. South Africa was made a full member of WONCA (World Organization of National Colleges and Academies of General Practice/Family Medicine) in 1972.

The South African Academy of Family Practice/Primary Care was founded in 1980. This organization was formulated because the general practitioner lost identity and autonomy within the College of Medicine. However, the College still remains the examining body for general practice, as well as being the home of the Faculty of General Practice. Entry into the College of Medicine is by examination only, whereas the Academy is open to all physicians in active general practice or similar occupations.

The present health care system is regulated by the Health Act of 1977. It serves to bring about greater co-ordination in the three-tier system. A large proportion of South Africans receive virtually free medical care from the State sector of the health service. However, as their incomes increase, they pay more for this service.

The South African Medical and Dental Council ensures standards of medical education and discipline. It keeps a register of all medical practitioners; a separate register is kept for registered specialists. This registration is a legalized requirement before being allowed to practice as a doctor in South Africa. The Council consists of elected members of the medical profession, as well as government appointees.

The Medical Association of South Africa is a voluntary Association and cares for the interests of physicians in all disciplines, with regard to fees, discipline, medicopolitical and many other areas. It advices Council with regard to serious breach in ethics affecting the medical profession.

The 7 university faculties of medicine graduate a total of approximately 1000 each year. The undergraduate course consists of 5 academic years; the 6th year is as a student intern and the final year as an intern. Following this, full registration takes place and the doctor can practice as a general practitioner. A vocational training scheme of 4–6 years, followed by a series of examinations at a fellowship level from the College of Medicine or a university is required to register and practise as a specialist (Fehrsen 1983).

The family practitioner is responsible for providing a service to those patients who elect to come under his care and, traditionally, contact is initiated by the patients. Patients have free choice of practitioner in the private sector.

PLACE OF PRIMARY HEALTH CARE

How it is organized

Primary health care has many definitions of its content and function. However, there are two main groups of primary care doctors:
1. The general practitioner in private practice.
2. Public sector clinic doctors and rural hospital doctors who have a greater involvement in what is today recognized as community medicine, surgery and obstetrics especially.

The private family practitioner practises solo, in partnership or in group practices.

The public sector doctor is usually a member of a health team, practising in a city or rural district hospital situation. Here, the primary health nurse is a vital member of the health team.

How it is financed

Private family physicians are independent, but the rural district hospitals, health clinics and community health care centres are financially endowed and controlled by government or provincial health departments.

Checks/controls of quality

Private practice is scrutinized by the South African Medical and Dental Council, as well as by the Disciplinary Committee of the South African Medical Association. The public have the right to complain about the quality of service and the fee structure.

The district hospitals, clinics and small rural hospitals are under the control and direction of the National Department of Health and provincial and local authorities.

Remuneration and incentives

About 80% of the White, Asian and Coloured communities and about 7% of the Black population belong to medical aid societies. These are sickness insurance schemes to which the member makes regular contributions and, in return, his family is covered for sickness benefits. These medical aid schemes are privately owned and contract to pay the doctor the fee as laid down in the statutory tariff of fees. Doctors do not necessarily have to contract with medical aid schemes but the advantages are that the fee is guaranteed and payment is made directly to the contracting doctor. Doctors can contract out and charge a private fee, but the medical aids will, reimburse the statutory tariff (Fehler 1972).

In the very near future, changes are envisaged in the medical fee structure (Table 22.1).

Table 22.1   Example of fees

	Statutory medical aid fees	Private fees
Consultation — in rooms	R 9.50	R18.00
Home visit — day	R19.00	R37.50
Home visit — night	R31.60	R50.00

*R1.00 = approximately 0.50 cents in US currency.

Patients can attend State-aided provincial hospitals and are charged R20.00 for any service. Pensioners and destitute are seen as a free service. Medicines are not usually provided, except for pensioners and the Black population.

Most State-subsidized provincial city hospitals are run by, and orientated for, specialists — very few general practitioners have appointments in these centres of medical education. In the rural areas, most hospital services are managed by general practitioners.

In the private sector, the incentives are the satisfaction of the independence of private practice, as well as the financial gain.

In the government-controlled hospitals and clinics, physicians have a fixed remuneration and have security in their job situation, with regular leave as well as many perks.

WHO DOES WHAT IN PRIMARY HEALTH CARE?

At the moment, 4 of the 7 medical schools have departments of family medicine with undergraduate and postgraduate teaching, with part-time teachers from active general practice. The extent of undergraduate teaching varies. Some departments have instituted an elective period. Some students spend a period of 1–4 weeks with an accredited general practitioner, this is probably their only exposure to private sector family medicine. Clerkships in public sector primary care vary from one school to the next.

The departments of family medicine have a service responsibility to emergency rooms, outpatients' departments and community clinics, associated with the university medical school.

Three of the departments of family medicine offer a postgraduate degree. The College of Medicine also offers a postgraduate diploma. These are all additional qualifications with no financial gain attached to them.

Much postgraduate education is conducted by the South African Academy of Family Practice/Primary Care. There are 7 regions in South Africa, and each region has regular monthly meetings or symposia, journal club meetings and weekend courses. Small groups have been formed where family practitioners, who do not take part actively in large meetings, are able to participate in these smaller groups, meeting regularly each month.

The College of Medicine, through the Faculty of General Practice, also offers regular video shows and discussions in some areas, as well as a tape-recording service.

The primary health care nurse is under the responsibility of the family practitioner or, in some instances, works directly with specialists involved in primary care, such as obstetricians or paediatricians.

At present, there are two professional bodies who take care of the traditional healers in South Africa — both issue certificates to their members and are governed by an extensive and detailed code of conduct (Karlsson & Moloantoa 1984).

Present and future roles of the team

Implementing a comprehensive national primary health care programme requires input from many disciplines in medicine from many government departments as well as the private sector. To meet the various needs the primary health care doctors will have to assume flexible roles to assure that their contribution will be most effective. Other health care team members will be drawn from related professions, people in planning and community representatives.

The success of any health care encounter depends not only on knowledge and skills abbut also on excellent communication. The advantage of sharing the same culture and languages is most important in the development of the primary health team (Wagstaff, 1984).

Nurses when trained in primary curative care are able to manage 80% of the problems of patients attending day clinics. The importance and value of the nurse in primary health care has been formally recognised, particularly if she shares the patients culture and language.

EDUCATION AND STANDARDS

The general practitioners receive their postgraduate training through the efforts of the Academy, the College of Medicine, continuing education courses run by universities and meetings of the Medical Association of South Africa.

At present, family practice consists of non-specialists. There is no limitation to the scope of practice, but they may be called upon to prove their competence to the South African Medical and Dental Council if a complaint is received.

The Academy, together with departments of family practice of the universities, and the Medical Association, are at present negotiating for official recognition for vocational training for family medicine.

COMMON DISEASE PROBLEMS AND PREVENTION

South Africa, a developed country within a third world developing country, is confronted with the usual Westernized diseases, but, in addition also with third world problems, such as malnutrition, cholera and infestations. Obesity and alcoholism are prevalent, as is essential hypertension, which is becoming more prominent in the urban Blacks. Diabetes is a very important illness in the Asian members of the community, reaching epidemic proportions.

Poverty, bad farming practices, droughts and the overuse of plant and soil resources contribute to the illnesses of the rural Black population.

It is important for a family practitioner, setting out to treat Blacks, to understand their customs and culture. The Blacks tend to be also concerned about the cause of their ailment and they also wish to know who made them ill. They frequently attend the Western scientific doctor, as well as the traditional healer.

More education, for both doctor and patient, is urgent to attempt to prevent illnesses.

PREVENTIVE ROLES FOR PRIMARY HEALTH CARE IN THE FUTURE

We feel that the opportunistic method of providing preventive and promotive health care as recommended by Stott (1983) is the ideal way of fulfilling this need in the community. For this, however, there are two preconditions: firstly, there should be a primary care facility within reasonable access of every person in the community and, secondly, people should make use of such facilities frequently enough for the opportunistic approach to be able to operate. There are many areas in the country in which these conditions apply and the challenge is to change the behaviour of doctors and other health workers in primary health care to give adequate attention to this area of prevention during the normal consultation process.

There are still many areas in the country, however, especially rural areas, where the service is not readily available to all people and where consultation rates are not high enough to make an immediate success of the opportunistic method. In these areas, we see a definite place for the cohort method and preventive teams going around to do, for instance, as weight surveillance and immunisation in children. As the service becomes more sophisticated and available they will, hopefully, be replaced by the opportunistic method, which is probably cheaper to deliver and more cost-effective in-the long run (Stott, 1983).

RELATING TO OTHER LEVELS

The increasing recognition, training and legislation for clinical nurses to act in the delivery of primary health care is gaining momentum, particularly in health centres and rural hospital areas. They are usually involved in health care teams, who are delegated and monitored by family physicians in the public sector. Legislation prevents such health teams from practising in the private sector, as the physician only can command a fee for work done by himself. Current political policy encourages private enterprise and there is much to debate about the privatization of health care.

PUBLIC INVOLVEMENT AND RELATIONS

The public today is more educated and are thus expectant of a high quality of care from the family physician. They are involved in forming societies, e.g. the diabetic or arthritic foundations where their meetings are frequently addressed by family practitioners.

HOW TO CORRECT THE INEQUALITIES AND MAKE THE BEST USE OF RESOURCES

The inequalities within the health care system in South Africa are historically related to the fact that the western health care system was initially developed only to serve the white community in the 19th century. Since the beginning of the 20th century, the community and government has slowly become aware that we have a responsibility to all within the country. This commitment to the whole population has been more evident since the early 1970s. There is, however, a massive backlog in getting an equitable distribution of manpower and resources.

The South African Academy of Family Practice/Primary Care is taking a leading role in trying to redistribute the doctors within the primary care sector. The first vocational training scheme started up at the beginning of 1985 is situated in an underserved community and the same is planned for the future expansion of this scheme. It is envisaged that this will assist with the distribution of doctors to areas of need.

There is also a greater intake of black medical students which will increase the numbers of doctors within the different cultural groups in the future. This is especially important in the context of primary care, in which the ideal is to have a doctor of first contact who is of the same community as oneself to enable the maximum quality of doctor-patient relationship to occur.

On a wider community basis, distribution of resources is ultimately dependent upon the distribution of political power within the community. South Africa is experiencing a period of political change in which more and more previously dispossessed communities are participating within the political process. So doing, we foresee that services will be relocated as political power becomes shared.

A tremendous opportunity still, however, remains for all those who wish to see a more equitable distribution of health care to get out into the underserved areas and, together with nurses and other health care workers develop the services and the abilities of the local population to provide an optimal primary health care service.

PRESENT PROBLEMS

There are many, such as:

1. Lack of vocational training for family medicine. Many leaders in the medical hierarchy are uninformed regarding family medicine and believe that the community physician and family physician are of the same discipline.

2. There is also a lack of the family physician's influence in the medical school: here the specialist orientates students to his way of thinking and, at times, has a solitary thought towards specialization.

3. In the private sector, family practitioners have to contend with the unethical behaviour of specialist colleagues who fail to communicate with the primary care doctor, either verbally or by letter, with regard to a patient referred for an opinion — at times they fail to refer the patient back to the original doctor (Fehler 1983). Referral to a specialist is not mandatory and the patient can approach a specialist directly. However, the specialist is ethically required to inform the family doctor of his findings.

4. The South African Medical Association, the Medical Council and university bodies are under the control of specialists or university professors, none of whom have knowledge of family medicine — thus the family physician has little influence on these bodies.

This is largely due to family practitioners' lack of interest in participating in medical politics.

5. The health care system is determined by economic, political, cultural, as well as social, circumstances. There is a marked maldistribution of manpower between the urban and rural population groups, the rich and poor, Black and White. The lack of Black physicians in the rural areas leads to underdoctored sections in the underprivileged areas, especially with regard to the private sector.

6. There is unequal competition between the private sector and the health care system, where the private practitioner is unable to practice as a full health team with paramedical services — government legislation prevents this.

7. Irregularity exists between the earning capacity of specialists and family physicians. Specialist fees for identical services are in the region of 66% in excess of family physician fees.

8. Fee structures encourage procedures and investigations and not good patient-oriented primary care.

FUTURE NEEDS FOR 2000

The main goals for the future are to co-ordinate all streams of primary care medicine, to accept the health team concept with a definition of the role of each worker, and to ensure that all planning is service-orientated (Nel 1984).

All universities should establish autonomous departments of family medicine and associate with the South African Academy of Family Practice/Primary Care and Faculty of General Practice of the College of Medicine of South Africa. Vocational training should be mandatory for practising family medicine.

Family practice must show its willingness to make primary and continuing care available to all the people of South Africa — Black, White, Coloured, rich and poor, urban, rural and tribal citizens.

Equality of status for family practitioners, alongside their specialist consultant colleagues is important.

Advances in scientific, technological and medical knowledge have led to the present era of increased specialization, but paradoxically it has made us aware that, at the present time and in the future, the patient's greatest need is for a patient-centred generalist to be the doctor of first contact. We need to learn how to train this kind of doctor and health care worker and structure the health care services in such a way that the developing principles of family medicine/primary care will be practised to the benefit of future patients (Stott 1983).

REFERENCES

Campbell G O, Seedat Y, Daynes G 1982 Clinical medicine and health in developing Africa. David Philip Publications, 1982. p xi.

Department of Foreign Affairs and Information 1981 Dynamic change in South Africa. Government Printer, Pretoria, p 67, 70

Department of Health, Welfare and Pensions 1979 Health data. DHWP, Pretoria, p 1

Fehler B M 1972 Cost of effective primary care from now to the year 2000. SA Medical Journal 23 November: 1541

Fehler B M 1983 Ethical behaviour of specialist colleagues. SA Medical Journal 64:153

Fehrsen S G 1983 Family practice in South Africa. In: Geyman J P, Fry J (eds) Family practice: Appleton Century Crofts, an International Perspective in Developed Countries. p 143

Gluckman H 1944 The provision of an organised national health service for all sections of the people of the Union of South Africa (Report of National Health Services Commission 1942–1944)

Karlsson E M Moloantoa K E M 1984 The traditional healer in primary care — yes or no? SA Journal of Continuing Medical Education (April) 2:43

Nel P O 1984 Community involvement in primary health care. SA Journal of Continuing Medical Education (April) 2:78

Official Yearbook of South Africa 1980/81 Chris van Rensburg Publications, Johannesburg, p 12, 556

Spencer I W F 1984 Primary care in South Africa. SA Journal of Continuing Medical Education (April) 2:21

Stott N C H 1983 Primary health care — bridging the gap between theory and practice. Springer-Verlag, Berlin,

Wagstaff L A 1984 The role of teams in primary health care. SA Journal of continuing Medical Education (April) 2:37.

Israel

INTRODUCTION

The patterns of the health services in Israel have evolved by a process of evolutionary change deeply rooted in the geographical and historical features of the country and in the moral and social philosophies of its people. Israel is situated on the eastern shore of the Mediterranean sea, between the desert and the sea. It is bordered by Lebanon in the north, Syria and Jordan in the east, and by Egypt and the Gulf of Eilat in the south. Its length from north to south is about 450 km and its maximum width is 66 km, covering an area of 27 000 km². The land is partially flat and partially mountainous. The Jordan Rift, beginning at the foot of Mount Hermon, contains the Sea of Galilee (212 metres below sea level) and the Jordan river, which flows into the inland Dead Sea, the lowest point on earth (394 metres below sea level), whose waters are the most important mineral resources of the country.

Climatically, there are two main seasons — a cold rainy winter and a hot dry summer. Israel's industry is based on a highly developed agricultural output, on the industrial processing of local and imported raw materials, and on highly technological electronic and computerized industries. The population (Central Bureau of Statistics 1983) numbers 4.2 million, of whom 55% were born in Israel, 25% in Europe or America, and 20% in Asia or Africa. Of these, 83% are Jews, 13% Moslems, 3% Christians, and 1% Druzes and other religions.

Historical perspectives

The earliest origins of man in Israel date to the Pleistocene period, perhaps over a million years ago. Archaeological and historical research has unearthed cities dating from the very dawn of civilization, and cultures whose writings, beliefs and traditions were to inspire three great monotheistic religions cradled in Jerusalem. The Holy Land, bequeathed to the Children of Israel, was situated on the crossroads of the major trade routes of the ancient world linking Asia, Africa and Europe and was destined, then as now, to serve sometimes as a bridge and sometimes as a wedge between warring empires and rival civilizations. Since Abraham left Ur in Chaldea near the Persian Gulf to fulfil his destiny in the Promised Land of Canaan, recorded Jewish history is punctuated by successive wars, expulsions, dispersions and returns from exiles. Nevertheless, throughout 4000 years of conquests and annexations, the Jews maintained their identity as a people (Shapiro 1963), and a remnant of the Jewish population, albeit extremely reduced in numbers, survived continuously in the Land of Israel supplemented by a trickle of immigrants from the countries of their dispersion (Bachi 1974).

Towards the end of the last century, when the first organized groups of Jewish settlers returned to rebuild their homeland, the biblical milk and honey had been transformed into parched deserts, eroded hills and malarious swamps. In the midst of primitive living conditions, poor nutrition and climatic rigours, the settlers fell easy victims to the malaria, typhoid, dysentry, bilharzia, trachoma and tuberculosis endemic in this region. Scarce medical facilities were hopelessly inadequate to stem the relentless toll of morbidity and mortality. In 1911, realizing the futility of individual efforts, the settlers formed collective agricultural settlements based on a distinctive socialist ideology, and banded together within the framework of the various labour unions to form small voluntary mutual aid societies, or Kupat Holim, for providing medical care to their families (Polliack 1976).

In 1922, the League of Nations initiated the British Mandate. This period was marked by extensive projects for soil reclamation, irrigation and swamp drainage accompanied by increasing immigration. The Mandatory government restricted its medical activities to public health measures and malaria control. Individual preventive and curative services were minimal and largely inaccessible to the Jewish settlers, who were thus obliged to supplement them by their own efforts. Kupat Holim expanded its services to provide increased medical and social benefits, especially in the rural and development areas where these facilities were sorely lacking. The Hadassah American Womens' Zionist Organization set up a chain of infant welfare clinics and school health services, especially in the towns, and established the first medical school and university hospital on Mount Scopus in Jerusalem.

The termination of the British Mandate in 1948, followed by the proclamation of an independent State of Israel, was the signal for an immediate declaration of war and invasion by the surrounding countries. While desperately fighting for its very existence, the country was immediately faced with the problems of staffing the government administrative services which had been abandoned by the withdrawal of the British Mandatory Authorities. It was also forced to cope with the immediate health needs of successive waves of refugees who poured into Israel from the concentration camps of war-ravaged Europe and the Middle East. During the first 3 years, over 650 000 refugees were admitted, exceeding in number the total Jewish population at that time. Vast reception camps were established, while medical and welfare facilities were feverishly expanded for treating the acute and chronic diseases, malnutrition, tuberculosis and mental disorders prevalent among the refugees.

This necessitated the urgent expansion of the existing services provided by Kupat Holim, the Ministry of Health and other Agencies (Grushka 1968). The immediate need to ensure the physical survivial of these refugees left little time for considering the implications of this explosive and unplanned expansion on the structure of the health services. Despite the incessant wars and economic crises, the small population of Israel struggled to absorb 1.5 million immigrants from over 60 countries into a social pressure-cooker into which dozens of cultural groups were smelted into the pluralistic society which forms today's population. At the same time, the country raced with frightening intensity through an accelerated process of urbanization, industrialization and modernization, which has catapulted it, somewhat prematurely, into ever-escalating living standards and the problems of the modern Welfare State. Many of the anomalies of the present health services can be traced to these historical events and social developments.

THE HEALTH SERVICE

The Ministry of Health bears overall authority for supervising the health care services, professional licensing and standards, public health measures, environmental and preventive health services. The Ministry, however, also directly operates its own hospitals, mostly inherited from the Mandatory government, which provide 38% of all hospital beds, as well as 70% of the maternal and child clinics and a large percentage of the mental health and geriatric services (Modan 1982).

The Kupat Holim Health Insurance Institution is the largest provider of health services in Israel, providing comprehensive prepaid health insurance and medical benefits to 80% of the total population (Doron 1982). These consist mostly of members of the General Federation of Labour and their families, including retired parents and dependents and also, by special arrangements, old-age pensioners, self-employed persons and over 100 000 social welfare recipients. In addition, Kupat Holim also builds and operates its own hospitals, comprising 35% of all general hospital beds, and an extensive network of primary health care clinics and medical facilities throughout the country. Its operative budget is derived from members and employers' contributions (60%), government participation (30%) and payments for services to other sick funds (10%) (Ron 1980). Each insured member contributes 4% of his salary, with a fixed maximum, to which his employer contributes an additional 5%. Benefits entitle all members to the full range of preventive, curative and rehabilitative services without further payment, except for nominal fees for prescription drugs, and graded copayment for prosthetic appliances and long-term nursing care. Dental treatment is not presently covered, but is increasingly available at considerably reduced rates.

Four small sick funds provide health insurance and primary medical facilities to some 16% of the population mainly in urban areas. About 4% of the population are without prepaid health insurance. The Hadassah Organization, the Malben Joint Distribution Committee, the Local Health Authorities and other voluntary and semivoluntary agencies provide additional extensive hospital facilities and other services, especially in projects for the elderly, the handicapped and other groups. The Ministries of Labour, Education and Social Welfare, and the National Insurance Institute are also involved in social insurance and related aspects of health care, including old-age pensions, occupational and accident insurance, and maternity and child benefits.

Israel is relatively well endowed with health manpower (Tulchinsky et al 1982). The present doctor:population ratio (1:480) is maintained by immigration and by 4 medical schools graduating 280 doctors annually (1: 13 000 population) after 6-year undergraduate programmes, followed by a mandatory internship year. The nurse:population ratio is 1:154, with 700 registered and practical nurses graduating annually from increasingly academic programmes in 17 nursing schools and 2 universities. The dentist:population ratio (1:1300) is supplemented by 80 graduates from 2 dental schools. There is currently one pharmacist per 1200 population, with an additional 60 graduating annually after completing 4-year study programmes. University affiliated schools for physiotherapy, occupational and speech therapists, dieticians and nutritionists are converting to 2–3-year degree programmes, while medical and laboratory technicians, radiographers, health educators and sanitation engineers are graduating in increasing numbers from university or practical programmes.

Primary health care services

Primary health care services for most of our population are administered through 15 Regional Offices, each serving about 200 000 people, and are based on an extensive network of over 1400 clinics built and operated by Kupat Holim in nearly every village, neighbourhood, town and city (Doron 1983). These clinics vary in size, structure and scope of activities, according to their location, function and the size of the population served.

Small urban and rural clinics are staffed by a family doctor and nurse and may include a small drug dispensary and dental services. In some areas, preventive services and maternal and child care are provided in separate facilities by the local health authority under the auspices of the Ministry of Health. In others, and especially in the rural areas, these services have been integrated and centralized in comprehensive health centres serving 2000–3000 residents of neighbouring settlements within a radius of 7–10 km (Yodfat 1970, Arnon 1971). Each settlement also maintains a nursing station. In the absence of a resident doctor, nurses may assume limited clinical responsibilities as 'nurse practitioners'.

Most urban clinics serve a community of 5000–20 000 people residing in close proximity, and are staffed by doctors, nurses, medical clerks and receptionists. Depending on the size of the clinic, these may be supplemented by medical social workers, allied health personnel, laboratory, radiological and other diagnostic facilities, a dispensing pharmacy and various medical and surgical specialists, to whom direct access may or may not be available.

Additional ambulatory consultative services are accessible by referral in regional clinics staffed by part-time consultants from the regional hospital. In recent years, regional home-care units have been established as an additional resource for the chronically ill, disabled or homebound. Emergency medical and ambulance services are located in the first aid stations of the Magen David Adom in each area, where a doctor is available when other services are closed.

The unchecked influx in the recent past of immigrant doctors from numerous countries with widely varying medical standards, clinical scope and proficiencies, led to diversion of those who 'fell off' the hospital ladder into the community clinics. As a result, many urban clinics are still staffed by 'general internists' treating only adults, and 'general paediatricians' treating only children. During the past decade, however, there has been a dramatic increase in the number of vocationally trained family physicians capable of providing medical care to all age groups. This has led to a rapid increase in the number of purpose-built urban clinics in which the family physician, the family nurse and sometimes a medical social worker, work together as a health care team. Each of these teams is responsible for a panel of 1500–2000 patients registered with the family physician, to whom direct access is available, usually on a walk-in basis.

In many teams, the nurse fulfils an expanded complementary role, facilitates health promotive and preventive behaviour, and participates actively in the management and follow-up of patients with long-term illness. The social worker is involved in individual casework, family crisis situations and mobilizing community resources. The work of the team has been facilitated by the introduction of problem-oriented medical records, age-sex registers and registers of long-term illnesses. Regular staff meetings are held, in which the paediatrician, school doctor or nurse, dietician, physiotherapist, occupational therapist, marriage counsellor, the home-care unit, or other health personnel often participate.

The doctors and allied health personnel are full-time salaried employees of the sick fund. Doctors' salaries are based on a capitation rate according to the number of registered patients, without incentive payments, except for higher per capita rates for infants and elderly patients, and higher salary grading for vocationally trained family physicians. In recent years, Kupat Holim has followed the smaller sick funds in contracting with part-time 'independent' doctors working from their own homes or rooms. Ancilliary staff and diagnostic facilities are, however, usually modest and often minimal in such premises. Overt private medical practice is not a feature of the health system, and is generally confined to specific clinical fields or patients 'shopping around', or seeking to bypass the inevitable queues and prolonged waiting times which characterize the freely accessible medical services.

The public and the Workers' Councils of the General Federation of Labour are well represented on Joint Supervisory Committees at central, regional and clinic levels of the medical services. Their representatives, however, reflect the spectrum of their political affiliations rather than the social or demographic distribution of the communities which they represent. Direct consumer participation is predictably limited by these constraints.

PRESENT HEALTH STATE AND PROBLEMS

There can be little doubt that Kupat Holim, the Ministry of Health and the other health agencies who have contributed to the development of health care, have brought immense personal, social and economic benefits to our country and to the health of its population. Morbidity patterns have undergone remarkable improvements (Central Bureau of Statistics 1983). The major tropical and infectious diseases still endemic in neighbouring countries have been virtually eradicated. Maternal mortality in all ethnic groups is almost zero. Infant mortality has declined from 22.7 per 1000 live births in 1970 (18.9 among Jews and 37.2 among non-Jews) to 13.9 (11.6 among Jews and 20.4 among non-Jews) in 1982. Birth rates have fallen to 22 and 33 per 1000 respectively. Crude death rates have declined to 6.9 per 1000 population (7.5 among Jews and 4.0 among non-Jews).

Life expectancy at birth for Jewish men and women (72.8 and 76.2 years respectively) and for non-Jews (70.8 and 73.2 years respectively) compare favourably with most developed countries. Extensive immunization, family planning, child development and parent education programmes are being expanded to improve child care. Improvements in the standard of living, as measured by crowding index, availability of consumer goods, percapita incomes, home ownership and years of schooling have also contributed to the improved health status of all sectors of our population.

Nevertheless, as in other industrialized countries, into the vacuum of reduced morbidity thus created, have flowed an ever-increasing range of previously unappreciated disorders: chronic degenerative diseases and disabilities of the middle-aged and elderly, the congenital and acquired handicaps of the young, mental disorders, road accidents, and a host of preventable disorders related to industrial hazards, food and environmental hygiene, and to the personal, psychosocial and culturally determined life styles and habits of our heterogenous population.

Today, our health services face considerable difficulties in adapting to these health needs in the face of spiralling health expenditure, duplication and fragmentation of services, and lack of co-ordination between the various elements and the numerous health authorities involved in their planning and provision. These problems have been compounded by blatant deficiencies in the organization of primary health care services, and the absence of cost-containment measures, which have contributed to their over-utilization and malutilization as expressed in an annual average of 10 doctor-patient contacts and 24 prescription items per patient. They have also contributed to increasing dissatisfaction among doctors and patients.

These difficulties have been further aggravated by a dispro-portionate distribution of medical manpower and budgets. Hospital costs now consume 46% of health expenditure, as compared with 40% in 1973. During the same period, the proportion of our total health budget allocated to ambulatory clinic and preventive health services had declined from 40% to less than 32% today. This ir-rational bias in budget allocation towards the hospital section has been a major factor in producing a crisis in medical care in Israel. This crisis was further fuelled by the medical schools, whose educational curricula were heavily oriented towards the hospital-based specialties. It was, therefore, inevitable that primary health care was eroded of its content and fell into disrepute in the eyes of the health authorities, the medical profession and the patients, and that serious doubts were raised as to the need for a generalist doctor in the highly specialized hospital-oriented framework of our medical services.

Nevertheless, the very factors which produced the crisis have also produced a backlash, which is now resulting in the renaissance of family medicine as an effective basis of the primary health care services. In 1953, the pioneer Health Centre was established in Kiryat Hayovel Jerusalem as a teaching unit for the University Department of Social Medicine. It provided integrated family and community-oriented health care by a team of physicians, nurses and allied health personnel (Kark 1974). Family medicine was already recognized as an independent medical specialty with a 2-year programme of vocational training in 1963 (Scientific Council 1963), thus preceding most, if not all other countries in this respect. Its status was, however, clearly inferior to that of other specialties, and it failed to attract local graduates.

A major impetus was provided in 1964 by the introduction of a revised curriculum for vocational training in family medicine (Polliack & Medalie 1969), and by the establishment within the Tel Aviv University Medical School of the first academic department of family medicine. In later years, academic departments were established in the medical schools in Jerusalem, Haifa and Beer Sheba, the latter with an innovative community oriented curriculum (Segall et al 1978). In 1975, with the introduction of mandatory examinations for all specialties, the first Board of Examiners in Family Medicine was appointed by the Scientific Council of the Israel Medical Association, followed by the establishment of the Israel Association of Family Physicians, which became a founder member of WONCA. In 1977, a Commission (Scientific Council 1977) strongly recommended the reorganization of primary health care services based on vocationally trained family physicians and health care teams. These recommendations were endorsed by Kupat Holim who, since then, has invested considerable budgets in expanding practice and training facilities for the rapidly increasing numbers of trainees and family physicians in its clinics.

The present vocational training curriculum extends over 4 years of postgraduate studies after completing the compulsory internship year. It consists of 27 months of rotating residencies in hospital wards, and 15 months in teaching practices under supervision of approved family physician tutors. It also includes a course of academic studies, provided on a day-release basis throughout the training period by the department of family medicine in each region. Vocational training is provided within the service framework of Kupat Holim, which employs the trainees. The content and standard of the programme are defined and supervized by the Scientific Council of the Israel Medical Association. Successful completion of the curriculum and the mandatory Board examinations leads to registration by the Ministry of Health as a 'Specialist in Family Medicine'.

FUTURE NEEDS TOWARDS THE YEAR 2000

Health needs based on priorities

Today, our population is cushioned against poverty, sickness, unemployment, handicaps and crises by means of extensive health services based on the principle that health care must be widely available according to patients' needs, rather than on their ability to pay for these services. Concomitantly, our prepaid medical services have snowballed to the dimensions of a major health industry, which has become prohibitively costly (8% of our gross national product) and increasingly fragmented, within an ever-widening maze of services in which the doctors no longer hold a controlling monopoly and in which the patients often flounder. The elderly and the chronic sick now constitute an ever-increasing percentage of our population. A society, better educated and informed than ever before, is expressing ever-increasing demands and expectations for better health and bigger medical miracles, and is less and less willing to accept the limitations of previously endurable discomforts and disorders.

Paradoxically, it is becoming increasingly clear that better health cannot be achieved by simply pumping more and more money into more easily available medical services. The frightening nightmare of health as a bottomless pit is increasingly apparent in the face of unchecked public 'demand', which exceeds objective 'needs', which inevitably exceed available resources. Health, in terms of complete physical, emotional and social wellbeing seems to be an ever-receding illusion and perhaps even a medical myth. Additional disillusionment has stemmed from the increasing realization that the modern technological hospital, while very effective in treating acute life-threatening and serious illness, has an unlimited capacity to consume immense budgets without necessarily producing corresponding benefits to health in terms of human wellbeing.

Integrated primary health care

The health needs and the scope and nature of the problems, disorders and diseases prevalent in the community differ from the highly selective conditions for which hospital resources are so essential. Although the content of primary medical care in the community includes portions of many medical disciplines, the clinical approach, diagnostic and management methods, and their application in the community setting, differ markedly from those of the hospital-based specialties (Fry 1966). Experiments, in this and other countries, to replace the family physician and the primary health care team with hospital 'outreach' programmes, or with various combinations of 'primary specialists' have proved extremely wasteful of medical manpower and budgets (Farell et al 1982). It seems neither logical nor desirable to facilitate direct patient access to highly qualified specialists whose specific training has fitted them to function optimally in a hospital or consultant setting, and whose involvement as 'primary practitioners' will inevitably lead to further fragmentation of the primary health care services (Sheps 1981).

There is, therefore, a growing recognition in Israel that the family physician and the allied health professionals in the primary health care team hold the key to economic, efficient and effective health care (Polliack 1983). Economic, because it is much cheaper than hospital-based or primary specialized services (Moren et al 1980); efficient, because it can protect the public from the dangers of fragmented medical care, and malutilization of expensive hospital facilities; effective, because it is a flexible service, capable of adaptation in response to changing health needs and priorities.

A community-oriented preventive approach

The integrative approach of the family physician and the primary health care team is especially appropriate in Israel in the face of a growing belief that further major achievements in the health of our population will depend mainly on the increasing implementation of preventive measures and health education. A community oriented preventive approach (Abramson et al 1981) is particularly applicable to diseases related to personal lifestyles and habits, long-term mental and physical disabilities, the control of communicable and nutritional diseases, occupational hazards, road accidents, and the personal and behavioural determinants of health and disease in our population.

Co-ordination, regionalization and decentralization

The provision of integrated, community-oriented primary health care also requires co-ordination of the various elements and levels of the health services based on the existing sick funds and health authorities. Regionalization of services, and decentralization of authority are particularly relevant to the primary health care services (Doron 1982), because the local level is more sensitive to the specific health needs in each community. It could also facilitate meaningful community participation in the implementation of the health services, and encourage cost awareness and containment.

Manpower development for primary health care

Effective primary health care services will require rational planning of manpower needs in relation to optimal ratios and distributions of family physicians and allied health personnel, and on developing valid information systems which could enable accurate projections of the needs in this respect. In Israel, manpower problems are not quantitative, but are qualitative in terms of the appropriate skills for doctors, nurses and allied health workers required for the performance of their tasks. Nor can the schools of medicine, and of allied health professionals remain indifferent or ambivalent to the needs of the society from which they derive their mandates and considerable budgets. Their educational objectives, teaching and research activities should first and foremost be directed towards meeting the health needs of the population, and the manpower requirements of the health services.

Undergraduate, continuing and vocational training

If family medicine and primary health care are to be presented as career choices to students, then there is an urgent need to allocate increased teaching facilities and resources towards these objectives on both undergraduate and postgraduate levels. A special responsibility also rests on the academic departments of family medicine. Unlike the more established and traditional medical disciplines, these are often camouflaged under a variety of names which seem to expose basic uncertainties as to their academic identities, ideological affiliations, and educational objectives. The manner in which we define, present and teach the practice and content of family medicine will have far reaching implications and eventually decide the future direction, content, scope and limitations of primary health care in the community.

If, however, our educational programmes are to be perceived as relevant by our students and trainees, then a considerable amount of teaching must be provided in the natural setting in which they will ultimately practise. While not denying the complementary role of hospital or university-based facilities or 'model' clinics, or of full-time academic teachers and researchers, it seems essential that academic family physicians and allied health profession tutors also serve as role models in the normal service setting, if they are to maintain credibility in the eyes of their students and colleagues. Continuing education and in-service training programmes for family physicians, nurses, social workers, health educators and allied health personnel should also be reviewed in relation to these principles and their relevance to primary health care. Much has been spoken about 'team work'. Few health professionals have received formal or practical training for working together as a multidisciplinary team.

Teaching facilities in the clinics

If family physicians and allied health workers are to participate effectively in academic and clinical teaching activities, then educational facilities and work systems in the clinics must be greatly improved. Despite initial efforts in this respect, work conditions in most of our 'teaching clinics' differ little from those in non-teaching clinics, and academic activities often clash with service commitments. Nor does the rigid bureaucratic structure of our organizational system encourage flexibility or adaptability at clinic levels. Hence, the quality of practice and teaching in these clinics depends mainly on the individual abilities and personal talents of the staff members to work and teach, despite the many constraints over which they have little control.

The solution to these and similar flaws in relation to manpower training would seem to depend on a recognition, by all concerned, that academic activities, clinical teaching and research are as much an integral part of the work of the family doctor and allied health professionals in the community clinics, as are their service commitments. There is, therefore, a need to co-ordinate the activities of the academic institutions and the health service authorities as legitimate partners in jointly planning, monitoring and developing high quality facilities in the clinics, so as to enable vocationally trained family physicians and allied health professionals to teach and practise on the academic and clinical levels for which they have been trained.

The challenge

While it is premature to assert that these principles and policy directions have been adopted or even universally accepted in Israel, the feasibility of their implementation has been amply demonstrated. The challenge posed by these needs is clear and unequivocable in relation to the future of primary health care in our country. On the acceptance of this challenge, may well depend the development of family medicine and, hence, the possibility of achieving the Alma-Ata objectives (World Health Organization 1978) in relation to better health care for the population of Israel by the year 2000.

REFERENCES

Abramson J H, Gofin R, Hopp C, Gofin J, Donchin M, Habib J 1981 Evaluation of a community program for the control of cardiovascular risk factors — the CHAD program in Jerusalem. Israel Journal of Medical Sciences 17: 201–212
Arnon A 1971 The Nehora health centre. The Family Physician (Israel) 1: 80–84
Bach R 1974 The population of Israel. The Hebrew University, Jerusalem, p 77
Central Bureau of Statistics 1983 Statistical abstracts. Ministry of Health, Jerusalem
Doron H 1982 Regionalization of health services in Israel. Israel Journal of Medical Sciences 18: 357–363
Doron H 1983 Developing concepts and patterns of primary care. Israel Journal of Medical Sciences 19: 694–697
Farell D L, Worth R M, Mishina K 1982 Utilization and cost effectiveness of a family practice center. Journal of Family Practice (USA) 15: 957–962
Fry J 1966 Profiles of disease. E & S Livingstone Ltd, London, p 4–15
Grushka T (ed) 1968 Health services in Israel. Ministry of Health, Jerusalem
Kark S L 1974 Community medicine and primary health. In: Epidemiology and community medicine. Appleton-Century-Crofts, New York
Modan B 1982 Current status of health services in Israel. Israel Journal of Medical Sciences 18: 337–344
Moren. J, Frazier T, Altman I, DeLozier J 1980 Ambulatory medical care — comparison of internists and family-general practitioners. New England Journal of Medicine 302: 11–16
Polliack M R 1976 The road to prepaid health care. Update (UK) 13: 694–696
Polliack M R 1983 Vocational training for family practice in Israel. Israel Journal of Medical Sciences 19: 783–786
Polliack M R, Medalie J H, 1969 Programme for specialization in family medicine. British Medical Journal iv: 487–489
Ron A 1980 Roles scope and current issues. Kupat Holim Health Insurance Institution, Tel Aviv
Scientific Council 1963 Manual for medical trainees. Israel Medical Association, Jerusalem
Scientific Council 1977 Report of commission on organization of medical services in the community. The Family Physician (Israel) 7: 342–354
Segall A, Prywes M, Benor D E, Susskind O 1978 University Center for Health Sciences, Ben-Gurion University of the Negev — an interim perspective. In: Katz F M, Fulop T (eds) Personnel for health care: case studies of educational programmes. WHO, Geneva, p 111
Shapiro H L 1963 The Jewish people — a biological history. UNESCO Publications, Paris
Sheps C G 1981 The modern crisis in health services — professional concerns and the public interest. Israel Journal of Medical Sciences 17: 71–79
Tulchinsky T H, Lunenfeld B, Haber S, Handelsman M 1982 Israel health review. Israel Journal of Medical Sciences 18: 345–355
World Health Organization 1978 Report of the international conference on primary health care Alma-Ata USSR. W H O, Geneva
Yodfat Y 1970 Teamwork in family medicine. The Family Physician (Israel) 1: 51–54

Nigeria

NATIONAL FEATURES

Geographical

Nigeria, a West African territory just north of the equator and east of the Greenwich meridian, can claim with justification to be a leading nation in the African continent.

Size. 357 000 square miles; equivalent to the areas of Belgium, France, Switzerland and Italy combined (Fig. 24.1).

Population. At the last reasonably accurate census in 1963, it was 54 million. Allowing for an estimated growth rate of 2.5% per annum, the population is now over 90 million. Every fifth African is a Nigerian. As there is little support yet for a slow-down in population growth, the total should be over 140 million by the year 2000.

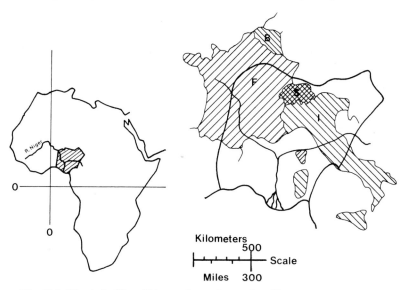

Fig. 24.1 Nigeria in West Africa, and superimposed on Europe.

Political

Nigeria became an independent Federal Republic within the British Commonwealth in 1960. The original Westminster type of constitution proved unstable, and the government is now a military one, though with a large element of appointed civilian involvement. Nigeria is divided into 19 states, reflecting the ethnic diversity of its peoples. English is the lingua franca and the language of all higher education, justice, commerce and health care administration. However, other languages, such as Hausa, Yoruba and Ibo, are widely spoken. The literacy rate is still low.

Resources

Nigeria was formerly a major exporter of hardwoods, tin, cocoa, palm-oil and groundnuts, with very little local industry. During the 1960s and 1970s oil became dominant, and now accounts for 95% of the revenue. Nigeria is a member of OPEC and the world's ninth largest producer. During the initial boom there was extensive investment in local industry, with phenomenal growth in the Federal capital, Lagos, and all the other State capitals, with an impressive network of well-engineered main roads between them. However, the oil-glut and attendant recession have led to a belated attempt to revive the agricultural sectors of the economy. Growth of food crops has lagged behind growth in the population, and rice, corn and wheat are now major imports. Investment in power, water supply and telecommunications has also not kept pace and the infrastructure for further development is shaky. The struggle for survival has led to widespread corruption, which the present military government is trying to contain. However, the regime is relatively liberal, and the people remain cheerful. Despite its problems, other nations in Africa look to Nigeria for leadership.

COMMON HEALTH PROBLEMS

Vital statistics

Statistics in Nigeria are not reliable. Registration of births and deaths is not compulsory, except in Lagos, and even there the figures are incomplete. Estimates are based on limited local surveys, generally associated with teaching hospitals. In 1980 the Federal Ministry of Health issued the following table (Table 24.1). The figures show that nearly half the population are children under 15

Table 24.1 Vital statistics; Nigeria compared with a typical developed country

Statistic	Nigeria	Developed country
Crude live birth rate per 1000 population	45	12
Crude death rate per 1000 population	20	10
Rate of natural increase of population (%)	2.5	<1
Median age (years)	18	27
Proportion of deaths occurring among under 6-year-olds (%)	50	6
Infant mortality rate per 1000 live births	120	10
Percentage of population under 15 years (dependency ratio)	45	25
Percentage of population 15–64 years (labour age-group)	52	67
Percentage of population 65 years and above (senior citizens)	3	12

Source for Nigeria: Federal Ministry of Health 1980 (in *Africa Health* 1983, vol. 6, 1, 23)

years of age, and it is in that age group that the heaviest morbidity occurs.

Disease prevalence

Poverty is still widespread, and K. T. Joiner, a consultant paediatrician in Ilorin, has highlighted the lot of children with a list spelling MISERY (Table 24.2).

Among adults, conditions like hypertension and diabetes appear as prevalent as in developed countries, but in many other ways the spectrum of disease is markedly different.

Tuberculosis. Still widespread in both rural areas and the periurban shanty towns, where partial self-medication leads to a high proportion of resistant cases.

Leprosy. Reports show a patchy prevalence. Igbo-Ora, in the west, 6 cases in 8 years. Abakaliki in the east, 300 new cases in a year. Control measures have not been well maintained.

Table 24.2 Paediatric health problems

M	—	Malnutrition, malaria, medications (traditional), modern living (hazards), malignant disease
I	—	Infections, infestations, ignorance, illiteracy and insufficient funds
S	—	Sickle cell disease and other major anaemias
E	—	Enteritis — dehydration
R	—	Respiratory infections
Y	—	Yellow neonate — neonatal jaundice

Source: K T Joiner (in *Africa Health* 1983, 6, 1, 23)

Onchocerciasis. Blindness in late cases with ocular invasion, common in the north, less common in the south. In the south there is increasing concern about the high proportion of cases with backache and other forms of musculoskeletal pain, previously unrecognized as being related to the disease. The disability causes loss of productivity among farmers in *Simulium*-infested river-basin areas. The many other endemic tropical diseases also take their toll.

Low dietary fibre related diseases. These 'diseases of civilization' are on the increase in urban areas. In the city of Onitsha on the banks of the Niger river, Iyi-Enu Hospital figures show that the prevalence of appendicitis now exceeds that of hernia, a situation very different from 30 years ago. White bread, sugar and highly processed foods are starting to replace the indigenous diet for city dwellers.

Road traffic accident deaths. The 10 countries in the world with the highest accident rates are all in Africa, and Nigeria heads the list. Increase in car ownership, poor vehicle maintenance, dangerous driving, and increasing use of drugs and alcohol, all contribute. Brewing is probably the fastest growing industry, despite the recession.

HEALTH CARE SYSTEM

Federal responsibilities

Health services to the public are essentially controlled at state level, but the federal Ministry of Health provides overall co-ordination through a National Council on Health, on which all state commissioners of health and their chief executives sit. The federal Ministry of Health takes direct responsibility for:

1. *Teaching hospitals*, inspection, approval and funding.

2. *Professional registration and standards* — through the Nigeria Medical Council, Nurses and Midwives Council and Pharmacy Board. Doctors trained overseas have to pass an assessment examination, run twice yearly by the Nigeria Medical Council, before being given Temporary Registration.

3. *Postgraduate training* — through the National Postgraduate Medical College of Nigeria. There is also the West African Postgraduate Medical College, responsible to the West African Health Community within the Economic Community of West African States (ECOWAS)

4. *Research, pharmaceutical quality control, port health, epidemiology* and many other national functions.

A Division of Primary Care has recently been recognized in the federal Ministry of Health to control the schools of health technology set up in every state, training a non-physician cadre of staff for primary health care (PHC) — community health Aides, assistants, supervisors and officers. The Division registers them when trained, and also co-operates closely with UNICEF and WHO in recommending their initiatives for implementation within State health services.

Sources of care

It is upon the state Ministeries of Health that provision of health care to the public is laid, but resources are inadequate. Non-governmental sources also give a major share. These include:

1. *Voluntary agency hospitals and health services.* Most of these are church-related and, up to 10 years ago, were providing one-third to one-half of all medical care, particularly in the rural areas. Though government services have now expanded more rapidly, there are still over 100 voluntary agency hospitals and health facilities registered with the Christian Health Association of Nigeria (CHAN). Some have pioneered important PHC work, such as the village health worker training programme at Garkida, Gongola State, or the action research done by Morley at Ilesha and Imesi in Oyo State in 1956–61, resulting in the growth chart and under-fives clinic system now commonly used in most countries of the world.

2. *Private sector medical services.* The first private doctors started up or established themselves during the 1914–18 war. By 1960 there were 84 in private practice. The sector is now growing rapidly and spreading from the big cities to smaller up-country towns. The development has partly been in reaction to government bureaucracy and in the hope of quicker financial gains, but there are many centres with excellent facilities, group practices or hospitals of up to 200 beds, and offering good comprehensive service.

Governmental sources, federal, state and local government, provide a full range of care, but coverage is still far from complete. At present it is believed that only one-third of the population in the country have access to modern health facilities. That leaves nearly 60 million dependent only on traditional healers, birth-attendants and bone setters — or nothing.

Levels of care

Patient-centred health care in Nigeria is generally considered at three levels — primary, secondary and tertiary, the secondary being the service given at district-type hospitals run by general duty medical officers. Community-centred care is related to all three levels but particularly to primary health care.

Tertiary care hospitals in Nigeria have increased in size and numbers more rapidly than the economy can stand. The first was Ibadan Medical School, started in 1948, with its fine new teaching hospital opened in 1956. Now there are 9 medical schools, and 4 or 5 more in various stages of preparation. A high proportion of the health budget is going on teaching hospitals.

By comparison the *secondary-care* general hospitals and maternity hospitals have received scant attention despite providing 90% of inpatient care in their 60 000 beds (Table 24.3).

Table 24.3   Health establishments

University teaching hospitals	9 with 5730 beds
General hospitals	694 with 44 208 beds
Maternity hostpitals, homes and centres	2289 with 15 455 beds
Health centres	685 with 3561 beds
Armed forces hospitals	18 with 2650 beds
Special hospitals (mental, ophthalmic orthopaedic, tuberculosis and leprosy)	49 with 4561 beds
Health clinics and dispensaries	3407

Source: Federal Ministry of Health 1980 (in *Africa Health* 1983, vol. 6, 1, 23)

Primary care received a big push in Nigeria's 1975–80 Development Plan with the launching of a major basic health services scheme. It proved far more costly to implement than originally envisaged. Primary care is not cheap when costs are multiplied to meet the needs of so many millions. The new cadre of health professional has come to stay, the community health personnel, at four levels — aide, assistant, supervisor and officer — and these should be a vital new resource, if their relationships with the nursing and medical professions work out satisfactorily in practice.

Manpower

The total numbers in health care are far below what is needed to provide modern health care for Nigeria's present population (Table 24.4). Efforts are being made, but they barely keep pace with the

Table 24.4   Health manpower

Medical practitioners	10 399 (12.0)
Dental practitioners	379 (0.4)
Pharmacists	2609 (3.0)
Nurses	29 962 (33.3)
Midwives	24 112 (27.7)
Community health officers	280 (0.3)

Figures in brackets denotes number per 100 000 population.
Source: Federal Ministry of Health 1980 (in *Africa Health* 1983, vol. 6, 1, 23).

population growth. Economic stringency makes rapid improvement difficult.

PLACE OF PRIMARY HEALTH CARE: WHO DOES WHAT?

While it is acknowledged that the policy of Health for All by the year 2000 means emphasis on primary health care, it is not proving an easy policy to implement. In a country where there are so few doctors much depends on what can effectively be done by non-physicians.

Non-physician PHC

Community health aides and assistants (CHA)

Primary school educated. Given course of 1 to 2 years, depending on pretest ability. Taught some clinic-based duties, like assistant nurses — recording temperatures, keeping simple records, weighing children and filling in a growth chart, administering medicines. Also taught community-based duties, like health inspectors — health education, hygiene, care of water supplies, etc. They are allowed to do some primary clinical consultations under the supervision of nurses, guided by a bulky volume of standing orders in the form of flow charts to cover all the eventualities they may meet. These standing orders were prepared by consultant physicians and nurse educators with experience of primary care, and they provide legal cover when doing what might otherwise be considered 'doctors' duties'.

Midwives and nurses

Nigeria has an excellent cadre of nurses and midwives, and there are six times as many of them as there are doctors. More community health is now included in their training curriculum. They cover much of normal midwifery, picking out high-risk cases for referral; also care for common conditions, immunization, family planning and nursing care in health centres and maternity homes.

Community Health Officers (CHO)

Extra training in clinical care and administration, and all the duties covered by the aides and assistants, given in university-sponsored courses to senior health personnel. In the south of Nigeria these are mainly senior health sisters, for whom the CHO qualification allows increased responsibility and promotion to take charge of a primary health centre. In the north of Nigeria most CHO candidates have come through the ranks of the rural health superintendents, as there are fewer nurses in the north. Only the exceptional ones come to the same standard. If a CHO is appointed to work in a primary or comprehensive health centre with a doctor, the job description says that, 'the doctor is to be responsible for medical duties; the CHO to be in administrative charge', but this arrangement has yet to be tested in practice.

Professional health educators

Diplomas and masters degreee courses can now be obtained from the Africa Regional Health Education Council (ARHEC) course in Ibadan by those with nursing or other type of health professional background. It is through these people, and from others with the right experience and motivation, that there may come another even more important source of primary health care, the village worker.

The part-time village (or primary) health worker

These are mature men or women, chosen by their village community, and given a very simple training as near to their homes as possible. In the model course run by ARHEC personnel at Idere, in relation to the Ibadan training, it has been found possible to teach farmers, petty-traders, drivers and others to manage 10 simple aspects of primary health care (Table 24.5). These may cover 80% of health problems in the village. It is hoped that those trained will continue with their usual occupation, receiving financial support from their communities for the hours spent on health work. They are not professionals and it should be possible to multiply numbers despite the economic situation.

Table 24.5 Ten elements of primary health care taught to village health workers in Idere

1. Malaria, treatment and prophylaxis
2. Childhood nutrition, prevention of malnutrition and anaemia
3. Water supplies, disposal of excreta, prevention of guinea-worm
4. Diarrhoea, use of oral rehydration
5. Conditions that can be prevented by immunization; childhood infections
6. Coughs, tuberculosis and leprosy .
7. Care of small wounds, prevention of tetanus; what to do in case of snake-bite
8. Recognition of the early effects of onchocerciasis, treatment and prevention
9. Care of women in pregnancy
10. Possibilities of family planning

Physician-run PHC

Doctors have an important place in primary health care. In many situations their role is more of supervisor, trainer, and leader of the health team.

Youth Corps doctors

In their first postregistration year all doctors in Nigeria are required to do a year of national service. For many this is in a rural hospital or health centre, often with the minimum of help from senior colleagues.

Medical officers

These may be in secondary-care hospitals, government or voluntary agency. The outpatient clinics of these hospitals provide primary care, mainly curative, but with some prevention if the doctor is so inclined. His duties may also include touring to fixed rural health centres and clinics staffed by CHAs or midwives. Few Nigerians are currently entering this type of work in the public service, and the government has been recruiting from overseas, mainly from Asia. The church-related hospitals still attract well-motivated missionary doctors and Catholic Sister-doctors, and are developing PHC outreach as well as hospital-based services. Mkar Christian Hospital, in Benue State, has an excellent system whereby communities can set up first aid posts, and send an aide for training at the hospital. If the work at the post grows, the community can apply for it to be upgraded to a maternity centre, and the government sends them a midwife. The hospital provides supervision now to over 70 centres, with a physician as full-time director of the scheme.

University Health Service

General practitioners provide care to what are, in effect, privileged communities. Standards are similar to those in developed countries. Most teaching hospitals also run general outpatient departments, staffed by general practitioners, but they are mainly concerned with sorting out cases for the specialist clinics.

Private practitioners

Private practitioners run clinics and hospitals of 10–200 beds, depending for finance largely on 'retainers' from institutions and industrial concerns; hence they are mainly in the cities and larger towns. Many have excellent, purpose-built premises and offer a comprehensive care, with immunization, under-fives clinics, family-planning, health education sessions, and curative service at reasonable prices. One such centre found that 40% of their patients defaulted on bills, but service was still given.

PHYSICIAN EDUCATION FOR PRIMARY CARE

Most Nigerian medical schools have a traditional-type curriculum, which includes community health, and involves a rural posting of 6–8 weeks. Lagos is experimenting with a new curriculum which has 9 months of primary care in the final year. This is not equated with general practice, and no general practitioners are involved in the clinical instruction. Calabar medical school is the only one to have a department of general practice, but that too is still feeling its way. After qualification, Nigerian doctors experience the same pressure to enter a specialty, as is felt by doctors in most countries of the world. It is only recently that the option of specializing in general practice has been open to them. The opportunity is being eagerly taken up, and this may, at last, prove a breakthrough and bring doctors into primary care.

The Faculty of General Medical Practice

All postgraduate education in Nigeria is co-ordinated under the umbrella of the National Postgraduate Medical College, with its headquarters in Lagos. This began in 1970, and now has 14 specialty faculties, including one for general medical practice. About 120 Foundation Fellowships in General Practice have been awarded by the College to the most senior practitioners with established reputations. A Board for the Faculty was set up in 1979, and a syllabus and structure of a 4-year residency programme worked out in 1980. Entry to the Faculty is now by examination only. The first GP registrars started in 1981, and by 1984 there were over 50 in training. The first 2 years are in an approved general hospital, maybe voluntary agency or government, rotating around the various sections, and filling in a clinical practice record book (log book), with space to record the hospital number of patients with each type of condition managed or operated upon. At the end of 2 years the candidate may sit the Part I finals examination (60% written, 40% oral/clinical), set and marked by Fellows of the Faculty, sometimes with an external examiner from the Royal College in the UK. The second 2 years are generally spent in a private sector practice or hospital, inspected and approved, but other primary care settings are being considered. At the Part II finals examination the candidate has to submit a case book/dissertation on a theme approved by the Faculty and of importance to the discipline of general practice in its Nigerian setting.

The introduction of the programme has widened the formerly accepted concept of general practice in Nigeria. It is not just private practice any more. Doctors in public service, working on a generalist basis, are also included. The medical officer in a district hospital has been shown to share the same ground. Primary and secondary care have been brought together, and the general practitioner is seen as the bridge between the non-physician primary care workers on one side, and the hospital-based specialists on the other. The GP's role has been defined by the Faculty as 'a front-line medical practitioner, or doctor of first-contact [i.e. first *physician* contact], who delivers comprehensive health care either privately or in public service'.

There is a Faculty of Public Health (or Community Health) within the Postgraduate College, but its programme tends to lead doctors into administrative or academic posts, e.g. head of a school of health technology, or as a director of port health. It does not produce the 'front-line doctors' which the country so urgently needs. It has to be seen whether the Faculty of General Medical Practice can be more successful. The first senior registrars to qualify are only just coming through — but signs are hopeful.

PRESENT PROBLEMS

The economy

The world-wide recession of the 1980s hit Nigeria badly despite its oil, and the need to cut back drastically on public services expenditure affected all areas of life, including the provision of drugs and supplies to hospitals and health centres. In-patients have often had to buy their drugs, dressings and even intravenous fluids from pharmacies outside at inflated prices. The military government is trying to improve the situation, but the problems are still great.

Village health worker supervision

Potentially these community-based health promoters are the key to spreading at least some basic elements of primary health care in a time of economic stringency. However, once back in their villages, their interest wanes and standards fall unless there is constant encouragement and supervision. At the heart of most successful programmes there has to be a strong and sympathetic leader with a charismatic personality. Methods of improving supervision are now the subject of enquiry and research.

Centralization of appointments in state capitals

Community health personnel, nurses and doctors in the public service are generally recruited and appointed by state health management boards in the state capital and are then moved out to small towns and rural areas wherever there may be a vacancy. Many come unwillingly to serve 'in the bush', and cannot wait to complete the year that is expected of them before they go back to the city again. Not unnaturally, motivation is poor and standards low. A switch to advertising specific posts, whether in city or in rural area, would lead to staff going where they *choose* to go. The public service needs much greater decentralization if there is to be any successful primary health care on the scale so urgently needed.

FUTURE NEEDS FOR NIGERIA

1. *Effective national policies* from the federal and state governments, for growth of more food, provision of more water, and a recognition of the dangers inherent in the use of more white bread and highly

refined foods, and the growing dependence on alcohol, tobacco and drugs.

2. *Greater priority for the production or importation* of a limited range of basic generic drugs; encouragement of economy of prescribing by both physicians and authorized non-physicians.

3. *Education for self-help*; greater use of the media for health education; encouragement of all village health worker training programmes.

4. *Allocation of more resources for health*; at present only 3% of GNP, though it can justifiably be said that expenditure on water and fertilizer, etc, is also a major contribution to health.

5. *Population growth control* is not a popular issue, but will have to come, or all plans to provide health for all by the year 2000 will be overwhelmed by the increasing numbers to be cared for.

CHALLENGES FOR THE NIGERIAN FACULTY OF GENERAL MEDICAL PRACTICE

1. Ensure that the successful beginning made is carried on. In particular, for finance from federal or other sources to maintain the academic base and study centre in Lagos, and develop branches in each of the main areas of the country.

2. Speed up the process of giving good general hospitals approval for training to match the rapidly increasing demand for places, and the need for more physicians of high quality and good motivation in primary and/or secondary care.

3. Engage in constant evaluation and research to ensure that the GP residency programme is relevant to the changing needs of Nigeria and in harmony with the programmes of other faculties.

4. Encourage the doctors who have received the training to move into work which is of significance in the development of primary health care, in both rural and urban areas, in co-operation with the whole primary health care team.

5. Press the universities to start general practice departments, or primary care departments with a proper place for general practice, in every medical school in the country, so that more doctors will come to see their future career in terms of general practice/primary care.

Acknowledgements

I am indebted to *Africa Health* 1983, vol. 6 for tables used in this chapter and to Professor E. A. Elebute, President of the National Postgraduate Medical College, Nigeria, for his valuable advice.

Zimbabwe

THE COUNTRY

The ancient land of Ophir and the kingdom of Monomotapa encompassed the land known from the 1890s as Southern Rhodesia, and Zimbabwe since 1980.

Zimbabwe is situated in Africa between the Zambesi and the Limpopo rivers (Fig. 25.1). To the east it is separated from low-lying Mocambique and the sea by a mountainous area rising to 2750 m (9000 ft). The western semiarid boundary is protected by progressively more arid country merging with the Kalahari desert.

Rainfall is seasonal, occurring in the summer months of November to March. There is a higher rainfall in the north and east, sufficient to grow cereal and other crops, and amounting to anything from 63–153 cm (25–60 in) per annum. In the south and west there is a lesser rainfall, and without irrigation the country is suitable only for cattle and game ranching.

On the higher central plateau, the most productive land, the climate is pleasant, of low humidity and with temperatures ranging from about 2°–35°C. In the river valleys of the north and south it is much hotter and humid, although the rainfall is less.

THE PEOPLE

At one time it was a land teeming with game and inhabited by a few short-statured steatopygeous hunters, the bushmen. During the great migration of the Bantu people southwards soon after the European renaissance, the bushmen were ousted by tribes of the Shona people. These were pastoral, with a shifting agriculture protected from slavery and invasion by the natural malarial and mountain barriers to the east. They mined and smelted iron for tools and weapons, and gold for trade with the Arabs, and later the Portuguese.

COUNTRIES OF SOUTHERN AFRICA

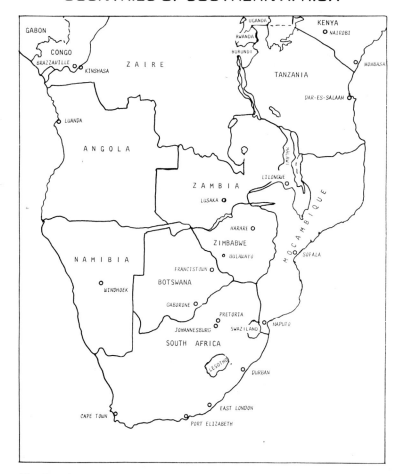

Fig. 25.1 Countries of southern Africa

In 1837 the Matabele tribe of the Zulu nation, which reached Natal during the Bantu migration, fled from their paramount King Chaka and settled in the southwest of the country. The Matabele tribe, a war-like pastoral nation, subjugated the Shona to the north, exacting tribute of grain, cattle, women, slaves, or death.

Missionaries followed a few years later, taking the route from Capetown. Quinine ensured survival, while their surgical ability and meagre pharmacopoea gained them friends.

The missionaries were closely followed by hunters and traders from the south. Their reports fired the scramble for Africa and in 1890 Cecil John Rhodes pre-empted other nations by obtaining an agreement with the King of the Matabele allowing his British South Africa Company to dig for metals and farm in Mashonaland.

The obvious intention of the settlers to remain and to limit Matabele hegemony fired two unsuccessful liberation wars in 1893 and 1896. For the next 90 years the country was known as Rhodesia, or Southern Rhodesia.

During this time, with the aid of black labour, the settlers created a thriving state with an enviable infrastructure and a sound economy based on agriculture, mining and manufacture. The white population grew to 270 000 by 1975, while the black increased from less than 500 000 to about 7 million.

As blacks became more educated, largely due to missionary effort, they resented the second class status imposed on them by imperceptive separatist laws.

White conservatism, slow to suffer change, stimulated an increasing guerilla freedom war. Sanctions, world opprobrium and Marxist guns and training ensured a political victory for the guerillas under Comrade Robert Mugabe.

THE HEALTH SYSTEM

Traditional

The traditional healer or *N'ganga*, educated by apprenticeship, or by dreams following a call, purports to communicate with ancestors through a trance or interpretation of patterns made by thrown bones or other artefacts. He does this on a fee-for-service basis when consulted for ill-health, disaster, crop failure or any threatening situation. The diagnosis, often ancestral wrath or the machinations of mischievous spirits, comes from ancestral spirits. The prescription may be herbal, but is often some form of penance; or preventively, the wearing of an amulet or the placing of charms about the entrance to the dwelling. By virtue of their knowledge of the nuances of culture, the N'ganga manage neuroses extremely well.

Midwifery may be conducted by traditional attendants for a living, but is more commonly carried out by elderly female relatives, who understand the process through personal experience.

The spiritually based concept of care is still entrenched, and even though many patients seek the symptomatic relief of biomedical care, it is still thought necessary to ascertain the spiritual reason for the illness in a separate consultation with the N'ganga.

Biomedicine

Following on the missionary medicine, which barely touched more than a fraction of the blacks, came the doctors attached to the settler group in 1890. By 1935 the country was peppered with small hospitals and satellite clinics. The mission hospitals dealt mainly with the blacks in rural areas, while the government hospitals had separated 'hotel' accommodation wards for whites and blacks, giving free treatment to the latter, with common service areas such as the operating theatres. Private practitioners dealt largely with whites, admitted when necessary to government hospital white wards, cared for by their own doctor.

Both groups had taught young men and women to perform various types of medical aide work on an informal basis to meet the needs of any individual area.

Intravenous arsenic, Prontosil (a sulphonamide) and later penicillin wrought such potent miracle cures that biomedicine gained credibility to the extent that all services were flooded, including the private sector which had grown in parallel with the others.

More help was needed. The orderlies began to be formally trained as 'medical assistants' to man the clinics feeding the hospitals from the more remote areas. Many specialized into microscopists, dental or pharmacy assistants, 'radiographers' and even 'anaesthetists'.

By 1950 the amount of work forced most doctors to stay in their hospitals to cope with the mounting volume of curative work. It became necessary to create preventive teams led by provincial medical officers of health with nurses and health inspectors reinforced by a new category of 'health assistants' trained in practical environmental and educative health matters. Token fees were introduced to discourage the frivolous.

In the mid-1950s, two large new hospitals were opened. They were better equipped than any other and contained specialist departments. The glut of applicants for district medical officer posts fell away and many such posts became unfilled vacancies.

The provincial medical officers of health had to assume the care of doctorless small hospitals and their satellite clinics, visiting each at intervals. The standard of peripheral care dropped as the central high technology medicine expanded, taking more and more of the health budget.

The medical school, which graduated its first doctors in 1968, had little impact as the new graduates specialized and stayed in the towns, entered city general practice, or left the country for good.

The peripheral health services were further hit badly by the guerilla war. Many government and mission hospitals and clinics had to close. When Zimbabwe came into being in 1980, it could, with justice, be said that the people of the rural areas were neglected.

By means of foreign aid and heavier taxation the new government started to expand the rural health service as fast as possible, training more medical and health assistants, and introducing a 'new' category — the village health worker (VHW).

Some of the district hospitals, formerly one-man stations, now have three or four doctors, many of whom are expatriates on short-term contracts, while others still have no resident medical officer. The district medical officers have been given back their preventive role in their own areas, to some extent directed and supported by an expanded number of provincial medical directors (formerly the provincial medical officers of health).

A health information system, based on the observations of village health workers, has been designed to reach upwards through rural clinics eventually to the Ministry of Health. A reverse support system from the referral hospitals and back eventually to the village health worker is envisaged.

Present problems

The expansion which took place was expensive, and continues to be expensive to maintain. Foreign aid and large tax returns have ceased. Established health units cannot be scrapped, and cuts in votes seem to hit the newer and projected ventures, despite political commitment.

HEALTH PROBLEMS (see also Chapter 10)

Common diseases

Nutrition: toddler malnutrition

Affecting 30% of preschool children, this problem is no better than it was 30 years ago, despite persistent health education. Although poverty plays a part, the main problem is the traditional spiritual concept of illness, which resists health education conducted in a mass manner. In a number of enclaves where the health education teams have adopted one-to-one methods, supported by a credible doctor or hospital known by the community to be doing a good curative job, the nutritional status of children approximates the best in the developed world.

Other malnutrition

Vitamin deficiency syndromes are seen less often today, but obesity and hypertension have increased enormously in the past decades. Non-insulin-dependant diabetes appears to be exploding. Vascular occlusive disease, while not yet common, is no longer a remarkable condition. There is accumulating evidence that these conditions may be related to deficiencies occasioned by the growing predilection for refined carbohydrate and cereal foods.

There is a high risk that we may yet see Western disease overlaying the, as yet, unconquered infectious and childhood nutritional problems.

Tropical disease

The two major locally occurring diseases are malaria and bilharzia. Curative measures for bilharzia on a large scale seem counterproductive for people who return to the same environment, certain to aquire an even greater worm load. Universal environmental control is presently impossible. It is very expensive and liable to be negated if not carried out by neighbouring countries at the same time. Impounded water schemes, essential for agriculture, compound the problem.

Drug-resistant malaria is a bogey which we are shortly to face, but the towns and highlands fortunately are relatively free of the disease. Part of this freedom is due to environmental change, while some is due to the continuing use of residual organochlorides in dwellings. The ecological implications are a subject of periodic heated debate.

Infectious disease

Diphtheria and poliomyelitis have been rare since the mid-1960s. The last smallpox case occurred in 1964.

Whooping cough still is a problem, despite immunization.

Tetanus is more commonly seen as a neonatal infection, often as a result of traditional practices of cord dressing. Immunization of the pregnant mother has helped to reduce the problem, and is part of an extended programme of immunization.

Measles control still eludes us, despite concerted efforts. The problem of the 'cold chain' has not been solved, and is more difficult because of the chain's extreme length from the manufacturer to the point of administration. The credibility of the health service suffers when an ostensibly immunized child dies of the disease a few months later; still a common happening.

Diarrhoeal disease is synergistic with toddler subnutrition, and awaits the more rapid development of clean water supplies. This is not quite so simple, as it has been noted that the diarrhoea of giardiasis often replaces that of the coliforms when relatively clean water replaces that from shallow wells and rivers.

Pulmonary tuberculosis, an acute fatal illness in the 1950s, is now more often a chronic cavitating disease. The superb control system of the 1950s and 1960s saw an increased incidence with a peak of 120 per 100 000 in 1960, dropping to 40 per 100 000 in 1970. Fragmentation of effort and war disruption, together with refugee migration from bordering countries, has seen a rise to 85 per 100 000 in the last years.

Cancer

This exists at the same level as elsewhere, though the patterns differ.

Migrant labour

Most black men seek work in the towns, leaving a rural family to care for their agricultural holding. Many consort with prostitutes, or may take a 'town wife', becoming responsible for two families. Alcoholism, sexually transmitted disease and psychosomatic illness, which are rife and increasing, may stem partly from the associated social disruption.

Spritual beliefs

The difficulty of persuading believers in a spiritual cause of illness that their ill health is amenable to personal rational action has already been mentioned. The credibility of the teacher must outweigh that of traditional wise persons and upbringing.

The extended family

This has been useful in that the care of the aged and infirm has previously been safely left to the extended family. However, it often inhibits productivity and ambition. A man who has energetically attempted to improve his family's income and life-style feels obliged to assist his extended family, to whom he has a great sense of loyalty. The help demanded frequently leaves him worse off than if he had been more slothful, so he is unwilling to persist.

Population control

It is difficult to persuade an agricultural people that they should deprive themselves of potential helpers on their peasant holdings, reduce their security in old age, and minimize the numbers of descendants to worship them after death, by limiting the size of families. To die without issue is to be condemned to annihilation after death.

Urban-based families, faced with competing costs, are more likely to accept the need for smaller families. Despite active family planning promotion, the rate of natural increase remains above 3% per annum. This cannot hope to be matched by a sustained economic growth. If such an increase persists, unemployment and poverty will also increase. The first physical barrier to be reached will be a dearth of water. These and other results of population explosive growth have profound implications for future health and quality of life.

The consultation

The enforced use of paramedicals to meet the demands of the people for medical help has led to their use in a clinical role, consulting, diagnosing and treating, often with extremely tenuous qualified supervision and support. Consultations are rituals in which a presenting complaint is met by a very short enquiry and the prescription of symptomatic or placebo medication. No attempt is made to formulate a proper definition of the patient's problem,

Table 25.1   Some Zimbabwe statistics

Land area	390 759 km²
Population (1982): rural 5 800 000 } total urban 1 700 000	7 500 000
Gross domestic product per head (1982) Z$1 = US$1,6	± US$ 400
(1983) Z$1 = US$0,8	± US$ 200
Registered medical practitioners (1984): rural based	±200
urban based	±915
total	1115
On specialist register	296
Registered dentists (1984)	120
Registered nurses (1984)	4090
Registered medical assistants (1984)	3300
Registered health inspectors (1984)	72
Registered health assistants (1984)	246
Total registered health professionals of all categories except village health workers (non-registrable)	14 000

and in many cases the 'clinician' is not sufficiently knowledgeable to make such a definition or to ascribe a cause.

In a recent study of clinic attenders, 99% of patients left having been given or prescribed some form of medication.

This can only lead to a reinforced belief that all problems require magic for their solution. This leads to dependance, and vast sums needlessly spent on 'cheap' drugs. In turn, people shop around for the 'clinician' with the most powerful magic — often the one who prescribed an injection or a highly coloured capsule. This will eventually lead to a loss of credibility of the health service; people turning back to older forms of magic, or the newer fringe medicine. Epidemiologically, if problems remain undefined, decisions for action will be based on faulty premises.

Thus, the high degree of credibility built by our more leisurely predecessors with their careful enquiry, the use of aids such as the simple microscope, and the application of rational management, will be lost. No matter how many health professionals are deployed, their contribution to improved health will be minimal or negative. (Table 25.1).

THE FUTURE

The road to advancement

Foreign aid that requires rigid structures and edifices as monuments to itself is counter-productive. When aid ceases, as it must, the maintenance of those structures and the purposes for which they were built collapse.

Though humanitarianism demands it, emergency food aid keeps many alive to produce children doomed to a miserable existence dependent on further food aid. The answer lies with Zimbabweans, although continued help may be required. A climate must be created to encourage self-reliance, dependent on our own effort. Highly prized education, health care and the ownership of property to develop productively should be dependent on effort. They should not be expected as general handouts, but as special provisions for the weak and helpless. This in turn implies a good deal of urbanization, leaving the countryside to fewer people. This cannot occur if there are no industrial and commercial developments, which in turn cannot occur unless entrepeneurs can visualize that the effort involved is worthwhile to themselves.

All this depends on a reversal of present trends. Government will have to divest itself of power and bureaucracy to a minimum consistent with good order, justice and peace, and the development of the infrastructure necessary for common advancement. This minimum government responsibility includes the will and ability to deal with matters which might militate against the public health in all its aspects.

Whether or not curative care is included as a public health responsibility or is left to individual private contract, attitudes must change if we are to contribute towards improved health.

CONTRIBUTIONS TO PRIMARY HEALTH CARE

How to achieve health for all by the year 2000?

The basic needs are political stability and economic growth so that every person is able to provide himself with adequate nutrition, adequate clothing and shelter. Once achieved other problems become minimal. High priority is a safe water supply to eradicate water-borne diseases, provide water for irrigation and an improved nutrition for the population.

An expansion of maternal and child care health programmes, so that all pregnant women have some antenatal care and a safe delivery is necessary, and an extended programme of immunization perfected.

Rural and district hospitals have to be expanded to provide support for more primary care clinics and many more village health workers. At present, too many resources are located in the urban centres, while the rural areas are very sparsely covered. Rural areas need to be made more attractive for doctors and nursing personnel. It is not sufficient to encourage them to work there for humanitarian reasons; doctors and nurses, like everyone else, have their own desires and ambitions and they have family commitments which attract them to the larger centres. To overcome this there should be financial inducements and improved conditions of work.

What other role can be played by the doctors and health workers in helping in the provision of primary health care? Firstly, the doctors should be trained as teachers so that they can instruct the paramedics to do much of the work which would conventionally be done by them in the Western world. Time spent in teaching paramedics is always difficult to find when running a busy district or rural hospital, but unless this is done, the doctors will become so overworked that it will be impossible for them to achieve anything.

The population in each area must be involved in improving their standard of living by educating them on all health matters. Here, once again, the doctors and paramedics have a large part to play as educators as well as physicians. The use of drama, the acting out of everyday situations and the resolutions thereof, are having favourable results. An advantage of the use of drama is that it attracts a large crowd, giving the immunization teams a chance to check and update the medical history of the people present, especially the children.

The use of appropriate technology, if carefully applied, could change the way of life of many millions of Zimbabweans, e.g. solar power can provide water heating and electricity.

REFERENCES

Population census 1982 Central Statistical office, Harare
Zimbabwe Medical, Dental and Allied Professions Council Registration Lists, August 1984
Zimbabwe Quarterly Digests of Statistics 1983–84

Saudi Arabia and the Gulf

In the West, where the tempo of change is relatively slow and where
the background cultural conditions are looked on as 'normal' by the
Westerner, it is sometimes difficult to perceive the influence of
history and geography on the development of medical services.
These influences can be seen more clearly by an expatriate in the
countries of the Gulf where the leap from traditional to modern
medicine has been made in less than two decades. Here, the inhos-
pitable terrain, poor communications and the traditional Islamic
culture have all posed problems to those who are trying to establish
modern health care systems in the region and it is only in recent
times that some solutions have been found.

The size of the Arabian peninsula (Fig. 26.1) is usually under-
estimated: Saudi Arabia, which occupies about four-fifths of the
peninsula, exceeds Western Europe in land area. Although the Gulf
is about the same latitude as Florida and Dharhan, the headquarters
of ARAMCO (the Arabian American Oil Company), is situated
nearly on the same latitude as Miami, the geography of the
surrrounding land masses and the pattern of prevailing winds have
made the countries around the Gulf semiarid or arid deserts, which
experience some of the highest climatic temperatures recorded on
Earth.

Table 26.1 lists the countries of Arabia and the six, usually
considered as, the Gulf states are indicated with an asterisk. Since
Saudi Arabia dominates in terms of size, population and rate of
development, it will be treated as typical of the Arab countries of
the Gulf and described in detail. Health care developments in the
other Gulf states will then be related to this.

Civilization is thought to have arisen in the countries of the
Fertile Crescent around the head of the Gulf about 10 000 years
ago. The Gulf itself has been one of the main centres of world trade
and commerce for at least 4000 years. An alternative route for trade
with the Indies depended on shipping the goods to the Yemen —

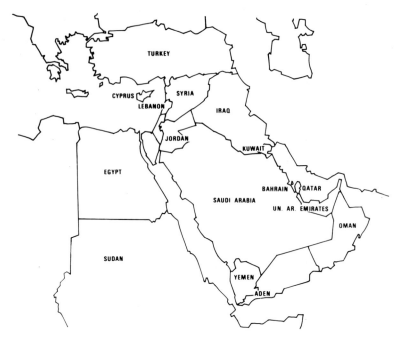

Fig. 26.1 The Arabian peninsula

the Arabia Felix of the Romans — and then carrying them by caravan along the Red Sea coast to the Mediterranean where they were distributed to Europe, the Levant and North Africa. Mecca, in Saudi Arabia, was a major centre on this caravan route and the Prophet, Mohammed, who founded Islam, was born there about

Table 26.1   Countries of the Arabian Peninsula

Country	Area (in sq. miles)	Population (in millions)	% Population urbanized 1960	1981	GNP per capita
Bahrain*	256	0.35			
Kuwait*	6877	1.56	72	89	20 900
Oman*	120 000	0.90	4	7	5920
Qatar*	4000	0.25			
Saudi Arabia*	927 000	9.30	30	68	12 600
United Arab Emirates*	33 000	0.80	40	73	24 660
Yemen Arab Republic (Yemen)	75 000	5.90	3	11	460
Yemen Peoples Democr. Rep. (Aden)	112 000	2.00	28	37	460

* Gulf States

1400 years ago. It was from the Arabian peninsula, after Mohammed's death that the great Arab conquests erupted over the following two centuries. Islam now influences all social and cultural institutions in the Gulf countries. The Haj, the pilgrimage to Mecca which all Moslems should make at least once in their lifetime, has ensured that Saudi Arabia remains the centre of the Moslem world. In 1984, more than two million people visited the holy places in Mecca during the course of one week. Such mass movements of people, especially in the past, have had a major influence on health and epidemics in the region. With the development of alternative sea routes to the East and with the introduction of alternative sources of the raw materials from the Indies, the Gulf declined in strategic importance until the discovery of oil in the early years of this century.

The first oil concessions in Saudi Arabia were granted in 1933 and oil was found in 1938. The Second World War hindered further development and the full potential of the oil fields was not recognized until the late 1940s. Now the Gulf is the major source of the petrochemicals on which the developed world depends and Saudi Arabia possesses about a quarter of the world's known reserves of oil. This is a mixed blessing since, on the one hand, the revenue from oil has allowed a rate of development which is unparalleled in the world but, on the other, it has made the Gulf of major strategic importance in international power struggles. Since 1980 the Gulf War between Iran and Iraq has slowed progress significantly, since it is absorbing resources — both human and material — that might have been devoted to the constructive development of the countries of the region. This has been aggravated by volatility of the price and demand for oil on the world market.

A number of city states along the south-western shore of the Gulf, ruled by emirs and sheikhs, formed relationships with Britain in the 19th century and these were formalized in treaties, whereby Britain took responsibility for defence and foreign affairs. During the 1930s oil was found in most of these sheikhdoms and this was developed after the Second World War. Financial strength led to a desire for independence and this was achieved in Kuwait in 1961, and in Bahrain and the United Arab Emirates in 1971. The oil revenues, the openness to foreign influence and the relatively small area and population of these states have allowed rapid development in all fields including the provision of health care. The British association with Oman was not so close as with the other states, the discovery of oil was later (1962) and, in general, development has

Table 26.2   Health indicators in countries of the Arabian Peninsula

Country	GPN per capita (US $)	Infant mortality rate		Life expectancy at birth (years)		Total fertility rate	% Child population 0–4 years
		1960	1981	1960	1981		
Kuwait*	20 900	90	33	60	70	5.9	19.23%
Oman*	5920	190	130	38	49	7.1	22.22%
Saudi Arabia*	12 600	190	110	43	55	7.3	18.28%
United Arab Emirates*	24 660	140	50	47	63	6.8	12.50%
Yemen Arab Republic (Yemen)	460	210	190	36	43	6.8	18.64%
Yemen Peoples Democr. Rep. (Aden)	460	210	140	36	46	7.0	20.00%
For comparison							
— Sweden	14 870	17	7	73	77	1.7	6.02%
— USA	12 820	26	12	70	75	1.8	8.01%

* Gulf States

been slower. The two Yemen Republics, in the south-west corner of the peninsula, are relatively poor in natural resources and remain underdeveloped (Tables 26.1 and 26.2).

The Kingdom of Saudi Arabia was established in 1932 by King Abdulaziz but significant change from the traditional way of life came only in the reign of King Faisal (1964–75), who demonstrated that a modernization programme need not compromise the strict observation of the Islamic values. Under his guidance, a series of 5-year development plans were devised

> to maintain the religious and moral values of Islam, to assure the defence and internal security of the Kingdom, to maintain a high rate of economic growth by developing economic resources, to maximize earnings from oil over the long term and conserve depletable resources, to reduce economic dependence on the export of crude oil, to develop human resources by education, training and raising the standards of health, to increase the well-being of all groups within the society and foster social stability under circumstances of rapid social change, and to develop the physical infrastructure to support the achievement of such goals.
>
> (Mostyn 1981)

The first Development Plan (1970–75) was devoted to securing the industrial base on which further progress was to be built. The Second Plan (1975–80) was directed at building the physical infrastructure for development — roads, airports, ports, a modern

communication system (telephones, postal service, television and
radio network), schools, universities, hospitals and health centres.
The Third Plan (1980–85) is directed toward developing the human
potential of the citizens, with emphasis on education and health,
and promoting self-sufficiency in food production. Unlike many
Utopian plans, it is remarkable how much has been achieved — the
industrial base is strong, the communication system is outstanding,
good educational facilities are available up to university level for
both male and female and a substantial share of the nation's
resources is being devoted to the development of health facilities.
The Ministry of Health is now avoiding the usual developing-
country pitfall of misplaced emphasis on secondary and tertiary
health care institutions and a very active programme for upgrading
primary care is under way.

Table 26.2 shows some health indicators for the Gulf Countries
contrasted with those of Sweden and the United States (Grant
1983). Statistics were not available for Bahrain and Qatar but they
are likely to be similar to those of Kuwait and the United Arab
Emirates (UAE). With regard to infant mortality in the league table
of countries, Kuwait and UAE are in the middle range, while Saudi
Arabia, Oman and the two Yemen Republics are in the very high
group. In such situations, the provision of effective primary health
care is likely to produce substantial benefit. In Saudi Arabia, progress is fast at present and the situation in 1984 is likely to be
substantially better than in 1981. It is striking that, while there are
fairly wide variations in infant mortality and life expectancy,
fertility rates and the percentage of children aged 0–4 years are
similar throughout the peninsula and the levels are those that would
be expected of developing countries with little evidence of birth
control.

The development of a Western style health care system has taken
place over the past 20 years. Table 26.3 demonstrates this for Saudi
Arabia (Gezairy H 1979, Ministry of Planning Kingdom of Saudi

Table 26.3   Health manpower and facilities in Saudi Arabia

	1959*	1970	1975	1980
Physicians	249	1172	3107	6461
Nurses	632	3261	6606	12 255
Hospitals		74	96	104
Hospital beds		9039	12 111	17 523
Clinics, dispensaries, etc.		591	782	1179

* This includes only Ministry of Health employees.

Arabia 1982). The provision of health care is divided between the Ministry of Health, the private sector and the other government agencies, such as the Ministry of Defence and Aviation and the National Guard. In 1979, almost 65% of health personnel were employed by the Ministry of Health, 15% by the private sector and 20% by the other government agencies (Sebai 1981). As is usual, the distribution of medical resources is uneven, with the Ministry of Health being responsible for most health care outside the large towns.

The other countries of the region have operated in the same time frame with Kuwait and Bahrain a few years ahead of the others. The policy of all the Gulf states is to provide free health care for their citizens. In general, the coastal regions of the Gulf and the Red Sea with their long-standing associations with other countries for trade and the pilgrimage were much more open to change than the traditionalist, conservative heartland of the peninsula, which was almost inaccessible to foreigners until recent years. The work of local healers, based on cautery, bone-setting, bleeding and herbal remedies described by Maloney (1982), would have been normal practice until the introduction of Western medicine.

The early philosophy of introduced medicine was strongly influenced by the ideas prevalent in the United States in the 1960s — that medicine should be specialist-dominated and hospital-based. General practice was either in hospital outpatient departments or in health centres. Private practitioners in the community were almost all 'specialists' and few would admit to being general practitioners. Expatriate doctors in the outpatient departments would screen large numbers of patients, offering either symptomatic remedies or immediate referral to a range of specialists in the same clinic.

The work in health centres in Saudi Arabia has been studied (Sebai et al 1980, Sebai 1981, Banoub 1982, Sebai 1982) and the findings showed many problems. The health centres were frequently in rented accommodation which was not designed to meet the needs of the service. The staff were almost all expatriate — Egyptian, Jordanian, Sudanese, Pakistani, Bangaladeshi, Filipino — with little real understanding of the local culture and many with a superficial grasp of Arabic. They had no vocational training for primary care, no programme of continuing education, and few had access to modern medical text books or medical journals. The medicine practised was largely curative, mainly symptomatic; the average consultation lasted two and a half minutes and the medical record consisted of a one line entry in a ledger. Maternity and child health services, such as antenatal care and immunization were almost non-existent. Home visiting was not permitted. While the centres were adequately staffed, there was no concept of a team approach to prevent disease or promote health and there was no attempt to involve the community.

Though such health centres still exist, the Saudi Ministry of Health has undertaken a radical programme to upgrade the present service to provide a true primary health care system. Many new purpose-designed health centres are being built. Eleven model health centres — one in each region — have been establish to allow experiments in the provision of health care and to demonstrate the quality of care expected. A new medical record system has been designed and field-tested in the model health centres. Experiments in the appropriate use of ancillary staff in community outreach have been undertaken. A programme of continuing education is being devised to reorientate doctors already in post and the Ministry is sending young doctors to participate in the family and community medicine residency (vocational) training schemes which have been established in the universities.

King Saud University, Riyadh, and King Faisal University, Dammam, both have active departments of family and community medicine. The impact of undergraduate teaching is now being felt and many young graduates have a much more positive attitude to primary health care. Both universities have started graduate residency training programmes. The Ministry of Defence and Aviation hospitals in Riyadh and Jeddah also have residency training and the programme in Riyadh has been assessed and approved by the Joint Committee on Postgraduate Training for General Practice of the United Kingdom. The Ministry of Health in Bahrain has a residency training programme in association with the American University of Beirut, while the Ministry of Health in Kuwait is developing links with Edinburgh University to train young Kuwaiti doctors there.

The lack of an appropriate higher qualification in family medicine/primary care gives rise to many difficulties. Some governments link advancement in government service to educational achievement. In Saudi Arabia, a doctor without an acceptable higher degree cannot move to the upper pay scales. Among our specialist medical colleagues in the Gulf Countries, primary care is not taken seriously and a suitable higher qualification would help to establish the academic respectability of the discipline in this region. Unfortunately, the established higher degrees in family medicine in the rest of the world are fairly culture-specific and do not relate well to practice in the Middle East. Plans are being made to introduce an 'Arab Board' examination in primary care, similar to the American Boards in family medicine. The date of introduction is not yet known. Until such time as a suitable degree is established, the various institutions promoting postgraduate training in family and community medicine will need to look to countries overseas for help.

Information related to health is difficult to obtain in the region. Population, mortality and morbidity statistics must all be suspect because of the problems in collecting the data. Table 26.4 shows morbidity data for 1983 from the Riyadh Al Kharj Hospital Programme of the Ministry of Defence and Aviation. This data is collected in a computer-based primary care information system and the table shows the rate of new diagnoses per thousand registered population at the mid-year. This corresponds roughly to the incidence rate. Doubts have been expressed as to how typical this population is, but the data compares reasonably well with the available census statistics in age and sex, and the social mix resembles that of urban Saudi Arabia though the economic status may be above average. The table compares the Saudi data with the data of the Second National Morbidity Survey in the United Kingdom. While there are similarities, especially in ranking, there are some striking differences. Both neoplasms and mental diseases seem much less common in Riyadh. The finding with regard to neoplasm is supported by other work. El Akkad (1982) draws attention to the low incidence of malignancy in Arabia in a paper on the development of a cancer service for the Kingdom. The observation regarding mental disease has also been made several times in the Kingdom, but the difference may be due to a failure to recognize psychiatric disorders, since there is a known tendency to somatize emotional problems in Arab cultures (Racy 1980, Kapoor 1983). The finding of such differences between societies can identify fertile fields for research.

Among the serious infectious illnesses, tuberculosis, schistosomiasis, brucellosis and trachoma are common enough to constitute significant public health problems. Urinary schistosomiasis and malaria are particularly prevalent in the Asir region of Saudi Arabia and the Ministry of Health has Malaria and Schistosomiasis Control Units operating in this area. Endemic malaria appears to have been eradicated from the Eastern Region. The ARAMCO epidemiology

Table 26.4 Comparison of the rate of diagnosis of new episodes in the Riyadh Al Kharj Hospital Programme, 1983, with patient consultation rate in the UK Second National Morbidity Survey, 1970–71

ICD-9 chapter	Disease or condition	UK 1970–71 Rate per 1000 registered patients	Rank	Riyadh 1983 Rate per 1000 registered patients	Rank
1	Infective and parasitic diseases	70.7	4	122.3	10
2	Neoplasms	12.0	17	1.9	16
3	Endocrine, nutritional and metabolic immunity disorders	26.0	11	25.8	13
4	Diseases of blood and bloodforming organs	12.1	14	7.8	15
5	Mental disorders	109.9	13	15.4	6
6	Nervous system and sense organ diseases	113.1	5	112.5	5
7	Diseases of the circulatory system	66.2	12	21.4	11
8	Diseases of respiratory system	260.7	1	402.5	1
9	Diseases of the digestive system	60.8	7	88.9	12
10	Diseases of the genitourinary system	74.8	9	67.6	9
11	Complications of pregnancy, childbirth and the puerperium	22.4	15	5.2	14
12	Diseases of the skin and subcutaneous tissue	113.3	8	86.0	4
13	Diseases of the musculoskeletal systemconnective tissue	91.3	6	90.4	7
14	Congenital anomalies	2.4	16	3.4	17
15	Certain conditions in the perinatal period	0.4	18	0.7	18
16	Symptoms, signs and ill-defined conditions	141.7	2	249.0	2
17	Injury and poisoning	82.5	10	53.2	8
18	Supplementary classification	138.9	3	152.5	3
	Total rate of diagnosis	1399.2		1506.5	
	Total population (number)	292 247.0		117 820.0	

unit (ARAMCO 1982) has recorded no case of local spread since 1975. In 1980 it became necessary, by royal decree for a child to be fully immunized — diphtheria, pertussis, tetanus, polio and measles — before a birth certificate could be issued and this has virtually eliminated acute polio.

With the control of infections, diseases related to life-style are likely to become more prominent. Road traffic accidents are now the commonest cause of death in adults in Saudi Arabia. Obesity and diabetes mellitus are frequent in the middle aged and may be related to change in dietary habits. Heavy smoking is very common, encouraged by the low price of cigarettes, but this is a relatively recent change in habit and no increase in chronic bronchitis, heart disease or lung cancer is yet detectable.

Certain problems remain which will affect primary health care in the short term. The general level of education and understanding of health and hygiene is low among many adults and this affects acceptance of, and compliance with, good medical care. While the rising standard of education throughout the region will reduce this problem in the future, it is likely to remain an important factor over the next 10 years. The task of attracting and training enough indigenous medical and paramedical staff is also formidable. This is especially so for female paramedical team members, since many people in this society do not yet accept that health care (other than as a doctor) is a proper activity for a respectable girl.

In 1982 the Secretariat General for the Council of Ministers of Health for the Arab Countries in the Gulf (1982) prepared a report on the future development of primary health care in the Gulf. This was very much in accord with the Declaration of Alma-Ata. It emphasized the importance of the preventive, promotive as well as the curative aspects and gave a commitment to developing a team approach to the provision of health care. Special importance was laid on appropriate training and continuing education of each of the team members.

If present trends continue, the countries of the Gulf will achieve the target of health care for all by the year 2000. If the 1982 report is implemented, the quality of primary health care will be very high indeed.

REFERENCES

ARAMCO Medical Department 1982 Malaria Epidemiology Bulletin: 28
Banoub S N Community health in Saudi Arabia. Primary health care in the
    Qasim region. Saudi Medical Journal Monograph no. 1: 59–70
El Akkad S Plans for cancer care in Saudi Arabia. Saudi Medical Journal
    3: 71–74
Gezairy H 1979 Health manpower in Saudi Arabia past, present and future.
    Middle East Journal of Anaesthesiology 5: 141–148
Grant J P 1983 The state of the world's children 1984. Oxford University Press,
    London

Kapoor O P 1983 Common chronic disease patterns in Arabian Gulf, Saudi Arabia and Yemen. S.S. Publishers, Bombay

Ministry of Planning Kingdom of Saudi Arabia 1982 Achievements of the first and second development plans 1390–1400 (1970–1980) Ministry of Planning, Riyadh

Moloney G E 1982 Community health in Saudi Arabia. Local healers of Qasim. Saudi Medical Journal Monograph No. 1: 87–98

Mostyn T 1981 Saudi Arabia. A MEED practical guide. Middle East Economic Digest, London

Racy J 1980 Somatization in Saudi women: a therapeutic challenge. British Journal of Psychiatry 137: 212–216

Sebai Z A, Miller D L, Ba'Ageel H 1980 A study of three health centres in rural Saudi Arabia. Saudi Medical Journal 1: 197–202

Sebai Z A 1981 The health of the family in a changing Arabia. Tihama, Jeddah

Sebai Z A 1982 Community health in Saudi Arabia. Primary health care in the district of Al Asiah. Saudi Medical Journal Monograph No 1: 71–76

Secretariat General for the Council of Ministers of Health for the Arab Countries in the Gulf 1982 Primary health care in the Arab countries in the Gulf. Riyadh (in Arabic)

South East Asia and Singapore

INTRODUCTION

In most developing countries in South East Asia, the national strategy to meet the goal of health for all by the year 2000 is based on primary health care as the main thrust. This is because only through primary health care can the health services be made universally accessible at a cost the community and the country can afford. It is unlikely that health services run along conventional lines could be expanded to meet the basic needs of the total population, because the human, physical and financial resources required would be too great. An overwhelming proportion of resources for the delivery of health care is concentrated in the urban areas, utilizing highly sophisticated technology servicing a small minority of the population. In addition to inadequate geographical coverage of the population, the extent of community support is also inadequate, even in areas which are accessible to health services.

The approach to health care to meet the requirement of health for all is no longer based on the traditional donor–recipient relationship, but based on a partnership or co-operative relationship between government agencies and the community. This new approach, which considers health development as an integral part of the overall socioeconomic development, calls for a new outlook, orientation and skills on the part of health and related staff who will have to develop qualities of leadership and managerial skills in order to facilitate and support the community development approach to health.

The past two decades have seen the evolution and development of health policies in this region aimed primarily to provide health care to improve the quality of life of our peoples. There has been a compelling need for innovative cost-effective approaches and methods to cope with the vast extent of current health needs aggravated by the sheer magnitude of the rural population. With the shift of emphasis toward comprehensive primary health care for our growing population, current health care delivery systems in South East Asia, with their inadequacies and resource limitations need to be improved and their health care services extended — the ultimate goal being the provision of high quality primary health care which is accessible, comprehensive and acceptable to both the patients and the community.

The term primary health care evokes a variety of concepts and definitions due to differences in perception, varying professional backgrounds and cultural norms, and also from the particular social and political systems. In recent years the countries in South East Asia have expressed acceptance and the intention to adapt the primary health care concept for their own respective national health programmes. The philosophy of primary health care is to promote and support basic health care at the grassroot level, with emphasis on community involvement and participation. Primary health care involves activities undertaken at the level of first contact of people with the health delivery system, namely:
1. Medical care of established diseases
2. Prevention of diseases and disabilities
3. Health promotion through health education
4. Rehabilitation services.

MODELS OF HEALTH CARE IN SOUTH EAST ASIA

A brief review of the models of health care delivery systems in South East Asia would show that primary health care assumes different forms in different countries. Great strides have been made to reinforce basic services in an effort to provide the total population with effective health care at a price they can afford. The countries of Vietnam, Kampuchea and Laos, although they form — together with Thailand — the Indo-China region in the centre of continental South East Asia, have been left out of this review because of local political and other problems.

I. Indonesia

Area (km^2): 1 919 413
Crude birth rate: 33.7 per 1000
Crude death rate 11.7 per 1000
Infant mortality rate 130 per 1000
Population: 147 490 298   (*Statistics for 1983*)
    The Indonesian archipelago is made up of more than 13 666

islands, but 5 large land masses dominate, namely Sumatra, Java, Kalimatan, Sulawesi and Iranian Java.

The major health problems are communicable diseases, nutrition, hygiene and sanitation, high mortality rate, population growth, low health knowledge and consciousness of people and economic factors. National development programmes have resulted in the restructuring of the provincial health organizations, the important focal point being on the community health services. The primary health care approach was suitably adopted and designated Village Community Health Development. The main objective was to develop every aspect of the individual and community resources to improve their well-being through the improvement of their health status. The village community health development activities are not carried out in several provinces as an integral part of community development as well as national development.

II. The Philippines

Area: 300 000 km^2
Crude birth rate: 30.8 per 1000
Crude death rate: 7.7 per 1000
Infant mortality rate: 30.7 per 1000
Population: 48 098 460   (*Statistics for 1983*)

The Republic of the Philippines is an archipelago composed of 7100 islands and has 3 major island groups, namely, Luzon in the north, the Visayas in the central part and Mindanao in the south.

The leading health problems are communicable diseases, malnutrition, environmental sanitation and chronic debilitating diseases like malaria and tuberculosis, as well as a high population growth rate. The responsibility for promoting adequate health services to the people is that of the government through the Ministry of Health. However, the system of health care delivery is divided between:

1. Public sector — government and government controlled agencies
2. Private sector — private hospitals, private clinics and private practitioners
3. Mixed sector — professional, private and other health related organizations
4. International health organizations.

The Ministry of Health maintains a network of hospitals at both district and provincial level, with larger regional medical centres for secondary and tertiary levels of health care. At the primary health care level, rural health units have largely contributed to the improved health status of the nation. With increasing demands of the rural health unit in recent years, the establishment of barrio (*barangay*) health stations increased recruitment of additional personnel, which included the local 'herb' practitioner (*herbalario*), the untrained indigenous midwife (*hilot*) and support from voluntary organizations have increased the outreach of the health services. This, together with community participation, has in no small measure met the primary health care needs of the country.

III. Thailand

Area (km²): 514 000
Crude birth rate: 22.8 per 1000
Crude death rate: 5.1 per 1000
Infant mortality rate: 70 per 1000
Population: 44 278 000   (*Statistics for 1983*)

The Kingdom of Thailand occupies about 514 000 km² in the centre of continental South East Asia. It is bordered by Kampuchea in the south-east, by Laos in the east and north-east, by Burma in the north, north-west and west, and by the Andaman Sea and Gulf of Thailand in the south. Of its population, 43% are under 15-years-old. About 75% of the population live in hamlets and villages.

Health services are provided by both the private and public sectors. The private sector provides curative medicine as well as family planning services, mainly in the metropolis of Bangkok and the 126 municipalities. Health services of the public sector are concentrated in the provincial areas. In addition, there is a variegated network of traditional medical practitioners and practices which is part of the traditional Thai cultural pattern. This takes care of more than half the population for its symptomatic problems. This is especially predominant in the rural areas, where other health services are neither available or not accepted by the people.

In order to correct the problem of inadequate coverage of health services, as well as to encourage community participation, several public health community centre projects have been undertaken. The main goals are an emphasis on:
1. Primary health care
2. Health services to the rural areas
3. Increasing manpower at all levels
4. Improved health planning and management

5. Availability of minimum essential medical care for the population.

Primary health care schemes are being implemented on a nation-wide scale to cover 50% of villages in the country in the next 20 years. District hospitals are also being built to cover all districts and these hospitals also function as health centres and midwifery clinics to provide basic medical care. Primary health care will rely on existing organizations set up in villages and will attempt to harness traditional medicine and practices and use community reserves like Buddhist temples and monks, village health volunteers and health communicators in the approach and solution of the health problems of the villages. Primary health care will be eventually a private system developed and executed by rural people themselves with the support of government agencies.

IV. Malaysia

Area (km^2): 329 749
Crude birth rate: 31.7 (PM), 29.4 (Sarawak), per 1000
Crude death rate: 5.2 (PM), 3.6 (Sarawak), per 1000
Infant mortality rate: 4.3 per 1000
Population: 13 435 588   (*Statistics for 1983*)

Malaysia was founded in 1963 and is now a federation of 13 states and a federal territory. Eleven states and the federal territory are located in Peninsular Malaysia (PM) and two states — Sarawak and Sabah — are in the Island of Borneo. Since 1971, the federal govern-ment has been wholly responsible for the administration of medical and health services throughout Malaysia. At the turn of the century the private sector comprised only of estate and mine hospitals set up by the rubber and mining industry, but as more local doctors became available, the number of general practitioners increased rapidly in the urban areas. At the time of Independence in 1957, the health services were urban-based, curative orientated, with complementary rural health programmes. There was also an acute shortage of local manpower at both professional and subprofessional levels. However, great strides have been made to rectify the imbal-ance in distribution of services between the rural and urban areas with greater emphasis on preventive services, stepped-up training of medical manpower locally and organization of national health programmes.

The highest priority has since been given to the rural health service — an integrated service providing preventive, promotive and personal health services. Special emphasis is placed on maternal and child care, basic ambulatory curative care, dental care as well as environmental sanitation. Patient care is designed on a centripetal system with primary medical care at the periphery, secondary medical care at the intermediate level and tertiary care at the centre, with appropriate referral systems. In spite of this health service infrastructure, 25–30% of the population are still on the fringes of development and are either underserved or unserved. Primary health care, or 'community health movement' (*Perkerakan Kesihatan Masyarakat*) as it is known in Malaysia, appears to be the answer. As total coverage of the rural population can only be achieved by 1990, mobile health teams in Penisular Malaysia and the flying doctor service in Sabah and Sarawak serve as an interim measure to cover the unserved population until the permanent health facilities are expanded to provide complete coverage.

V. Singapore

Area (km^2): 618
Crude birth rate: 17.3 per 1000
Crude death rate: 5.3 per 1000
Infant mortality rate: 11.6 per 1000
Population: 2 413 945   (*Statistics for 1983*)

The Republic of Singapore comprises the main island and about 50 offshore small islands. The population density is 3954 persons per km^2, making Singapore one of the most densely populated countries in the world. The population is multiethnic, comprising 76% Chinese, 15% Malays, 7% Indians/Pakistanis and the remaining 2% others. 70% of the population are living in modern public housing estates. The development of satellite towns has eliminated most of the rural areas in Singapore. In 1983, the literacy rate was 84% and the number of persons above the age of 60 was 7%, a figure projected to 10% by the year 2000.

Primary health care in Singapore is undertaken by the Government Primary Health Care Services and the private general practitioners (Fig. 27.1). In the public sector it is provided at considerably reduced rates through government subsidy, while in the private sector on a fee-for-service basis. In 1980 it was estimated there were 14 million consultations, of these 10 million (70%) were handled by private practitioners and 4 million (30%) by government clinics. By the year 2000, these consultations are projected to reach 20 million per year.

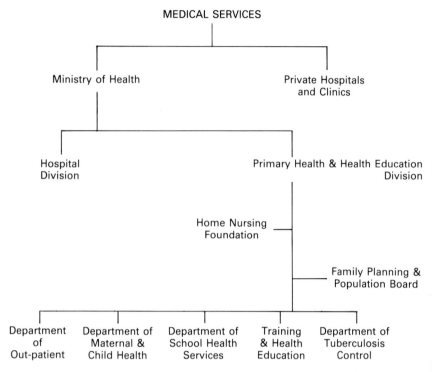

Fig. 27.1 Organization of the medical services of primary health care in Singapore

The doctor of first contact, namely the primary care physician both in the public and private sectors, therefore, completely manages today more than 90% of health problems, regardless of age and sex. This he does only with practical experience acquired over a period of time, with no vocational training whatsoever, unlike his counterparts in the various specialties.

It is estimated that there are 2200 medical practitioners. These include family physicians (primary care doctors and general practitioners), specialists (secondary and tertiary care doctors), doctors not in active practice and housemen. The active doctor population is approximately 97.7% of which number 43% are primary care doctors and family physicians. The average physician–population ratio of all physicians is 1:1200.

General practitioners and outpatient department doctors are the principal providers of primary care. In addition, a large number of physicians, obstetricians and gynaecologists, paediatricians and surgeons are not in exclusive consultant practice, but undertake

SOUTH EAST ASIA AND SINGAPORE 351

primary care broadly within their specialty. Private specialists find it difficult to exist on consultant practice alone because of lack of referrals from general practitioners, and general practitioners are reluctant to refer to specialists who are also in primary care.

It is possible for a young doctor to start a general practice immediately after housemanship. As a result standards are uneven. General practice has become equated with private 'shop-house' practice confined to episodic care of those who can pay. Private general practitioners, operating on a fee-for-service basis paid for in most instances personally by the patient, are not within the reach of poorer people, whose only recourse would be to seek treatment from government outpatient departments or traditional medicine healers. The tendency is to economize by coming only for periods of illness and to avoid continuing care with its preventive element.

The striking feature of the system of health delivery in Singapore is the rigid separation of government health services from those rendered by the private sector. The growth of the private sector in medicine has been striking, lagging only slightly behind the government sector. The work of the private sector in medical care is almost entirely curative.

THE FUTURE

Primary health care in a modern environment as in Singapore should evolve an advanced system of health care to bring to bear advanced technology and skills to the health problems of the community. The approach is to be family-based and community-oriented. It does not promise to be a cheap solution to safe-guarding the health of a community but it will certainly be the most cost-effective, representing the most efficient way to utilize health resources. However, very little, if any, attention has hitherto been paid to the specific training of the family doctor at either the undergraduate or graduate levels of medical education in the Asian countries. The founding of academies and colleges of general practitioners in South East Asian countries in recent years, with aims and goals identical to those of academies and colleges in developed countries, have helped to define this new area of specialization and to advocate for the training of a new generation of doctors in the practice of primary care. This means that our medical schools should recognize the importance of primary care and improved systems of health care delivery. They should redirect their curricula and teaching programmes toward primary comprehensive health care and reorganize sufficiently to provide substantial exposure to family physicians and family practice at the undergraduate level. This should enable the medical student to learn about the family physician's special attitudes and skills and be taught in the context of the family physician as he applies the discipline in patient care. The College of General Practitioners in Singapore believes that those entering family medicine/general practice should be trained by design to be competent and cost-effective; thereby enabling the trained family physician to utilize costly medical facilities more effectively than his untrained counterparts, making fewer referrals to specialists and hospitals, as well as the economic use of expensive investigations and drugs. The provision of improved health services would enhance the quality of life and accelerate social and economic development by reducing the loss of working hours through illness and also increasing labour productivity, both qualitatively and quantitatively.

Primary care must be the central axis on which the health services of the nation revolve. Only a very small proportion of sick people need the expensive technology of the hospitals, a fraction that can and must diminish with effective care at the primary level.

There is, therefore, an urgent need for special structured training of the graduate entering primary medical care services. With his newly acquired knowledge and skills, as well as clinical training in the principles and practice of primary medical care, he should be better able to serve the needs of his patients and community and to extend primary, continuing, comprehensive medical care to more people than any other field in medicine. His training seems the logical foundation for a cost-effective health care delivery system.

FURTHER READING

Fernandez V L, 1979, New horizons in primary health care in South East Asia
Geyman J P 1978 The modern family dcotor and changing medical practice
Katoumura H, Maruchi N, Togo M 1977 Health aspects of community
    development in South East Asia
Raja Kumar M K et al, 1979: Specialization in primary health care. College of
    General Practitioners (Malaysia)
The future general practitioner. A working party, 1972 Royal College of General
    Practitioners

Sri Lanka

NATIONAL FEATURES

Sri Lanka an island rich in natural splendour, packed into an area of 65 610 km² is situated east of the southern most part of India across 40 km of shallow ocean. Its extreme length of 445 km and greatest width of 225 km could be travelled in a day by road or rail (Fig. 28.1).

The entire coast has palm-fringed beaches beyond which the greatest part of the country is low lying and flat except in the south central area where the scenary changes immediately to green valleys, rolling hills and a few mountain ranges that could boast of a few spectacular peaks 2150–2450 m (7000–8000) ft in height. The scenic beauty is enhanced by many waterfalls and several rivers which radiate out of the hills, the longest being 334 km. Along their course down to the coast some of these rivers have been diverted into reservoirs for purposes of agriculture and hydro electric power.

Being a tropical island most of Sri Lanka is warm and dry (mean temp. 25° — 28°C), while the hill country enjoys a cool temperate climate (14.5°–24°C). Rainfall is seasonal (ranges 100–500 cm — 40–200 in — in dry–wet zones) and is ushered in by monsoonal winds. Such climatic conditions favour the rich vegetation and the variety of wild life found specially in the forest areas, where a few national parks have been set aside for the conservation of fauna and flora.

Sri Lanka has a long history of ancient civilization that flourished long before Europe. The original inhabitants were the Veddhas, a group that is almost extinct now. The present population of nearly 15 million (14.85 m in 1981) (Department of Census and Statistics 1982), comprising several races, are descendants of settlers since the 6th century B.C. The majority community the Sinhalese (73.3%) are descendants of Aryan settlers from North India who were the first to arrive, and they developed the Sinhala language. The second

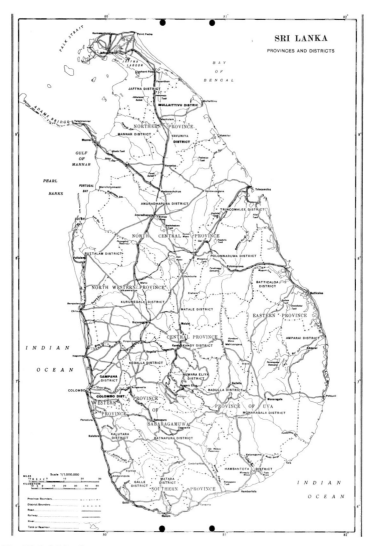

Fig. 28.1 Sri Lanka

largest community the Tamils (18.8%) are the descendants of Tamils from South India. The Muslims (7.44%) are descendants of Arab and Malay traders who settled here, and the Burghers and Eurasians (0.34%) are the only descendants of West Europeans, although the Dutch, Portuguese and British in succession colonized and ruled Sri Lanka (Ceylon) since 1505.

In 1948 Sri Lanka gained political independence and became a Democratic Socialist Republic in 1972. The country has a parliamentary system of government, an Executive President and a Parliament consisting of members elected by the people.

Although Western influence on society and culture have been considerable, the people of this country have a distinct culture and customs which have been influenced very much by Buddhism since its advent in 247 B.C. Society built up of closely linked family units, has occupation-based caste distinction, as a basis of stratification, but the impact of this is softening fast.

Religion, which is a significant facet of life, has a profound influence on their *culture*, and is given an important place in social and political life. The majority of the Sinhalese are Buddhists and the Tamils are Hindus, but there are Christians among both races and the Muslims profess their own faith. The people have also always been inclined to want ritual and ceremony.

The people of Sri Lanka place great value on education and have achieved a literacy rate of 85%. Education beginning in temples has a history of almost 2500 years, and now education is given free in schools and up to the universities. The national languages are Sinhala and Tamil, while English is very widely used by a significant proportion of the educated classes, specially in the professions.

The country's income over the years has been from agricultural sources. Although in later years, to meet the growing needs of the people, the economy has been diversified mainly through industrial development, tea, rubber and coconut exports still remain the main foreign exchange earners. Also in recent times, the country's economy has been boosted by developments in agriculture and hydroelectric power following on the Mahaweli River Diversion Project.

HEALTH CARE

The earliest records of health care institutions in Sri Lanka date back to 400 B.C. during the time of the Sinhalese kings. Ayurvedha was the system of medicine practised then, and has continued over the years. The ayurvedha practitioner still remains a respected member of the community and plays a significant role in the delivery of health care specially in rural areas. The government, seeing the need to integrate ayurvedha into the national health care system, created a Ministry of Indigenous Medicine in 1980 and now several ayurvedha hospitals and dispensaries have been established.

Table 28.1   DHS health facilities in Sri Lanka

Group	Type of institution	n	Level of care
1	Teaching hospitals	5	Tertiary, secondary
	Provincial hospitals	7	and
	Special hospitals	16	primary health care
2	Base hospitals	17	
	District hospitals	114	Secondary and
	Peripheral units	110	primary health care
3	Rural hospitals	112	Primary health care
	Maternity homes and		
	central dispensaries	102	
	Central dispensaries	338	
4	Health units	106	

Source: Ministry of Health 1983a

Much later, western medicine was introduced to Sri Lanka during the British rule and the Civil Medical Establishment of 1798 became the Civil Medical Department in 1858, from which has evolved the present Department of Health Services under the Ministeries of Health and Teaching Hospitals. Table 28.1 (Ministry of Health 1983a) shows the medical institutions and health units that function under the Department of Health Services.

The evolution and development of health care services in the country would not be complete without referring to the dramatic improvement in the health indices especially in the last four decades as shown in Table 28.2 (Ministry of Health 1983b).

Besides the Government's health care system, there developed from the early years, a private sector service based on western medicine provided by general practitioner/family doctors. In spite of the lack of government support, this service has survived and is developing fast and even expanding into rural areas.

In addition to the above, practitioners of homeopathy and acupuncture make a small contribution to health care.

Table 28.2   Health indices

	Birth rate (per 1000)	Death rate	Infant mortality rate (per 1000 births)	Maternal mortality rate	Life expectancy (years)
1945	36.6	21.9	140	16.5	42.7
1981	28.0	6.0	34.4	0.8	68.2

Primary health care

The people of Sri Lanka have free access to all the primary health care facilities in the country as shown in Table 28.3.

Table 28.3 Primary health care facilities

| | System of medicine practised | | |
	Western	Ayurvedha	Others
Government	Outpatient departments dispensaries and health units	Outpatient department and dispensaries	—
Private	General/family practices	General practices	General practices

The care provided at most of these places is almost fully curative except at the government health units which provide mainly preventive care.

The primary health care providers are many. Junior hospital doctors provide care at the outpatient departments of the big hospitals, while assistant medical practitioners, who have a 2–3 years training programme, do the same at peripheral institutions, but sometimes at bigger hospitals too.

Medical officers of health units are more experienced doctors and they work together with public health inspectors, public health nurses and family health workers to provide preventive care.

General practitioner/family doctors provide mostly curative-oriented care, but they quite often fulfil their role as personal doctor to individuals and families, and do their best to integrate curative and preventive aspects of care.

Ayurvedha practitioners again provide curative care but in the rural areas they also fulfil a role of being family physician and counsellor.

The providers of curative care would mainly deal with the common diseases/disease problems, such as upper respiratory tract infection (URTI) and urinary tract infection (UTI), skin problems, diabetes, hypertension, backache, dyspepsia, and headache, which are relatively simple, and the same as anywhere else. However, not too uncommonly, they encounter also diseases like filaria, malaria, diarrhoeal disease, acute viral hepatitis, typhoid fever and worm infestations.

Preventive care provided by the health team is also similar to that in other countries. This package includes maternal and child health care, school health care, immunization, family planning care, environmental care and control of communicable disease, tied up with health education. In addition, Sri Lanka has special disease control programmes for malaria, filaria, tuberculosis, leprosy, venereal disease, cancer, rabies and diarrhoeal disease.

Recent developments in the field of primary health care in Sri Lanka by Government proposals are relevant to 'Health for all by the year 2000'.

The main feature of the proposed primary health care structure would be a complex of graded health centres (Ministry of Health 1983c). This complex would consist of:

1. A basic functional unit, the Gramodaya Health Centre manned by a family health worker, responsible for delivery of essential health care to a cluster of villages to an average to a population of about 3000.

2. A subdivisional health centre serving a population of 20 000 in the charge of a registered assistant medical practitioner with at least two public health inspectors.

3. A divisional health centre serving a population of 60 000 in charge of a medical officer, who will be the manager for the entire complex, staffed by other medical officers and nursing and community health teams.

This complex, which parallels the decentralized administration of the country, would function in close co-operation with the national health development network, which includes all health-related sectors of the Government. The complex would also try to harness maximum participation from the community.

Education/training

If we look back into Sri Lankan history, at developments in education/training of providers of health care of the Western system of medicine, we find them running parallel to developments in the health care system itself.

The first medical school on a London-type model was set up in Colombo in 1870 and this was closely followed by a School of Nursing in 1878. Later, in 1926, the first Health Unit of South East Asia was set up in Sri Lanka and by 1928 this became the training centre for primary health care personnel.

Presently in Sri Lanka the following institutions play a part in education/training of the providers of primary health care.

University faculties of medicine	(5)
Postgraduate Institute of Medicine	(1)
Schools of nursing	(9)
National Institute of Health Sciences	(1)
Health unit training centres	(8)

However, education/training of doctors for primary health care has been more population orientated than person orientated. The medical school's teaching in community health includes lectures during third year in medical school and a field programme during the community medicine clerkship of three weeks. Very recently a week has been added on to this clerkship, to be devoted to a general practice attachment of three days and a seminar conducted by general practitioners.

At postgraduate level, the Postgraduate Institute of Medicine has among its many courses of study, an MD in community medicine, and a diploma in family medicine, which is conducted by a Board of Study, largely represented by the College of General Practitioners of Sri Lanka.

The National Institute of Health Sciences is responsible for training of members of the community health team and assistant medical practitioners. The Institute also conducts orientation programmes in community health for medical officers and training programmes for teachers, in addition to its research activities.

The ayurvedha practitioners have schools of ayurvedha medicine for their training, but a large number of these traditional practitioners set up in practice after a period as understudy to another. More recently there have been a number of programmes for training ayurvedha practitioners for preventive health care.

The problems

Many are the problems of such complex primary health care services as in Sri Lanka. Although in terms of accessibility they could be called satisfactory, there are major disparities in regional coverage, when only 20% of the resources are available to the areas where 80% of the people live.

Most of the services are curative orientated and there is no single unit that provides integrated and comprehensive care for individuals/families in the community on a continuing care basis. Also there is hardly any liaison between these services and no integration of their functions.

There has been no system of patient registration or organized referral and, as result, there is bypassing of the small institutions and the lower levels of care. The people, not knowing the use of the many and varied health care facilities around them, do a lot of 'doctor shopping' and find themselves in a 'medical maze'.

Community participation in health development is sadly lacking. There are voluntary groups involved in health activities, but these come up and disappear like mushrooms, in haphazard manner, without being of continuing support to the existing national health care system.

Availability of personnel for primary health care has been another big problem, perhaps because it has never been a very attractive career choice and also, in recent times, because of better prospects abroad. The primary care providers of the government sector have not had many incentives for working in the community, away from the glamour and excitement of the hospitals. Sometimes the lack of basic living facilities in some areas have been a major constraint to attracting personnel.

Those providers of care in the private sector have their own problems too. They have to organize the service they provide, investing in staff, equipment, records, etc. Their income depends on the fees they get for service. It is therefore understandable that these circumstances could lower the standards of care.

Primary care providers on the whole have not been very enthusiastic in engaging themselves in teaching or research, as involvement in these would lower their chances of enhancing a modest income, and therefore a lot of valuable material for research in primary care is lost.

FUTURE NEEDS

The problems stated above should spell out some of the future needs. Sri Lanka has the potential to develop primary health care to a very satisfactory level, but like any developing country much more could be desired in the way of health care resources. Therefore, it is even more necessary that what is available is distributed equitably, and used rationally and appropriately, by instituting a system of patient registration and organized referral.

The country would need to develop and utilize all the primary health care services of both Western and traditional systems of medicine, as the people appreciate certain values in each of them and have their own ideas of using them, but they should be so organized to complement each other, not overlap or duplicate.

Although, at present, it has been necessary to use paramedical health personnel to provide primary health care, with only a backup of doctors, before long the literate and increasingly sophisticated people would seek a doctor at first contact who would provide integrated primary health care on a continuing care basis. Therefore, the need would arise to have properly trained general practitioners/family doctors, spreading into the rural areas, either singly or in groups. Whether they be employed in government or private sectors, they could work with the health team and take much responsibility for health care of the community.

Education and training of doctors for the future would need changes in the undergraduate curriculum to give more emphasis to integrated primary health care, and also the continuing development of vocational training.

Finally, if a better primary health care service is to fulfil its promise, a sound system of medical recording would need to be developed, to back up research in primary health care, which is very much needed in Sri Lanka.

REFERENCES

Department of Census and Statistics 1982 Sri Lanka Year Book 1982, Sri Lanka
Ministry of Health 1983a Project document — improvements to the health care delivery system, primary health care infrastructure development, revised edn. Government of Democratic Socialist Republic of Sri Lanka
Ministry of Health 1983b Health bulletin. Government of Democratic Socialist Republic of Sri Lanka
Ministry of Health 1983c Country resources utilization review revised edn. Government of Democratic Republic of Sri Lanka

PART THREE

Towards 2000

Towards 2000: the advancing years

We are now nearly at the half-way point between the declaration of Alma-Ata and the year 2000 with its goal of health for all. What can we learn about the problems we face and how can we manage to overcome them? And what does health mean? The WHO's own definition is 'a state of complete physical, mental and social wellbeing and not merely an absence of disease'. How far could the peoples of the world move to that? In this final chapter we look at these problems and the work to be done. We look too at the responsibilities, not just of the health care professionals, but of governments and communities.

PROBLEMS

In the first part of this book, some of the key issues in the Alma-Ata Declaration were examined. In the second part, the state of primary health care in some selected countries was described. In spite of national differences, common themes have emerged. Many so-called developed countries have much to learn from developing countries and no single country can be satisfied that it is clearly on target for the year 2000.

Basic human needs

Medical services cannot achieve much in the absence of basic human necessities — safe water supplies, sanitation, adequate food and housing. There is much to be done, and in Chapter 10, Morley has highlighted the plight of children in some of the less developed countries.

The tragedy of people dying of starvation in Africa in the last few years has highlighted the difficulties faced by those countries and the need to find means of solving the underlying food supply problems. Ironically, some of those countries who have managed to feed their citizens comparatively well now have problems of surfeit from excessive consumption of saturated fats, sugar and salt.

Population, poverty and unemployment

Uncontrolled population growth continues in parts of the world. But even in some of those developed countries that have managed to control their growth, there are now new difficulties with unemployment and poverty due to industrial technological developments and economic changes.

Primary and secondary health care

Tensions between primary and secondary care persist. With limitations in resourcing health care, governments have to decide increasingly between funding developments in primary or in secondary care. Whilst both are essential, there is often inappropriate bias towards funding secondary care. It is easier to point to a new body-scanner or new hospital than to more community nurses, houses for the elderly or health promotion and disease prevention as evidence of improvement. It is also much easier to be swayed on decisions by a small group of specialists than by a larger and more diffuse collection of general practitioners. Decisions must be taken independently on the basis of community need. The tragedy has been not only that many of the developed countries have had the balance skewed but that many less developed countries have copied this model slanted towards high technology medicine with uncertain cost benefits.

Countries vary widely in the amount of money they devote to health care and how far this care is funded from central taxation, health insurance, or by the individual consumer at the time of service. Can we be sure that individual poverty, chronic disease and handicap do not influence the right to receive care and that available resources are managed equably and efficiently?

Prevention and curative medicine

The potential for combining prevention with curative medicine is slowly being realized. But it requires changes in attitude and approach by doctors and nurses to realize the benefits of combining the two as part of normal day-to-day primary health care.

The health team

We now know many of the reasons why some primary health teams do not work, or do not exist at all. The difficulties are often attitudinal and rooted in status and education. Failure to collaborate leads to waste and unnecessary suffering.

Community participation and self-help

Doctors and nurses cannot achieve health for all without the active participation of the consumers, both as individuals and as part of their communities. There is need to encourage more responsible self-care and to understand the benefits when patients and professionals achieve real partnership. There is also a need for professionals in the developed world to understand that personal health beliefs and attitudes are no less important or relevant than they are in developing countries.

Data and information

Too little is known about what goes on in primary health care and with what good or bad outcomes. Many of the statistics of mortality and morbidity are too crude and other information unavailable. General practitioners and family physicians must accept that they have to provide continuing reliable information for better planning, use of resources and care.

Lack of manpower planning because of absence of data on needs has led to excessive numbers of doctors in some countries and too few in others.

Inappropriate medical education and leadership

Time and again we see that our problems — primary versus secondary care, urban versus rural care, inadequate prevention, poor teamwork, lack of data and failure to encourage patient participation — can be traced directly to inappropriate medical education and political and professional leadership. A fragmented specialist: dominated undergraduate curriculum encourages the needs of patients to be seen in isolated pathological terms and fails to integrate them into the wider context of individual people in their own communities. The heirarchical teaching hospital model of care often hinders professionals from different disciplines from working effectively together and with their patients. Nor does a curriculum, which is based for the most part in an institutionalized setting, help students to look outside at the problems in the environment and in the community.

PRIMARY HEALTH CARE

Primary health care is the key in the pursuit of Health for All. It is capable of relating closely to the community in a flexible and responsive way. It can deal with the majority of day-to-day problems and select those patients who need secondary or tertiary care. It includes self-help and family care, and care by auxiliaries, nursing and paramedical professionals, traditional and alternative medicine practitioners and well-trained general practitioners and family physicians.

Its goals, in addition to care and relief and comfort of the sick, must include health promotion and maintenance, disease prevention, rehabilitation, care of the physically and mentally handicapped and chronically ill, elderly and dying.

It has to be available, accessible, efficient and effective.

How far are the countries described in this book achieving such goals and what are their priorities for 2000?

Developing countries

In Zimbabwe, Nigeria, Latin America and Sri Lanka prominent problems are lack of any effective system of PHC. Although many have paper schemes in theory, in practice they exist haphazardly, poorly planned and supervized and with uneven controls. Lack of resources adds to frustrations of the people as well as the health workers leading to low morale, low initiatives and low enthusiasm for the future. Life expectancy is significantly less than in the developed world.

Traditional medicine is a major source of health care in these countries. Western medicine has to live with and accept it as something the people want and respect.

Developed countries

In developed countries there are sophisticated and discrete problems. In South Africa, USA, Australia and others there are tensions between general practitioners/family physicians and specialists. There is no clear demarcation in primary medical care in these countries and there are many physicians competing with each other, creating duplication and no consistent continuity. of patient care. South African general practitioners appear to be struggling to rise above a sense of inferiority in their relations with specialists, in spite of the fact that they have a joint college and association.

In Canada, questions on the place of active obstetrics and surgery are under review. Many practitioners are withdrawing from such work and leaving it to specialists.

In Netherlands, Finland and Norway, governments have given strong support to primary health care, moving resources from hospitals to community and now are waiting to see what general practitioners make of these new opportunities.

USSR has unique problems of surfeit. It has the highest world rates of primary health workers per population, but most are women with low professional status. The challenges are of quality rather than quantity.

Israel has built up a comprehensive primary health care system largely run by trade unions — an impressive achievement from scratch since 1948. However, there are problems of waste, poor organization and national hyperinflation.

Saudi Arabia, with its new wealth, appears to be approaching PHC in a logical manner, without falling into the trap of investing excessively in hospitals and high technologies.

China is an example of how PHC cover has been achieved with very few modern facilities using basic health workers in and from the community.

In contrast, in New Zealand there are too many general practitioners working in a fragmented system for the wrong rewards.

In the United Kingdom, although there has been a National Health Service for nearly 40 years, with primary care occupying a central place, there are signs of problems as resources become scarcer and choices have to be made. Here the potential is large for developing primary health care, with a registered and identifiable population cared for by a team that includes patients as well as professionals.

PLANS

What needs to be done?

Realistic objectives

Targets for PHC: 2000 should be set down. They should be agreed at all levels of care by consensus of public, professional, administrative and government representatives. They must be within forseeable resource limits. They must include disease prevention, health promotion as well as treatment of disease and specify:

1. *Deployment and controls* of available services, manpower and facilities
2. *Processes and methods* to be used
3. *Outcomes* to be achieved and measured
4. *Budgets, resources and economies* available and required.

Work plans

Once objectives have been agreed then *plans* have to be produced, which are flexible, allowing local interpretation.
Plans should include:

1. Provision of PHC services that are as universally available and accessible as possible
2. Development of teamwork, that takes account of skills, training and experience
3. Built-in checks and measures of quality and outcomes
4. Allocation of leadership, responsibilities, directives and controls to individuals or groups.

Data and information

Optimal use of available resources can only be achieved if there are useful and reliable data and information, derived from a recording system that does not impose undue strains on the recorders. Although modern computer data technology will produce the best results, it is by no means essential and much can be collected through simple pen and paper recording.

Profiles

Data useful only to statisticians will not be enough. Regular feedback of applicable information to all involved in PHC is necessary.

Annual data profiles of work patterns, processes and outcomes might be produced for each person, family, PHC worker (including physicians), practice or unit, district, regional and country and compared with others at the same levels.

In this way differences and similarities can be pin-pointed, reasons considered and possible corrective actions taken.

For example indices already available in the *British National Health Service* can provide profiles for each general practitioner on his rates per population of:

1. Immunizations
2. Cervical cytology
3. Obstetric services
4. Night visits
5. Contraceptive services
6. Prescribing patterns and costs.

It is also possible to produce profiles of patients with chronic disease, consultation rates, referrals to hospital specialists and use of diagnostic facilities. With registered populations, practices with age-sex registers and disease indexes can monitor a wide range of practice activities.

New technologies

The introduction of microcomputers is making it possible to handle information derived from large numbers of patients, and to help the primary care physician in his everyday decision making.

Management

Primary health care is in urgent need of more effective management systems in clinical and operational fields, since many of the deficiencies are not ones of lack of knowledge, but of application of available knowledge. All of the activities listed require skilled management to achieve results.

ACTIONS

Whose responsibility is Health for All?

Governments

Clearly, governments cannot escape a major share of responsibility, even in those countries where primary care operates on a mainly private fee for service basis. Health care is expensive and therefore governments must be certain that all those in need can obtain their share of appropriate care. This means achieving a balance of services throughout the country, and not allowing urban areas to be overprovided for, at the expense of rural areas. It means achieving the right balance between primary and secondary care that is genuinely related to need. It means establishing effective monitoring and controls and making adequate finance and other resources available.

Communities

We have noted the trend to greater participation by communities and consumers in their own care and the likely benefits when that happens. Local communities should encourage such development and become acquainted with problems of resources and balancing needs against wants. In the long run, enlightened consumers may make the most significant changes in the health care they receive.

The professionals

Some professionals view, with anxiety and trepidation, pressures from governments on the one hand and from consumers on the other, and with some good reason. If primary care physicians and nurses are to preserve an appropriate measure of clinical freedom they have to be more sensitive to some of the issues raised in this book. They cannot expect unlimited resources and must take responsibility for making the best use of what there is. They must learn to be more effective in their work and to be prepared to demonstrate that effectiveness. They must sort out the problems of basic education and they must learn to work with each other for the common good.

A framework

A clear framework is necessary now, which should include:
1. Objectives (including deployment, processes and methods and outcomes)
2. Priorities
3. Allocation of resources
4. Plans (including teamwork and leadership workers)
5. Data-collection and analysis
6. Profiles
7. Development of new technology.

Time table

The three quinquennia till 2000 A.D. serve as useful time points.
1. *1986–1990*
   Prepare objectives and plans
2. *1990–1995*
   Implement plans with built-in assessment and evaluation
3. *1995–2000*
   Amend and adjust to meet changing needs.

CONCLUSION

We are right to be concerned about the future. If we want to see the emergence of primary health care as the central answer to Health for All in 2000, we must look for leadership.

The *World Health Organization* has made an impressive start and has challenged all those concerned to think carefully.

National colleges and academies of general practice/family medicine and professional nursing organizations should be pressing their own members, governments and the public for the necessary changes.

Individual family practices throughout the world should be asking themselves how far they are on target for 2000 and setting an example of progress.

WONCA itself, in the year of its 11th world conference in London, should be asking itself how far its aims are those of Health for All. The theme of its scientific programme is dedicated to the people of the world as it looks Towards 2000.

Index

Accidents, 55, 56, 72, 195, 312, 342
Acupuncture, 177, 216
Adult-to-adult relationship, 84
Africa Regional Health Education
    Council (ARHEC), 316
Alma-Ata Declaration, v, vi, ix, 6–10,
    14, 16, 18, 21, 24–25, 39, 69,
    86–87, 365
Alternative medicine, 216
American Academy of Family
    Physicians, 228
American Academy of General Practice,
    231
American Board of Family Practice,
    224–225
American Medical Association (AMA),
    221, 226
Anaemia, 62
Antenatal care, 73
Arabia, 333–343
    health indicators, 336
Arterial disease, 71
Arthritis, 62
At risk groups, 47–48
Australia, 29, 119, 137, 151–169, 368
    anticipated changes, 166–168
    changing needs, 160–161
    community expectations, 160–161
    complexity of health care system,
        161–162
    costs, 159–160
    cultural and social features, 151
    disease patterns, 157–159
    economic features, 152
    education and training, 155–157
    fee structures, 164
    future needs, 166–168
    general practitioners, 154
    geographical features, 151
    health system — evolution and
        format, 152
    history, 151

morale of medical profession, 162–163
national features, 151–152
need for health policy, 166
present problems and issues, 159–166
prevention, 157–159
primary health care, 153–155
quality assurance, 165–166
survey of standards and fees, 163–164
technology in general practice,
    164–165
Australian Medical Association (AMA),
    163, 165
Auxiliaries, 121–122

Bahrain, 335, 337, 338
Barefoot doctors, 81, 266
Basic human needs, 365–366
Bilharzia, 327
Birth rate, 54
Birth weights, 135–136
Breast feeding, 62, 142
British Holistic Medicine Association,
    108
British Medical Association (BMA), 36,
    216, 285
British Postgraduate Medical
    Federation, 108
Brucellosis, 340

Canada, 29, 119, 237–247, 369
    changing needs, 238–239
    education and training, 238, 239, 244
    future needs, 245–246
    future patterns, 240–243
    general practitioners, 239–240
    health care system, 238–240
    historical background, 238
    patient input into decisions, 245
    payment of medical service, 243–244
    standardization of services, 242–243
Canadian Medical Association, 238,
    242, 244

375